AF764255

Cancer Treatment and Research

Series Editor
Steven T. Rosen
Robert H. Lurie Comprehensive
Cancer Center
Northwestern University
Chicago, IL
USA

For further volumes, go to
http://www.springer.com/series/5808

Cord Sturgeon
Editor

Endocrine Neoplasia

Springer

Editor
Cord Sturgeon
Northwestern University
Feinberg School of Medicine
Section of Endocrine Surgery
Chicago, IL, USA
csturgeo@nmh.org

ISSN 0927-3042
ISBN 978-1-4419-0856-8 e-ISBN 978-1-4419-0857-5
DOI 10.1007/978-1-4419-0857-5
Springer New York Dordrecht Heidelberg London

Library of Congress Control Number: 2009940800

© Springer Science+Business Media, LLC 2010
All rights reserved. This work may not be translated or copied in whole or in part without the written permission of the publisher (Springer ScienceþBusiness Media, LLC, 233 Spring Street, New York, NY 10013, USA), except for brief excerpts in connection with reviews or scholarly analysis. Use in connection with any form of information storage and retrieval, electronic adaptation, computer software, or by similar or dissimilar methodology now known or hereafter developed is forbidden. The use in this publication of trade names, trademarks, service marks, and similar terms, even if they are not identified as such, is not to be taken as an expression of opinion as to whether or not they are subject to proprietary rights.
While the advice and information in this book are believed to be true and accurate at the date of going to press, neither the authors nor the editors nor the publisher can accept any legal responsibility for any errors or omissions that may be made. The publisher makes no warranty, express or implied, with respect to the material contained herein.

Printed on acid-free paper

Springer is part of Springer Science+Business Media (www.springer.com)

Preface

Endocrine neoplasms are fascinating tumors. Rare but usually dramatic diseases caused by the unchecked elaboration of hormones from endocrine fascinomas have been favorites of generations of medical students and professors alike. From an oncologic standpoint, endocrine tumors, even those arising from the same tissues, represent an amazingly heterogenous group of mostly indolent tumors (such as aldosteronoma or papillary thyroid cancer), with an occasional tumor of extraordinary malignant potential (such as adrenocortical carcinoma or anaplastic thyroid cancer). A detailed understanding of the biology of these tumors has allowed us to select the proper steps in treatment, before, during, and after surgery. There are many textbooks covering the subject of endocrine surgery, ranging from the comprehensive or specialized text to the abbreviated handbook. The purpose of this book is to describe the biology of disease and, within that context, discuss the proper clinical management of the endocrine tumors of the thyroid, parathyroid, pancreas, and adrenal glands.

The book is divided into five sections addressing neoplasms of the thyroid, parathyroid, adrenal gland, neuroendocrine pancreas, and multiple endocrine neoplasia. Experts from the United States, Canada, and Australia have contributed chapters addressing both the biology of endocrine tumors and the clinical management of disease. Recent discoveries regarding the genetic underpinnings of disease are highlighted. Updated consensus guidelines were used for clinical recommendations. The management of complex and often confusing clinical problems is discussed in detail.

Endocrine Neoplasia is a comprehensive, updated, and clearly written text covering the diseases for which endocrine surgical expertise is often needed. We look towards advances in the science and the art of endocrine surgery to continuously improve outcomes for our patients. The goal of this text was to provide a detailed description of both the underlying science of disease as well as the art of clinical management.

I would like to acknowledge the hard work of all the contributors to the text as well as the editing and production team at Springer. I would also like to acknowledge the inspiration that I have received from countless patients with diseases of endocrine neoplasia whom I have had the privilege to treat. Last, but not least, special thanks are due to my family, Jane, Kate, and Cassidy, for their support and patience which helped to make this book possible.

Chicago, USA Cord Sturgeon

Contents

Contributors

Sally E. Carty
Professor of Surgery, Chief of Endocrine Surgery, University of Pittsburgh School of Medicine, Pittsburgh PA USA

Anthony J. Chambers
Fellow in Endocrine Surgery and Surgical Oncology, University of Calgary and Tom Baker Cancer Centre, Calgary, Alberta Canada

Herbert Chen
Professor of Surgery, University of Wisconsin, Madison, WI USA

Shih-Ping Cheng
Department of Surgery, Mackay Memorial Hospital, Taipei Taiwan

Alan P. B. Dackiw
Assistant Professor of Surgery, Section of Endocrine Surgery, Johns Hopkins University School of Medicine, Baltimore, MD USA

Gerard M. Doherty
NW Thompson Professor of Surgery, University of Michigan, Ann Arbor, MI USA

Quan-Yang Duh
Professor of Surgery, University of California San Francisco, San Francisco, CA USA

Dina M. Elaraj
Assistant Professor of Surgery, Section of Endocrine Surgery, Northwestern University Feinberg School of Medicine, Chicago, IL USA

Clive Grant
Professor of Surgery, Department of Surgery, Mayo Clinic, Rochester, MN USA

Adrian Harvey
Endocrine Surgical Fellow, Cleveland Clinic Foundation, Cleveland, OH USA

Electron Kebebew
Senior Investigator, Head of Endocrine Oncology, National Cancer Institute, Surgery Branch, Bethesda, MD USA

Kaitlyn J. Kelly
Resident in Surgery, Department of Surgery, University of Wisconsin, Madison, WI USA

Steven K. Libutti
Professor of Surgery, Vice Chairman, Department of Surgery; Director, Montefiore-Einstein Center for Cancer Care.Bronx, NY USA

Goswin Y. Meyer-Rochow
Royal North Shore Hospital, Kolling Institute of Medical Research, University of Sydney, Sydney, NSW Australia

Jacob Moalem
Assistant Professor, University of Rochester Medical Center, Rochester, NY USA

Jeffrey F. Moley
Professor of Surgery, Chief, Endocrine and Oncologic Surgery Section, Associate Director, Siteman Cancer Center, Washington University School of Medicine, St. Louis, MO USA

Janice L. Pasieka
Clinical Professor of Surgery and Oncology, Department of Surgery, Foothills Medical Centre, Calgary Canada

Anathea C. Powell
Clinical Fellow, Tumor Angiogenesis Section, Surgery Branch, National Cancer Institute, National Institutes of Health, Bethesda, MD USA

Hsin-Chieh Jennifer Shen
National Cancer Institute, National Institute of Health, Bethesda, MD USA

Wen T. Shen
Assistant Professor of Surgery, University of California San Francisco, San Francisco, CA USA

Stan B. Sidhu
Clinical Associate Professor of Surgery, Department of Endocrine and Oncology Surgery, Royal North Shore Hospital, St. Leonards, NSW Australia

Rebecca S. Sippel
Assistant Professor of Surgery, Department of Surgery, University of Wisconsin, Madison, WI USA

Patsy S.H. Soon
Bankstown Hospital and University of New South Wales, Kolling Institute of Medical Research, Kensington, University of Sydney,
NSW Australia

Insoo Suh
Resident in Surgery, Department of Surgery, University of California
San Francisco, San Francisco, CA USA

Amber L. Traugott
Resident in General Surgery, Washington University School of Medicine,
St. Louis, MO USA

Kimberly Vanderveen
Fellow in Endocrine Surgery, Mayo Clinic, Department of Surgery, Rochester,
MN USA

Michael W. Yeh
Assistant Professor of Surgery, David Geffen School of Medicine,
University of California, Los Angeles, Los Angeles, CA USA

Linwah Yip
Assistant Professor of Surgery, University of Pittsburgh School of Medicine,
Pittsburgh, PA USA

Ali Zarrinpar
Resident in Surgery, Ronald Reagan UCLA Medical Center, Los Angeles,
CA USA

Part I
Thyroid

Chapter 1
The Biology of Thyroid Oncogenesis

Insoo Suh and Electron Kebebew

Introduction

Over the past 20 years, our understanding of the molecular biology of thyroid cancer has advanced significantly. These new insights have in turn unleashed a vast potential for clinical application across the diagnostic, prognostic, and therapeutic spectrum. A classic example of this is the identification of the RET proto-oncogene responsible for hereditary medullary thyroid cancer (MTC), which has led to earlier diagnosis by genetic screening, and thus better patient outcomes. It is one of the few hereditary cancers for which at-risk individuals can be identified by genetic testing and be advised a prophylactic thyroidectomy, as they will certainly develop MTC over their lifetime.

Thyroid cancer is the most common form of endocrine cancer, with over 35,000 new cases expected to be diagnosed in the United States in 2008. Of these, approximately 95% are well-differentiated tumors of follicular cell origin (papillary, follicular, Hürthle cell), 4–5% are MTCs which originate from the parafollicular or calcitonin (C) secreting cells, and 1% or less are undifferentiated or anaplastic thyroid cancer (ATC). Unlike the RET proto-oncogene that is responsible for hereditary MTC and is present in 75% of sporadic MTC as a somatic mutation, many genetic alterations, commonly in the mitogen signaling pathway, have been identified in thyroid cancer of follicular cell origin. This suggests that most thyroid cancers of follicular cell origin are genetically heterogeneous. This chapter will focus on the key genetic and epigenetic changes associated with most thyroid cancers of follicular cell origin, the clinicopathologic associations observed, and their possible clinical application to the management of thyroid cancer. In addition, the emerging theory of the role of stem cells in the etiology of thyroid cancer will be discussed.

E. Kebebew (✉)
Surgery Branch, National Cancer Institute,
10 Center Drive, Room 4W–5952, Bethesda, MD 20892–1201
e-mail: kebebewe@mail.nih.gov

C. Sturgeon (ed.), *Endocrine Neoplasia*, Cancer Treatment and Research, vol 153,
DOI 10.1007/978-1-4419-0857-5_1, © Springer Science+Business Media, LLC 2010

Common Genetic Alterations

Papillary thyroid cancer (PTC) and follicular thyroid cancer (FTC) are the two main thyroid cancer subtypes that are derived from follicular epithelial cells. Together, they account for the vast majority of thyroid cancer cases. Recent discoveries have shed new light on the genetic foundations behind PTC and FTC development, many of which involve the activation of the mitogen-activated protein kinase (MAPK) signaling pathway (Fig. 1.1). This pathway is activated by growth factors

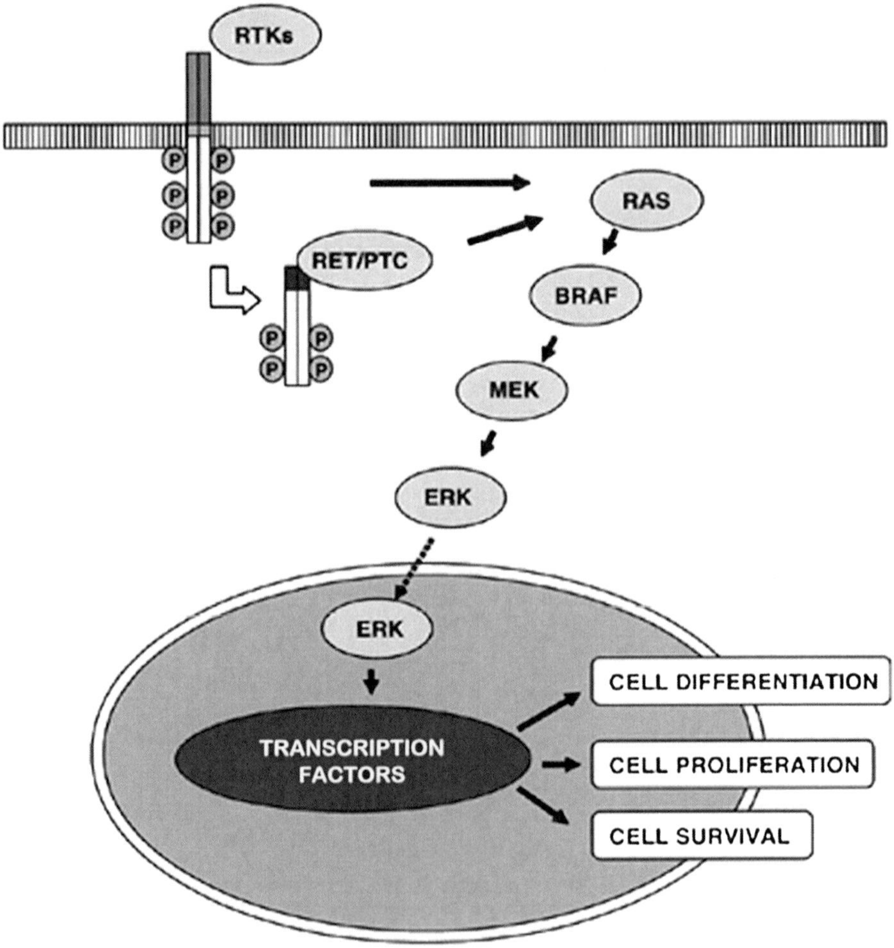

Fig. 1.1 The mitogen-activated protein kinase (MAPK) signaling pathway, activated by the binding of growth factors to receptor tyrosine kinases (RTKs), such as RET and TRK, leading to an intracellular phosphorylation cascade involving the activation of RAS, BRAF, MAPK/ERK kinase (MEK), and extracellular signal-regulated kinase (ERK) proteins. Activated ERK translocates into the nucleus and regulates the transcription of genes responsible for cell differentiation, proliferation, and survival (From Nikiforov 2008, used with permission.)

binding to cell-surface transmembrane tyrosine kinase receptors; this in turn causes an intracellular signaling cascade that ultimately regulates the intra-nuclear transcription of genes responsible for cell proliferation, differentiation, migration, invasion, and survival. The relevance of the MAPK signaling pathway is underscored by the finding that up to 80% of PTCs carry activating genetic changes of at least one of four MAPK-related genes – BRAF, RET/PTC, RAS, and TRK [1].

Despite its importance, the MAPK pathway activation does not appear to be the sole mediator of follicular cell-origin thyroid cancers. In particular, the mutational profile of FTC is largely distinct from that of PTC, with a higher rate of activating RAS (HRAS, KRAS, NRAS) mutations and a PAX8/PPARγ chromosomal rearrangement [2, 3]. This may, in part, be due to the preferential activation of another distinct signaling cascade known as the phosphatidylinositol 3-kinase/protein kinase B (PI3K/AKT) pathway. The PI3K/AKT pathway, like the MAPK pathway, also involves a progressive series of phosphorylation reactions starting with a transmembrane protein kinase. This cascade ultimately leads to the activation of AKT, which in turn phosphorylates proteins both in the cytosol and in the nucleus. Downstream targets of AKT regulate apoptosis, proliferation, cell-cycle progression, cytoskeletal integrity, and energy metabolism [4].

Constitutive activation of AKT has been demonstrated to be an important mechanism in the pathogenesis of FTC. This was first discovered when an inactivating germline mutation of PTEN, an inhibitor of AKT activation, was found to be responsible for Cowden's syndrome, in which 50% of patients develop follicular thyroid neoplasms. An analogous somatic PTEN mutation is responsible for only 6–8% of sporadic FTCs; however, AKT activation appears to be important in sporadic FTC independent of PTEN inactivation, possibly via RAS- or PAX8/PPARγ-mediated mechanisms. The PI3K/AKT pathway also appears to play a central role in PTC and FTC progression, possibly by upregulation of genes involved in epithelial-to-mesenchymal transition, such as osteopontin [4].

ATC, the most aggressive and lethal of thyroid tumors, is often thought to be derived from differentiated follicular cell-origin cancers under the "multi-hit" theory of carcinogenesis, and is associated with several other distinct mutations, but is almost always positive for p53-inactivating mutations [5]. Table 1.1 lists the most common genetic alterations associated with thyroid carcinogenesis. We will discuss the most common and important of these genetic changes below.

BRAF

The BRAF gene is located on chromosome 7q23, and encodes a 95 kDa cytoplasmic protein that belongs to the RAF family of serine/threonine kinases. Activation of BRAF by phosphorylation occurs downstream of the membrane or cytoplasmic receptor, which in turn relays signals through the MAPK pathway [6]. Somatic mutations in BRAF have been found in a wide variety of human cancers, and have mostly been confined to exons 11 and 15 [7]. In the thyroid, BRAF mutations

Table 1.1 Common genetic alterations in thyroid carcinogenesis

Mutation	Prevalence (%)	Resulting phenotype(s)	Main molecular function
BRAF	30–80	PTC	MAPK pathway activation
RET/PTC	5–35	PTC	MAPK pathway activation
	55–85	Radiation-induced PTC	
RAS	20–50	FTC, fvPTC, FA	MAPK and PI3K-Akt pathway activation
TRK	5–10	PTC	MAPK pathway activation
PAX8/PPARγ	35–60	FTC	Unknown
PTEN	<10	PTC, FTC, ATC	Tyrosine phosphatase inactivation
	80	Cowden's disease (germline)	
RET	75	MTC	MAPK pathway activation
	100	Familial MTC, MEN2 (germline)	
p53	20–80	Undifferentiated thyroid cancer, ATC	Tumor suppressor
β-catenin	25–65	Undifferentiated thyroid cancer, ATC	Cadherin subunit, Wnt pathway regulation

PTC papillary thyroid cancer, *FTC* follicular thyroid cancer, *fvPTC* follicular variant of PTC, *FA* follicular adenoma, *ATC* anaplastic thyroid cancer, *MTC* medullary thyroid cancer

generally tend to occur in exon 15 at the T1799A position, which results in an amino acid change from valine to glutamate in the kinase domain. This results in a conformational change in the CR2 activation loop of the BRAF protein, which leads to higher ERK1/2 kinase activity and constitutive MAPK activation. This V600E mutation accounts for almost all of the BRAF mutations found in thyroid cancer, though other mutations have been reported, such as A1801G point mutations, tandem TG1800AA mutations, and AKAP9-BRAF rearrangements [8, 9]. No germline BRAF mutation has yet been identified and is likely to be lethal [10].

The BRAF V600E mutation is the most common mutation in PTC, with an estimated prevalence of 45% [11–14]. There are some geographic and ethnic variations in prevalence; for example, rates in Korean patients are reportedly as high as 86% [14], whereas children and patients with a history of radiation exposure have much lower rates [15, 16]. Its prevalence also depends on the specific subtype of thyroid cancer, from higher rates in classical PTC and tall cell variants, to low rates in the columnar variant, and usually no presence in FTC [17, 18]. It is also found in poorly-differentiated ATCs, and usually in tumors with coexisting well-differentiated PTC [19, 20]. BRAF mutation is generally mutually exclusive of the other main genetic changes associated with PTC, such as RET/PTC, TRK1, and RAS [1]. This exclusiveness is one of the more distinctive characteristics of the genetics of PTC, because it suggests that a single genetic alteration may be sufficient to drive follicular cell transformation and carcinogenesis. Transgenic mouse models of the BRAF V600E mutation lead to thyroid cancer that recapitulates human PTC and progresses to poorly differentiated thyroid cancer [21].

Most investigators, but not all, have reported that the presence of BRAF V600E mutation in PTC is associated with more aggressive clinical behavior of these tumors. In general, BRAF appears to be associated with older age, male gender, extrathyroidal invasion, regional lymph node metastasis, higher overall stage, and recurrence [16, 22, 23]. The reasons for these associations are unclear, but one possible explanation lies in the apparent inability for BRAF mutation-positive tumors to take up radioiodine, leading possibly to ineffective radioactive iodine ablative treatment. Indeed, expression of thyroid-specific iodine-transfer genes, including TPO, NIS, Tg, and pendrin, are decreased in V600E-positive PTCs [24–27]. An alternative reason could be that BRAF mutation is associated with increased angiogenesis and local invasion, which are associated with increased expression of MMP3, MMP9, and MMP13 after BRAF mutant transfection [28].

RET/PTC

The RET gene is located on chromosome 10q11.2, and encodes a transmembrane tyrosine kinase. Glial cell-derived neurotrophic factor (GDNF) is the main ligand for RET; however, other ligands such as neurotrophic growth factor can activate RET through inter-receptor signal transduction. Ligand binding leads to the activation of RET and downstream MAPK signaling.

The relationship between RET and MTC was first established in 1993, when a germline activating point mutation in RET was identified in families with MEN 2A and familial MTC [29]. It has since become well-established that several distinct germline point mutations in RET are the cause of the MEN 2 and familial MTC syndromes, with immediate clinical benefit in the form of accurate genetic testing for at-risk families.

In the thyroid, RET is generally more highly expressed in parafollicular cells and not in follicular cells. This is because RET is preferentially expressed in neuronal tissue and parafollicular cells originate from the neural crest cells. However, the discovery of another type of RET genetic alteration causing constitutive activation in follicular cells was reported in 1987 [30]. In this case, the 3′ coding region of RET was rearranged and fused to the 5′ region of the H4 gene by virtue of their proximity, causing a self-dimerization and constitutive activation similar to what occurs with point mutations in the RET proto-oncogene in MTC. Over time, several other similar activating rearrangements have since been discovered in thyroid cancers of follicular cell origin and have been collectively referred to as RET/PTC rearrangement. The most common types are known as RET/PTC1 (fusion of RET and H4) and RET/PTC3 (fusion of RET and RFG), which compose over 90% of RET/PTC rearrangements; however, over 12 other types of RET/PTC rearrangements have been reported [31]. Ectopic RET/PTC expression was found to transform cells in culture and cause thyroid carcinomas in transgenic mice; its activation also caused a downregulation of expression of thyroid-specific genes [32]. Its mechanism appears to be MAPK pathway-dependent in that the silencing of BRAF in PTC cells reverses the effects of RET/PTC, suggesting cross-talk between the BRAF and RET/PTC signaling pathways [33–35].

RET/PTC rearrangements have a variable prevalence of 20–40% and are almost exclusively present in PTC. RET/PTC1 is associated with radiation exposure (up to 80% prevalence) and childhood cancers (40–70%) that resulted from the Chernobyl reactor meltdown [36–38]. However, some investigators have found these mutations in Hürthle cell variants of PTC and thyroid tissues with lymphocytic thyroiditis [39, 40]. RET/PTC rearrangements appear to be an early event in PTC carcinogenesis, on the basis of their presence in occult PTCs [41]. RET/PTC-positive PTCs have been associated with a younger age of onset, higher rate of lymph node metastases, classic histology, and perhaps a more favorable prognosis [17]. RET/PTC1 tends to be found in slowly growing indolent cancers, whereas RET/PTC3 is usually found in solid PTC variants with a more aggressive tumor phenotype [38, 42, 43]. However, the association between RET/PTC rearrangements and aggressive tumor phenotypes is controversial.

RAS

The RAS proto-oncogenes – comprised of H-RAS, K-RAS, and N-RAS – encode three distinct membrane-associated GTP binding proteins. These proteins are located on the inner surface of the cell membrane, and are activated after GTP binding to their docking sites on codon 12/13 of exon 1; their regulation occurs via an autocatalytic GTPase that has a docking site domain on codon 61 of exon 2. RAS-mediated activation plays a key role in G protein-coupled receptor tyrosine kinase signal transduction, including the MAPK and PI3K/AKT pathways. Most activating point mutations in RAS occur either in codon 12/13, which increases an affinity to GTP, or in codon 61, which inactivates the inhibitory GTPase.

Unlike in the case of BRAF or RET/PTC, RAS mutations occur both in benign and malignant thyroid tumors of follicular cell origin, but with variable frequency [44]. In PTCs, RAS mutations are relatively infrequent (10% of cases), but almost always tend to be present in follicular variants of PTC and are usually KRAS mutations [45, 46]. RAS mutations are much more common in FTCs, with a 40–50% prevalence [2, 47, 48]. In addition, some studies have also reported a higher rate of RAS mutation in poorly differentiated thyroid cancers and ATCs [49]. Despite this, RAS mutations are also common in benign follicular adenomas, in some studies at a higher rate than in FTCs [3]. The clinical significance of this higher rate is unknown. Nevertheless, the presence of RAS mutations in histologically confirmed cancers has been associated with more aggressive disease and poorer prognosis, especially when RAS mutations coexist with mutations in genes that encode G stimulator proteins [50, 51].

TRK

The TRK proto-oncogene is located on chromosome 1q22 and encodes the receptor for nerve growth factor. Similarly to RET/PTC, TRK undergoes oncogenic activation by chromosomal rearrangement to the 5′ region of another gene. Several types of rearrangements have been reported, depending on the subtype of TRK. TRK-T1 and TRK-T2 are formed through intrachromosomal rearrangement of TRK with the 5′ region of the TPR gene, whereas TRK-T3 is formed by interchromosomal rearrangement with the TAG gene. TRK-T1 is the most common rearrangement, and all of TRK rearrangements generally occur only in PTC and at a low rate (6–20%) [52].

PAX8/PPARγ

PAX8 is a transcription factor that is expressed at higher levels in follicular thyroid cells, and regulates the expression of thyroid-specific genes [53]. The PAX8/PPARγ oncogene is formed by a chromosomal translocation 5(2;3)(q13;p25) that leads to the fusion of PAX8 to domains A to F of PPARγ, a nuclear hormone receptor that regulates cell proliferation and differentiation. The resulting fusion protein is found predominantly in FTC, with a prevalence of 26–63% on the basis of immunohistochemical studies [53, 54]. Tumors with this mutation tend to be in younger patients, smaller in size, and more frequently associated with vascular invasion. The mechanism by which PAX8/PPARγ leads to FTC development is not well understood, but may either involve the competitive inhibition of wild-type PPARγ or a deregulation of normal PAX8 function in follicular cell differentiation [55, 56].

P53

P53 is one of the most common tumor suppressor genes, with inactivating point mutations found in up to 50% of human cancers. P53 is located on chromosome 17p13 and encodes a 53 kDa protein, which acts as a key cell-cycle regulator in response to DNA damage. Only 10% of all thyroid cancers harbor the P53 mutation; most of these tumors are poorly-differentiated and ATCs (75%), with mutations in exons 5 through 8 [5, 57, 58]. P53 mutations tend to be late events in the progression from differentiated-to-undifferentiated carcinoma. P63 and P73, which are isoforms of P53, have also been reported to play a role in thyroid carcinogenesis [59].

Epigenetic Mechanisms

Epigenetic changes refer to modification of gene expression, usually in the form of gene silencing, which occurs as a result of mechanisms that do not fundamentally alter the underlying genomic DNA sequence. This term encompasses a variety of mitotically heritable mechanisms that are designed to play important roles in normal eukaryotic processes, including embryogenesis, differentiation, and genomic imprinting. Advances in molecular biology techniques in the past two decades have allowed investigators to demonstrate that epigenetic changes also play a significant role in the pathogenesis of cancer.

There are three established epigenetic mechanisms – DNA methylation, histone modification, and nucleosome remodeling. DNA methylation, by far the most studied and characterized, refers to the methylation of cytosine residues in CpG dinucleotide-rich areas, known as "CpG islands," within the promoter region of a gene. The methylation effectively prevents further transcription of the gene, silencing its expression as well as that of any number of other downstream genes. Histone modifications occur via covalent reactions (usually deacetylation and methylation) at specific lysine residues of histone proteins, which cause the histone to more tightly bind and compact the DNA sequence within the chromatin structure, and thus prevent the ability of the gene(s) at this site to be transcribed. Nucleosome remodeling refers to a variety of ATP-dependent polypeptide complexes that appear to play roles in local noncovalent chromatin modification and transcriptional repression. These three mechanisms may occur independently of one another, but recent evidence increasingly suggests that they appear to intimately interact with one another to cause the silencing of cancer-related genes [60].

DNA Methylation

The study of DNA methylation and thyroid cancer has largely focused on the inactivation of two different groups of genes – classic tumor suppressor genes and thyroid-specific functional genes [61]. The tumor suppressor genes that are silenced via promoter methylation encompass a wide variety of regulatory functions. For instance, p27KIP1, p16INK4A, and CDKN2A are genes that encode inhibitors of cyclin-dependent kinase, which regulates cell-cycle progression. These genes are methylated in thyroid cancers but not in benign thyroid tumors [62, 63]. The commonly dysregulated MAPK pathway in thyroid cancer of follicular cell origin is regulated by a complex interplay of cell-surface and intracellular tumor suppressor genes, such as RASSF1A and FGFR2. The protein product of RASSF1A lacks enzymatic activity but contains a Ras association domain, and appears to play a role in blocking MAPK pathway activation; its silencing through promoter methylation has been reported in PTC, FTC, and ATC, as well as in numerous other solid-organ cancers [64, 65]. FGFR2 is a key inhibitor in fibroblast growth-factor-mediated MAPK activation, and is methylated in several thyroid cancer cell lines [66]. Cell adhesion also plays a critical role in tumor invasiveness and metastatic potential, and thyroid carcinomas may carry methylated genes that inhibit genes that promote cell–cell adhesion molecules such as CDH1 [67].

The process of normal thyroid follicular cell function – namely the TSH receptor-mediated iodide uptake and production of thyroid hormone – is also targeted and silenced by DNA methylation. The TSH receptor gene, as well as the sodium iodine symporter (NIS) and pendrin, has been shown to be methylated and down-regulated in thyroid carcinomas, especially in poorly differentiated tumors [68–70]. These findings may help explain why aggressive thyroid cancers often lose the ability to take up iodine, leading to failures in treatment with radioactive iodine.

DNA gene-promoter methylation status has also been shown to be associated with the presence of known genetic alterations that occur in thyroid cancer. BRAF is an example of this phenomenon. A recent study has shown that PTC specimens with methylated tumor suppressor genes, including TIMP3, SLC5A8, DPK, and RARβ2, had a significantly higher percentage of BRAF mutations and also predicted a greater degree of clinical aggressiveness [71]. This suggests that inactivation of these tumor suppressor genes can contribute to BRAF-mediated thyroid carcinogenesis in PTC. The methylation of RASSF1A, another MAPK pathway inhibitor as mentioned above, often occurs in concert with PTEN methylation in FTC [72, 73]. These examples demonstrate that DNA methylation events can be varied and multiple, and can occur in combination or as a result of genetic alterations that have an established role in thyroid carcinogenesis, and therefore likely influence thyroid cancer initiation and or progression. Table 1.2 lists the wide array of genes known to be methylated in thyroid cancer.

The role of DNA methylation in thyroid cancer is complex because this mechanism is not only integral to carcinogenesis, but also to normal cellular function. For instance, MAGE-A3/6 is a tumor-promoting gene that belongs in a family of genes known as "cancer/testis antigens" because of its overexpression in testicular germ cells, placenta, and several malignancies. Methylation-mediated silencing of MAGE-A3/6 has been shown to occur in normal thyroid tissues, whereas overexpression was found in thyroid cancer tissues and cell lines [74]. Further evidence of the contradictory role of DNA methylation lies in studies of global 5-methylcytosine content in thyroid cancers, which show an overall *decrease* in genome-wide methylation [75]. The mechanisms by which normal methylation processes are disrupted, and local hypermethylation leads to global hypomethylation across the cancer genome, are still poorly understood.

Other Epigenetic Mechanisms

Histone deacetylase (HDAC) is a principle enzyme involved in histone modification leading to gene silencing. Its action frees the histone's positively charged lysine residues at the N terminus, causing the histone to more strongly bind its associated negatively charged DNA and cause tighter chromatin compaction with resultant blockage of DNA transcription. Histone deacetylation has only recently begun to be studied in thyroid cancer. Most studies have examined the role of HDAC inhibitors in the recovery of expression of genes that regulate the cell cycle and normal thyroid function. Specifically, histone deacetylation appears to increase P53-inhibitory P27 gene expression, as well as loss of expression of NIS, TPO, Tg,

Table 1.2 Genes that are epigenetically silenced by DNA methylation in thyroid cancers

Gene	Normal function of encoded protein
DAPK	Calcium/calmodulin-dependent serine threonine kinase; acts as a tumor suppressor via proapoptosis
FGFR2	Tyrosine kinase receptor that competitively binds FGF; acts as a tumor suppressor by downregulating the MAPK pathway
NIS	Sodium/iodide symporter; transports iodide from blood into thyroid cells through basal membrane
p16	Competitive binder of CDK-4 and -6; acts as a tumor suppressor by blocking cell-cycle progression at G1/S phase
PTEN	Phosphatase; acts as a tumor suppressor by dephosphorylating PIP3 with resultant downregulation of the PI3K/AKT pathway
RARβ2	Retinoic acid receptor, acts as a tumor suppressor by regulating the growth of epithelial cells
RASSF1A	Signaling protein, acts as a tumor suppressor probably by inhibiting the Ras pathway
RIZ1	Nuclear protein methyltransferase; acts as a tumor suppressor by binding Rb
SLC5A8	Sodium/iodide symporter; transports iodide into thyroid cells through apical membrane; also acts as a tumor suppressor via proapoptosis
SLC26A4	Sodium/iodide symporter; transports iodide into thyroid cells through apical membrane
TIMP3	Tissue inhibitor of metalloproteinase via binding of Zn-binding site; acts as a tumor suppressor by inhibiting growth, angiogenesis, and invasion
TSHR	TSH receptor; binds TSH in the upstream regulation of iodide-dependent thyroid hormone formation

and RARβ [76, 77]. Other epigenetic mechanisms involving nucleosomal remodeling include noncovalent modifications in the SWI-SNF chromatin remodeling complex, as well as the nucleosomal remodeling complex NuRD, both of which have been shown to play important roles in the development of several solid-organ cancers, such as those of the lung, breast, prostate, pancreas, and kidney [78]. We are not aware of any studies thus far that have examined the role of these mechanisms in a thyroid cancer model.

Role of Stem Cells in Thyroid Cancer

The acceleration of stem cell research in the last 10 years has yielded exciting ideas about the role of stem cells in a variety of disease states. One of the most prominent of these ideas has become known as the cancer stem-cell hypothesis, which states that cancer begins with and is maintained by a small proportion of cancer cells that exhibit stem-cell-like properties. This theory is not mutually exclusive with others; in fact, it incorporates the idea that relevant mutations and other genetic changes occur within these stem cells first. Indeed, some of the most canonical genes involved in stem cell maintenance, including WNT and Sonic hedgehog, have been found to be overexpressed in many human cancers [79].

Side populations of stem cells in the thyroid gland were first postulated in 1992 [27], but were identified in thyroid cancers only recently – in 2007 [80]. In this study of several thyroid cancer cell lines, up to 0.25% of cells were found to have gene expression profiles distinct from the rest of the population, showing upregulation of stem-cell maintenance genes such as ABCG2, MYC, JUN, FZD5, HES1, and JAG1. Whether these cancer stem cells originate from normal stem cells, progenitor cells, or mature differentiated thyroid cells is still debatable. A recent theory postulates that the cells of origin may determine the histological subtype of thyroid cancer; for example, ATC would arise directly from an undifferentiated stem cell, whereas a well-differentiated PTC would arise from a bipotential stem cell [81]. This is, however, unproven and requires further study, but would have important clinical ramifications for treatment of aggressive thyroid cancers.

Clinical Applications

Much of what has been discovered about the molecular basis of thyroid oncogenesis is being evaluated for clinical applicability in patients with thyroid cancer. While the management of patients with thyroid neoplasms is well-established, two unresolved areas are being actively investigated: (1) distinguishing benign from malignant thyroid neoplasms that are indeterminate, suspicious, or nondiagnostic on fine needle aspiration (FNA) biopsy, and (2) treating recurrent or metastatic thyroid cancers that are refractory to conventional therapy (consisting of surgical resection, radioiodine ablation, and TSH suppression).

Improvements in FNA Cytology-Based Diagnoses

Cytology from FNA biopsy is currently the most accurate preoperative test for diagnosing thyroid masses. However, significant limitations of this method include its inability to determine malignancy in follicular or Hürthle cell neoplasms, as reflected by approximately 30% of FNA biopsies that are found to be indeterminate or nondiagnostic. To address this concern, several investigators have evaluated whether genotyping for the most common thyroid cancer-related mutations using FNA samples would improve the diagnostic accuracy of FNA cytology.

Until recently, most studies on FNA samples have been retrospective and focused predominantly on the BRAF V600E mutation, which was found to have 16–42% sensitivity and 100% specificity for PTC in patients with indeterminate or suspicious FNA biopsy results [82–85]. Recently, a prospective study examined the mutation status of BRAF, RET/PTC1, RET/PTC3, and NTRK in 132 patients with indeterminate or suspicious FNA diagnoses, on the basis of the rationale that at least one of these mutations would be present in up to 80% of definitive PTC cases. The results showed a 100% positive predictive value for cancer and a 98% negative predictive value.

However, only 7 (5%) of the 132 samples had histologically confirmed cancer diagnoses, limiting the power of these results [86].

Recently, microarray-based technology has enabled genome-wide gene expression profiles to be examined in cancer tissues. One application of these profiles has been to identify heretofore unrecognized genes that are differentially expressed between cancerous and benign tissue samples. Several groups have identified a wide variety of differentially expressed genes from microarray profiling of thyroid cancers, and some were able to validate their accuracy as diagnostic markers of malignancy [87–91]. Most of these genes have no known functional relevance to thyroid oncogenesis, but may serve as useful diagnostic and prognostic markers.

Novel Targeted Therapies

Most thyroid cancers are papillary or follicular carcinomas; i.e., they are of follicular cell origin. Most are well-differentiated and curable with surgical resection, radioactive iodine administration, and TSH-suppressive thyroxine supplementation. However, 10–15% of patients develop or present with poorly differentiated cancer, which is associated with loss of thyroid-specific functions such as iodide uptake and thyroglobulin production, which renders these tumors unresponsive to current therapy regimens. Similarly, MTC is derived from parafollicular C cells and thus do not take up radioactive iodine, leaving surgery the only, often insufficient, treatment option for this aggressive disease. Clearly, there is a need for novel therapies for this subset of patients. There is promise, however, because the advances in our understanding of thyroid oncogenesis, as detailed above, have led to the development of several candidate agents targeting specific genes or molecules that have been associated with thyroid carcinogenesis [44, 92].

Kinase Inhibitors

The relevance of the MAPK signaling pathway in thyroid carcinogenesis is underscored by the number of potential MAPK-targeted kinase inhibitors currently under evaluation. Many are still in preclinical study phases, such as the tyrosine kinase inhibitors PP1 and PP2, RAF kinase inhibitors AAL-881 and LBT-613, and MEK inhibitor CI-1040 [44]. We will focus on three MAPK inhibitors that have undergone relatively more extensive evaluation – sorafenib, vandetanib, and sunitinib.

Sorafenib (BAY 43-9006) was an agent specifically engineered to target RAF kinases, but was subsequently found to have potent activity against other kinases, including VEGFR-2, VEGFR-3, PDGFRβ, FLT-3, and c-KIT [93]. Several clinical trials have demonstrated this agent's efficacy in a variety of cancers, particularly hepatocellular carcinoma and renal cell carcinoma [94]. In thyroid cancer, sorafenib was found to have significant antitumoral properties in both in vitro and in vivo models, with effective inhibition of both wild-type and V600E-mutant BRAF activity [95]. Recently, a phase II clinical trial of orally administered sorafenib in 30 patients with metastatic iodine-refractory thyroid cancers showed a significant clinical benefit rate of 77% and a median progression-free survival of 79 weeks, which represents a significant advance over current chemotherapy regimens [96].

Vandetanib (ZD6474) is another orally administered kinase inhibitor that specifically inhibits VEGFR-2 and effectively blocks RET tyrosine kinase. Because of the importance of both genes in thyroid oncogenesis, preclinical studies first established that vandetanib blocks signaling and inhibits growth in thyroid carcinoma cells carrying RET/PTC or MEN-associated RET point mutations [97]. Some patients with advanced familial MTC seem to have some benefit from vandetanib therapy; [98] a phase II trial is currently underway to more definitively evaluate its effects in this patient population. As with sorafenib, vandetanib has also been shown to have antitumoral properties in other cancer models, but phase II clinical trials thus far show clinical efficacy in only non-small cell lung cancer.

Another multikinase inhibitor, sunitinib (SU11248) inhibits the RET/PTC tyrosine kinase, and thus would theoretically be of benefit in a significant subset of PTC [99]. Phase I trials demonstrated an acceptable safety profile, but multiple clinical studies have revealed significant hypothyroidism as a side effect [100]. This issue is being addressed and followed as this drug has moved to phase II trials in patients with unresectable iodine-refractory differentiated thyroid carcinoma.

PPARγ Agonists

Despite the unclear role of PAX8/PPARγ mutations in thyroid oncogenesis, the wild-type PPARγ gene is known to regulate cell growth and differentiation. Recent in vitro and in vivo studies have shown that PPARγ agonists such as troglitazone and rosiglitazone lead to growth inhibition, redifferentiation, and apoptosis in PPARγ-positive thyroid cancers. These actions may be mediated by the p27 or c-myc apoptosis pathways [101–103]. Rosiglitazone is currently in clinical trials for patients with advanced or metastatic thyroid cancer.

Epigenetic Modulators

Because epigenetic modifications are by definition reversible, there has been much interest in the role that reversing agents can play in thyroid cancer treatment in conjunction with radioiodine therapy. DNA methyltransferase inhibitors such as azacitidine (5-azacytidine) and decitabine (5-aza-2′-deoxycytidine) have been shown in several in vitro studies to redifferentiate thyroid carcinoma cells and restore iodine-dependent thyroid function [70]. HDAC inhibitors such as trichostatin A and sodium butyrate show similar in vitro effects, and in combination with DNA methyltransferase inhibitors, may have additive effects for redifferentiation [77, 104, 105]. Furthermore, HDAC inhibitors appear to inhibit cancer cell proliferation via cell-cycle arrest and apoptosis, possibly via re-expression of the tumor suppressor gene p27KIP1 [106]. Clinical trials are currently underway for several epigenetic-modulating agents – azacitidine, decitabine, depsipeptide (FK228), and SAHA (suberoylanilide hydroxamic acid) – in the treatment of radioiodine-refractory thyroid cancer.

Conclusion

There continues to be significant progress in understanding thyroid carcinogenesis on a genetic and molecular level. Modern molecular techniques and novel theories of cancer development have influenced our approaches to the heterogeneous nature of thyroid cancer. Although genetic alterations in BRAF and RET are certainly important in thyroid oncogenesis, other mechanisms such as epigenetic alterations and stem cell propagation appear to play significant roles as well. Ultimately, progress in understanding the molecular basis of thyroid cancer should improve the diagnostic and therapeutic management of patients affected by this disease.

References

1. Kondo T, Ezzat S, Asa SL (2006) Pathogenetic mechanisms in thyroid follicular-cell neoplasia. Nat Rev Cancer 6:292–306
2. Lemoine NR, Mayall ES, Wyllie FS et al (1989) High frequency of ras oncogene activation in all stages of human thyroid tumorigenesis. Oncogene 4:159–164
3. Nikiforova MN, Lynch RA, Biddinger PW et al (2003) RAS point mutations and PAX8-PPAR gamma rearrangement in thyroid tumors: evidence for distinct molecular pathways in thyroid follicular carcinoma. J Clin Endocrinol Metab 88:2318–2326
4. Shinohara M, Chung YJ, Saji M, Ringel MD (2007) AKT in thyroid tumorigenesis and progression. Endocrinology 148:942–947
5. Ito T, Seyama T, Mizuno T et al (1992) Unique association of p53 mutations with undifferentiated but not with differentiated carcinomas of the thyroid gland. Cancer Res 52:1369–1371
6. Joneson T, Bar-Sagi D (1997) Ras effectors and their role in mitogenesis and oncogenesis. J Mol Med 75:587–593
7. Davies H, Bignell GR, Cox C et al (2002) Mutations of the BRAF gene in human cancer. Nature 417:949–954
8. Xing M (2005) BRAF mutation in thyroid cancer. Endocr Relat Cancer 12:245–262
9. Moretti S, Macchiarulo A, De Falco V et al (2006) Biochemical and molecular characterization of the novel BRAF(V599Ins) mutation detected in a classic papillary thyroid carcinoma. Oncogene 25:4235–4240
10. Xing M (2005) The T1799A BRAF mutation is not a germline mutation in familial nonmedullary thyroid cancer. Clin Endocrinol (Oxf) 63:263–266
11. Puxeddu E, Moretti S, Elisei R et al (2004) BRAF(V599E) mutation is the leading genetic event in adult sporadic papillary thyroid carcinomas. J Clin Endocrinol Metab 89:2414–2420
12. Chung KW, Yang SK, Lee GK et al (2006) Detection of BRAFV600E mutation on fine needle aspiration specimens of thyroid nodule refines cyto-pathology diagnosis, especially in BRAF600E mutation-prevalent area. Clin Endocrinol (Oxf) 65:660–666

13. Kimura ET, Nikiforova MN, Zhu Z, Knauf JA, Nikiforov YE, Fagin JA (2003) High prevalence of BRAF mutations in thyroid cancer: genetic evidence for constitutive activation of the RET/PTC-RAS-BRAF signaling pathway in papillary thyroid carcinoma. Cancer Res 63:1454–1457
14. Kim TY, Kim WB, Rhee YS et al (2006) The BRAF mutation is useful for prediction of clinical recurrence in low-risk patients with conventional papillary thyroid carcinoma. Clin Endocrinol (Oxf) 65:364–368
15. Kumagai A, Namba H, Saenko VA et al (2004) Low frequency of BRAFT1796A mutations in childhood thyroid carcinomas. J Clin Endocrinol Metab 89:4280–4284
16. Nikiforova MN, Ciampi R, Salvatore G et al (2004) Low prevalence of BRAF mutations in radiation-induced thyroid tumors in contrast to sporadic papillary carcinomas. Cancer Lett 209:1–6
17. Adeniran AJ, Zhu Z, Gandhi M et al (2006) Correlation between genetic alterations and microscopic features, clinical manifestations, and prognostic characteristics of thyroid papillary carcinomas. Am J Surg Pathol 30:216–222
18. Trovisco V, Vieira de Castro I, Soares P et al (2004) BRAF mutations are associated with some histological types of papillary thyroid carcinoma. J Pathol 202:247–251
19. Begum S, Rosenbaum E, Henrique R, Cohen Y, Sidransky D, Westra WH (2004) BRAF mutations in anaplastic thyroid carcinoma: implications for tumor origin, diagnosis and treatment. Mod Pathol 17:1359–1363
20. Nikiforova MN, Kimura ET, Gandhi M et al (2003) BRAF mutations in thyroid tumors are restricted to papillary carcinomas and anaplastic or poorly differentiated carcinomas arising from papillary carcinomas. J Clin Endocrinol Metab 88:5399–5404
21. Knauf JA, Ma X, Smith EP et al (2005) Targeted expression of BRAFV600E in thyroid cells of transgenic mice results in papillary thyroid cancers that undergo dedifferentiation. Cancer Res 65:4238–4245
22. Trovisco V, Soares P, Preto A et al (2005) Type and prevalence of BRAF mutations are closely associated with papillary thyroid carcinoma histotype and patients' age but not with tumour aggressiveness. Virchows Arch 446:589–595
23. Xu X, Quiros RM, Gattuso P, Ain KB, Prinz RA (2003) High prevalence of BRAF gene mutation in papillary thyroid carcinomas and thyroid tumor cell lines. Cancer Res 63:4561–4567
24. Giordano TJ, Kuick R, Thomas DG et al (2005) Molecular classification of papillary thyroid carcinoma: distinct BRAF, RAS, and RET/PTC mutation-specific gene expression profiles discovered by DNA microarray analysis. Oncogene 24:6646–6656
25. Mitsutake N, Miyagishi M, Mitsutake S et al (2006) BRAF mediates RET/PTC-induced mitogen-activated protein kinase activation in thyroid cells: functional support for requirement of the RET/PTC-RAS-BRAF pathway in papillary thyroid carcinogenesis. Endocrinology 147:1014–1019
26. Riesco-Eizaguirre G, Gutierrez-Martinez P, Garcia-Cabezas MA, Nistal M, Santisteban P (2006) The oncogene BRAF V600E is associated with a high risk of recurrence and less differentiated papillary thyroid carcinoma due to the impairment of Na+/I- targeting to the membrane. Endocr Relat Cancer 13:257–269
27. Durante C, Puxeddu E, Ferretti E et al (2007) BRAF mutations in papillary thyroid carcinomas inhibit genes involved in iodine metabolism. J Clin Endocrinol Metab 92:2840–2843
28. Mesa C Jr, Mirza M, Mitsutake N et al (2006) Conditional activation of RET/PTC3 and BRAFV600E in thyroid cells is associated with gene expression profiles that predict a preferential role of BRAF in extracellular matrix remodeling. Cancer Res 66:6521–6529
29. Mulligan LM, Kwok JB, Healey CS et al (1993) Germ-line mutations of the RET proto-oncogene in multiple endocrine neoplasia type 2A. Nature 363:458–460
30. Fusco A, Grieco M, Santoro M et al (1987) A new oncogene in human thyroid papillary carcinomas and their lymph-nodal metastases. Nature 328:170–172
31. de Groot JW, Links TP, Plukker JT, Lips CJ, Hofstra RM (2006) RET as a diagnostic and therapeutic target in sporadic and hereditary endocrine tumors. Endocr Rev 27:535–560
32. Santoro M, Chiappetta G, Cerrato A et al (1996) Development of thyroid papillary carcinomas secondary to tissue-specific expression of the RET/PTC1 oncogene in transgenic mice. Oncogene 12:1821–1826

33. Knauf JA, Kuroda H, Basu S, Fagin JA (2003) RET/PTC-induced dedifferentiation of thyroid cells is mediated through Y1062 signaling through SHC-RAS-MAP kinase. Oncogene 22:4406–4412
34. Melillo RM, Castellone MD, Guarino V et al (2005) The RET/PTC-RAS-BRAF linear signaling cascade mediates the motile and mitogenic phenotype of thyroid cancer cells. J Clin Invest 115:1068–1081
35. Mitsutake N, Knauf JA, Mitsutake S, Mesa C Jr, Zhang L, Fagin JA (2005) Conditional BRAFV600E expression induces DNA synthesis, apoptosis, dedifferentiation, and chromosomal instability in thyroid PCCL3 cells. Cancer Res 65:2465–2473
36. Elisei R, Romei C, Vorontsova T et al (2001) RET/PTC rearrangements in thyroid nodules: studies in irradiated and not irradiated, malignant and benign thyroid lesions in children and adults. J Clin Endocrinol Metab 86:3211–3216
37. Tallini G, Santoro M, Helie M et al (1998) RET/PTC oncogene activation defines a subset of papillary thyroid carcinomas lacking evidence of progression to poorly differentiated or undifferentiated tumor phenotypes. Clin Cancer Res 4:287–294
38. Rabes HM, Demidchik EP, Sidorow JD et al (2000) Pattern of radiation-induced RET and NTRK1 rearrangements in 191 post-chernobyl papillary thyroid carcinomas: biological, phenotypic, and clinical implications. Clin Cancer Res 6:1093–1103
39. Chiappetta G, Toti P, Cetta F et al (2002) The RET/PTC oncogene is frequently activated in oncocytic thyroid tumors (Hurthle cell adenomas and carcinomas), but not in oncocytic hyperplastic lesions. J Clin Endocrinol Metab 87:364–369
40. Sheils O, Smyth P, Finn S, Sweeney EC, O'Leary JJ (2002) RET/PTC rearrangements in Hashimoto's thyroiditis. Int J Surg Pathol 10:167–168; author reply 8–9
41. Sugg SL, Ezzat S, Rosen IB, Freeman JL, Asa SL (1998) Distinct multiple RET/PTC gene rearrangements in multifocal papillary thyroid neoplasia. J Clin Endocrinol Metab 83:4116–4122
42. Thomas GA, Bunnell H, Cook HA et al (1999) High prevalence of RET/PTC rearrangements in Ukrainian and Belarussian post-Chernobyl thyroid papillary carcinomas: a strong correlation between RET/PTC3 and the solid-follicular variant. J Clin Endocrinol Metab 84:4232–4238
43. Basolo F, Giannini R, Monaco C et al (2002) Potent mitogenicity of the RET/PTC3 oncogene correlates with its prevalence in tall-cell variant of papillary thyroid carcinoma. Am J Pathol 160:247–254
44. Nikiforov YE (2008) Thyroid carcinoma: molecular pathways and therapeutic targets. Mod Pathol 21(Suppl 2):S37–S43
45. Namba H, Rubin SA, Fagin JA (1990) Point mutations of ras oncogenes are an early event in thyroid tumorigenesis. Mol Endocrinol 4:1474–1479
46. Ezzat S, Zheng L, Kolenda J, Safarian A, Freeman JL, Asa SL (1996) Prevalence of activating ras mutations in morphologically characterized thyroid nodules. Thyroid 6:409–416
47. Suarez HG, du Villard JA, Severino M et al (1990) Presence of mutations in all three ras genes in human thyroid tumors. Oncogene 5:565–570
48. Motoi N, Sakamoto A, Yamochi T, Horiuchi H, Motoi T, Machinami R (2000) Role of ras mutation in the progression of thyroid carcinoma of follicular epithelial origin. Pathol Res Pract 196:1–7
49. Vitagliano D, Portella G, Troncone G et al (2006) Thyroid targeting of the N-ras(Gln61Lys) oncogene in transgenic mice results in follicular tumors that progress to poorly differentiated carcinomas. Oncogene 25:5467–5474
50. Garcia-Rostan G, Zhao H, Camp RL et al (2003) Ras mutations are associated with aggressive tumor phenotypes and poor prognosis in thyroid cancer. J Clin Oncol 21:3226–3235
51. Goretzki PE, Lyons J, Stacy-Phipps S et al (1992) Mutational activation of RAS and GSP oncogenes in differentiated thyroid cancer and their biological implications. World J Surg 16:576–581; discussion 81–82
52. Bongarzone I, Vigneri P, Mariani L, Collini P, Pilotti S, Pierotti MA (1998) RET/NTRK1 rearrangements in thyroid gland tumors of the papillary carcinoma family: correlation with clinicopathological features. Clin Cancer Res 4:223–228

53. Kroll TG, Sarraf P, Pecciarini L et al (2000) PAX8-PPARgamma1 fusion oncogene in human thyroid carcinoma [corrected]. Science 289:1357–1360
54. Nikiforova MN, Biddinger PW, Caudill CM, Kroll TG, Nikiforov YE (2002) PAX8-PPARgamma rearrangement in thyroid tumors: RT-PCR and immunohistochemical analyses. Am J Surg Pathol 26:1016–1023
55. Gregory Powell J, Wang X, Allard BL et al (2004) The PAX8/PPARgamma fusion oncoprotein transforms immortalized human thyrocytes through a mechanism probably involving wild-type PPARgamma inhibition. Oncogene 23:3634–3641
56. Reddi HV, McIver B, Grebe SK, Eberhardt NL (2007) The paired box-8/peroxisome proliferator-activated receptor-gamma oncogene in thyroid tumorigenesis. Endocrinology 148:932–935
57. Olivier M, Eeles R, Hollstein M, Khan MA, Harris CC, Hainaut P (2002) The IARC TP53 database: new online mutation analysis and recommendations to users. Hum Mutat 19:607–614
58. Jossart GH, Epstein HD, Shaver JK et al (1996) Immunocytochemical detection of p53 in human thyroid carcinomas is associated with mutation and immortalization of cell lines. J Clin Endocrinol Metab 81:3498–3504
59. Malaguarnera R, Vella V, Vigneri R, Frasca F (2007) p53 family proteins in thyroid cancer. Endocr Relat Cancer 14:43–60
60. Jones PA, Baylin SB (2007) The epigenomics of cancer. Cell 128:683–692
61. Kondo T, Asa SL, Ezzat S (2008) Epigenetic dysregulation in thyroid neoplasia. Endocrinol Metab Clin North Am 37:389–400, ix
62. Khoo ML, Beasley NJ, Ezzat S, Freeman JL, Asa SL (2002) Overexpression of cyclin D1 and underexpression of p27 predict lymph node metastases in papillary thyroid carcinoma. J Clin Endocrinol Metab 87:1814–1818
63. Elisei R, Shiohara M, Koeffler HP, Fagin JA (1998) Genetic and epigenetic alterations of the cyclin-dependent kinase inhibitors p15INK4b and p16INK4a in human thyroid carcinoma cell lines and primary thyroid carcinomas. Cancer 83:2185–2193
64. Schagdarsurengin U, Gimm O, Hoang-Vu C, Dralle H, Pfeifer GP, Dammann R (2002) Frequent epigenetic silencing of the CpG island promoter of RASSF1A in thyroid carcinoma. Cancer Res 62:3698–3701
65. Xing M, Cohen Y, Mambo E et al (2004) Early occurrence of RASSF1A hypermethylation and its mutual exclusion with BRAF mutation in thyroid tumorigenesis. Cancer Res 64:1664–1668
66. Kondo T, Zheng L, Liu W, Kurebayashi J, Asa SL, Ezzat S (2007) Epigenetically controlled fibroblast growth factor receptor 2 signaling imposes on the RAS/BRAF/mitogen-activated protein kinase pathway to modulate thyroid cancer progression. Cancer Res 67:5461–5470
67. Rocha AS, Soares P, Seruca R et al (2001) Abnormalities of the E-cadherin/catenin adhesion complex in classical papillary thyroid carcinoma and in its diffuse sclerosing variant. J Pathol 194:358–366
68. Xing M, Tokumaru Y, Wu G, Westra WB, Ladenson PW, Sidransky D (2003) Hypermethylation of the Pendred syndrome gene SLC26A4 is an early event in thyroid tumorigenesis. Cancer Res 63:2312–2315
69. Neumann S, Schuchardt K, Reske A, Emmrich P, Paschke R (2004) Lack of correlation for sodium iodide symporter mRNA and protein expression and analysis of sodium iodide symporter promoter methylation in benign cold thyroid nodules. Thyroid 14:99–111
70. Venkataraman GM, Yatin M, Marcinek R, Ain KB (1999) Restoration of iodide uptake in dedifferentiated thyroid carcinoma: relationship to human Na+/I-symporter gene methylation status. J Clin Endocrinol Metab 84:2449–2457
71. Hu S, Liu D, Tufano RP et al (2006) Association of aberrant methylation of tumor suppressor genes with tumor aggressiveness and BRAF mutation in papillary thyroid cancer. Int J Cancer 119:2322–2329
72. Alvarez-Nunez F, Bussaglia E, Mauricio D et al (2006) PTEN promoter methylation in sporadic thyroid carcinomas. Thyroid 16:17–23
73. Pfeifer GP, Dammann R (2005) Methylation of the tumor suppressor gene RASSF1A in human tumors. Biochemistry (Mosc) 70:576–583

74. Milkovic M, Sarcevic B, Glavan E (2006) Expression of MAGE tumor-associated antigen in thyroid carcinomas. Endocr Pathol 17:45–52
75. Feinberg AP, Tycko B (2004) The history of cancer epigenetics. Nat Rev Cancer 4:143–153
76. Cras A, Darsin-Bettinger D, Balitrand N et al (2007) Epigenetic patterns of the retinoic acid receptor beta2 promoter in retinoic acid-resistant thyroid cancer cells. Oncogene 26:4018–4024
77. Furuya F, Shimura H, Suzuki H et al (2004) Histone deacetylase inhibitors restore radioiodide uptake and retention in poorly differentiated and anaplastic thyroid cancer cells by expression of the sodium/iodide symporter thyroperoxidase and thyroglobulin. Endocrinology 145:2865–2875
78. Sansam CG, Roberts CW (2006) Epigenetics and cancer: altered chromatin remodeling via Snf5 loss leads to aberrant cell cycle regulation. Cell Cycle 5:621–624
79. Thomas D, Friedman S, Lin RY (2008) Thyroid stem cells: lessons from normal development and thyroid cancer. Endocr Relat Cancer 15:51–58
80. Mitsutake N, Iwao A, Nagai K et al (2007) Characterization of side population in thyroid cancer cell lines: cancer stem-like cells are enriched partly but not exclusively. Endocrinology 148:1797–1803
81. Zhang P, Zuo H, Ozaki T, Nakagomi N, Kakudo K (2006) Cancer stem cell hypothesis in thyroid cancer. Pathol Int 56:485–489
82. Salvatore G, Giannini R, Faviana P et al (2004) Analysis of BRAF point mutation and RET/PTC rearrangement refines the fine-needle aspiration diagnosis of papillary thyroid carcinoma. J Clin Endocrinol Metab 89:5175–5180
83. Cohen Y, Rosenbaum E, Clark DP et al (2004) Mutational analysis of BRAF in fine needle aspiration biopsies of the thyroid: a potential application for the preoperative assessment of thyroid nodules. Clin Cancer Res 10:2761–2765
84. Rowe LR, Bentz BG, Bentz JS (2006) Utility of BRAF V600E mutation detection in cytologically indeterminate thyroid nodules. Cytojournal 3:10
85. Jin L, Sebo TJ, Nakamura N et al (2006) BRAF mutation analysis in fine needle aspiration (FNA) cytology of the thyroid. Diagn Mol Pathol 15:136–143
86. Sapio MR, Posca D, Raggioli A et al (2007) Detection of RET/PTC, TRK and BRAF mutations in preoperative diagnosis of thyroid nodules with indeterminate cytological findings. Clin Endocrinol (Oxf) 66:678–683
87. Barden CB, Shister KW, Zhu B et al (2003) Classification of follicular thyroid tumors by molecular signature: results of gene profiling. Clin Cancer Res 9:1792–1800
88. Finley DJ, Zhu B, Barden CB, Fahey TJ 3rd (2004) Discrimination of benign and malignant thyroid nodules by molecular profiling. Ann Surg 240:425–436 discussion 36–37
89. Mazzanti C, Zeiger MA, Costouros NG et al (2004) Using gene expression profiling to differentiate benign versus malignant thyroid tumors. Cancer Res 64:2898–2903
90. Weber F, Shen L, Aldred MA et al (2005) Genetic classification of benign and malignant thyroid follicular neoplasia based on a three-gene combination. J Clin Endocrinol Metab 90:2512–2521
91. Kebebew E, Peng M, Reiff E, McMillan A (2006) Diagnostic and extent of disease multigene assay for malignant thyroid neoplasms. Cancer 106:2592–2597
92. Kundra P, Burman KD (2007) Thyroid cancer molecular signaling pathways and use of targeted therapy. Endocrinol Metab Clin North Am 36:839–853, viii
93. Wilhelm SM, Carter C, Tang L et al (2004) BAY 43–9006 exhibits broad spectrum oral antitumor activity and targets the RAF/MEK/ERK pathway and receptor tyrosine kinases involved in tumor progression and angiogenesis. Cancer Res 64:7099–7109
94. Ng R, Chen EX (2006) Sorafenib (BAY 43–9006): review of clinical development. Curr Clin Pharmacol 1:223–228
95. Salvatore G, De Falco V, Salerno P et al (2006) BRAF is a therapeutic target in aggressive thyroid carcinoma. Clin Cancer Res 12:1623–1629
96. Gupta-Abramson V, Troxel AB, Nellore A et al (2008) Phase II trial of sorafenib in advanced thyroid cancer. J Clin Oncol 26(29):4714–4719

97. Carlomagno F, Vitagliano D, Guida T et al (2002) ZD6474, an orally available inhibitor of KDR tyrosine kinase activity, efficiently blocks oncogenic RET kinases. Cancer Res 62:7284–7290
98. Herbst RS, Heymach JV, O'Reilly MS, Onn A, Ryan AJ (2007) Vandetanib (ZD6474): an orally available receptor tyrosine kinase inhibitor that selectively targets pathways critical for tumor growth and angiogenesis. Expert Opin Investig Drugs 16:239–249
99. Kim DW, Jo YS, Jung HS et al (2006) An orally administered multitarget tyrosine kinase inhibitor, SU11248, is a novel potent inhibitor of thyroid oncogenic RET/papillary thyroid cancer kinases. J Clin Endocrinol Metab 91:4070–4076
100. Wong E, Rosen LS, Mulay M et al (2007) Sunitinib induces hypothyroidism in advanced cancer patients and may inhibit thyroid peroxidase activity. Thyroid 17:351–355
101. Ohta K, Endo T, Haraguchi K, Hershman JM, Onaya T (2001) Ligands for peroxisome proliferator-activated receptor gamma inhibit growth and induce apoptosis of human papillary thyroid carcinoma cells. J Clin Endocrinol Metab 86:2170–2177
102. Martelli ML, Iuliano R, Le Pera I et al (2002) Inhibitory effects of peroxisome poliferator-activated receptor gamma on thyroid carcinoma cell growth. J Clin Endocrinol Metab 87:4728–4735
103. Park JW, Zarnegar R, Kanauchi H et al (2005) Troglitazone, the peroxisome proliferator-activated receptor-gamma agonist, induces antiproliferation and redifferentiation in human thyroid cancer cell lines. Thyroid 15:222–231
104. Zarnegar R, Brunaud L, Kanauchi H et al (2002) Increasing the effectiveness of radioactive iodine therapy in the treatment of thyroid cancer using Trichostatin A, a histone deacetylase inhibitor. Surgery 132:984–990; discussion 90
105. Wischnewski F, Pantel K, Schwarzenbach H (2006) Promoter demethylation and histone acetylation mediate gene expression of MAGE-A1, -A2, -A3, and -A12 in human cancer cells. Mol Cancer Res 4:339–349
106. Mitsiades CS, Poulaki V, McMullan C et al (2005) Novel histone deacetylase inhibitors in the treatment of thyroid cancer. Clin Cancer Res 11:3958–3965

Chapter 2
Evaluation of the Thyroid Nodule

Dina M. Elaraj

Epidemiology

Thyroid nodules are very common in the general population. The prevalence of palpable thyroid nodules is only approximately 4–7%, but the prevalence of ultrasound-detectable nodules is between 19 and 67% [1]. Twenty to forty-eight percent of patients with apparently solitary thyroid nodules palpated on physical exam will have additional sonographically detectable nodules [2, 3]. Thyroid nodules are more common in women than in men by a ratio of about 4 to 1, and increase in frequency with age and with decreasing iodine intake [4]. Thyroid nodules are also more common in patients who have a history of head and neck irradiation, developing at a rate of about 2% per year compared with 0.1% per year in patients without a history of significant radiation exposure [5].

The great majority of thyroid nodules are benign, with the differential diagnosis including simple or hemorrhagic cysts, colloid nodules, follicular adenomas, or thyroiditis [6]. The overall risk of malignancy in a thyroid nodule is 5–10% [7]. While thyroid nodules are relatively common in the general population, in contrast, thyroid cancer is relatively uncommon with an expected annual incidence in the United States (U.S.) of 37,340 cases in 2008, constituting only 2.6% of all cancers and only 0.3% of cancer deaths [8]. The incidence of thyroid cancer has increased 2.4-fold in the U.S. over the last 30 years, from 3.6 per 100,000 in 1973 to 8.7 per 100,000 in 2003 [9]. Thyroid cancer is more common in women than in men by a ratio of about 3 to 1, and has now become the sixth most common cancer in women [8]. While thyroid cancer is more common in women, mortality rates from thyroid cancer are higher for men; this is thought to be related to an older age at diagnosis in men [10].

D.M. Elaraj (✉)
Section of Endocrine Surgery, Northwestern University Feinberg School of Medicine, 676 N. St. Clair St, Suite 650, Chicago, IL 60611, USA
e-mail: delaraj@nmh.org

C. Sturgeon (ed.), *Endocrine Neoplasia*, Cancer Treatment and Research, vol 153,
DOI 10.1007/978-1-4419-0857-5_2, © Springer Science+Business Media, LLC 2010

The goal of the thyroid nodule evaluation, therefore, is to identify and surgically treat patients with malignant thyroid nodules, while avoiding surgery in patients with benign, asymptomatic thyroid nodules.

Diagnostic Evaluation

Most patients present with an asymptomatic nodule which is self-discovered, found incidentally on an imaging study, or palpated by a physician on routine physical exam. A small percentage of patients manifest signs or symptoms due to compression, invasion into adjacent structures, or metastatic disease. The evaluation of the patient with a thyroid nodule should begin with a detailed history and risk factor assessment. Physical examination should focus on findings that are more often associated with a malignant process. Thyroid function studies and cervical ultrasonography are recommended for all patients. Fine needle aspiration (FNA) biopsy is the simplest, most accurate, and cost-effective method to establish a diagnosis.

Risk Factor Assessment

The risk of malignancy in nodular thyroid disease varies depending on factors such as gender, age, and personal and family history. Increased suspicion is associated with male gender, age <15 or >45 years, nodule size >4 cm, history of radiation exposure, and personal or family history of conditions known to be associated with thyroid cancer [5].

In addition to increasing a patient's risk for developing thyroid nodules, a history of radiation exposure, particularly in childhood, increases a patient's risk of developing thyroid cancer [11]. Multiple studies have shown an increase in the number of thyroid cancers diagnosed in children who lived within a 150 km radius of Chernobyl, in adult survivors of the atomic bombings of Hiroshima and Nagasaki, and in patients who received head and neck radiotherapy in childhood for the treatment of conditions such as enlarged tonsils, an enlarged thymus, tinea capitis, or acne [12, 13].

A family history of thyroid cancer also increases a patient's risk of thyroid cancer. While only 3% of thyroid cancers are heritable, there are multiple syndromes that are associated with an increased risk of papillary or medullary thyroid cancer. A family history of papillary thyroid cancer in two first-degree relatives increases the risk of thyroid cancer three- to ninefold, and these families are likely part of a familial nonmedullary thyroid cancer (FNMTC) kindred [14, 15]. Other syndromes associated with papillary thyroid cancer include familial adenomatous polyposis (FAP) and its variant, Gardner's syndrome (both due to a mutation in the *APC* gene), Cowden's syndrome (also known as multiple hamartoma syndrome, due to a mutation in the *PTEN* gene), and Carney complex (due to a mutation in the

PRKAR1A gene) [5, 16]. Familial syndromes known to be associated with medullary thyroid cancer include multiple endocrine neoplasia types 2A and 2B (MEN-2A and B), and familial medullary thyroid cancer (FMTC), all due to a mutation in the RET gene [17]. Eliciting a personal or family history of conditions which are known to be components of the above syndromes, therefore, is an important part of the risk factor assessment of a patient with a thyroid nodule.

In addition to evaluating a patient's personal and family history, other factors that may increase the risk or suspicion of thyroid cancer should be assessed including recent onset, rapid rate of growth, dysphagia, hoarseness, male gender, and age [18].

Physical Examination

A detailed physical exam is done, with particular attention to voice quality, characteristics of the nodule, and the adjacent nodal basins. Hoarseness raises the concern for recurrent laryngeal nerve invasion by an aggressive thyroid cancer. Firmness or consistency of the nodule is not particularly reliable in discriminating benign from malignant processes as some benign processes can be heavily calcified and firm and some papillary cancers can be cystic or soft. Fixation of the nodule to adjacent or overlying structures, or the presence of (especially ipsilateral) cervical or supraclavicular lymphadenopathy substantially increases the probability of cancer. Deficits in neurologic function should be carefully sought and documented, particularly for those nerves that pass through the central and lateral cervical compartments of the neck. Characteristics of syndromic endocrinopathies should be evaluated. Cutaneous lichen amyloidosis, usually in the intrascapular area, may be found in patients with MEN-2A. Medullary thyroid cancer, mucosal neuromas, and marfanoid habitus are almost universally present in patients with MEN-2B beginning in infancy or early childhood. Elevated blood pressure might raise the suspicion for pheochromocytoma in the correct clinical context. Pheochromocytoma must always be treated before thyroid surgery is performed.

Laryngoscopy

Many clinicians perform mirror or fiberoptic laryngoscopy on a routine basis for all patients with thyroid pathology, while others perform these tests more selectively. Several reports have concluded that routine preoperative laryngoscopy should be done on all patients with thyroid cancer [19, 20]. This practice is supported by the fact that some patients with compensated recurrent laryngeal nerve palsy will have a normal voice. Discovery of a preoperative vocal cord paralysis suggests that there is extrathyroidal extension of the tumor and may change the operative technique and postoperative expectations of the patient. Most experts, however, recommend laryngoscopy only for symptomatic patients or for patients who have previously undergone thyroid or parathyroid surgery. Many clinicians employ laryngoscopy selectively because of the paucity of compelling evidence to recommend for or against routine laryngoscopy. All patients with hoarseness, history of vocal cord paralysis, or prior neck surgery should undergo preoperative laryngoscopy to evaluate for recurrent laryngeal nerve palsy [21].

Diagnostic Tests

Multiple organizations including the American Thyroid Association (ATA), National Comprehensive Cancer Network (NCCN), American Association of Clinical Endocrinologists and Associazione Medici Endocrinologi (AACE/AME), and Society of Radiologists in Ultrasound (SRU) have published guidelines for the evaluation and management of thyroid nodules [5–7, 22]. The following is an approach based on aspects of several of the above consensus guidelines.

Imaging

All patients with palpable thyroid nodules should be evaluated by cervical sonogram. Ultrasonographic features generally thought to increase the suspicion of thyroid cancer include microcalcifications, irregular borders, and central hypervascularity. The sensitivity and specificity of these features are not very high, when considered independently. The SRU guidelines report a sensitivity of 26–59% and specificity of 86–95% for microcalcifications, a sensitivity of 17–78% and specificity of 39–85% for irregular margins, and a sensitivity of 54–74% and specificity of 79–81% for central hypervascularity [22]. The presence of more than one of the above features, however, increases the probability that a thyroid nodule represents a malignancy. The presence of a hypoechoic nodule in conjunction with at least one of the above independent risk factors was able to identify 87% of malignancies in one study of 494 consecutive nonpalpable thyroid nodules [23]. Figure 2.1 illustrates a hypoechoic 1.2 cm thyroid nodule with microcalcifications and irregular borders on ultrasound which was a papillary thyroid cancer. Cervical sonography is the imaging study of choice for the evaluation of thyroid nodular disease.

Computed tomography (CT) and magnetic resonance imaging (MRI) are useful to assess size, substernal extension, and relationship of a large thyroid nodule or goiter to surrounding structures or when adjacent tissue invasion is suspected. Cross-sectional imaging is not recommended for the routine evaluation of a thyroid nodule, however, because of low resolution of small nodules, and because the iodine load from intravenous contrast is considered undesirable if the patient might have differentiated thyroid cancer.

Fluorodeoxyglucose positron emission tomography (FDG-PET) is very effective in identifying many primary and metastatic thyroid cancers. Although PET scanning

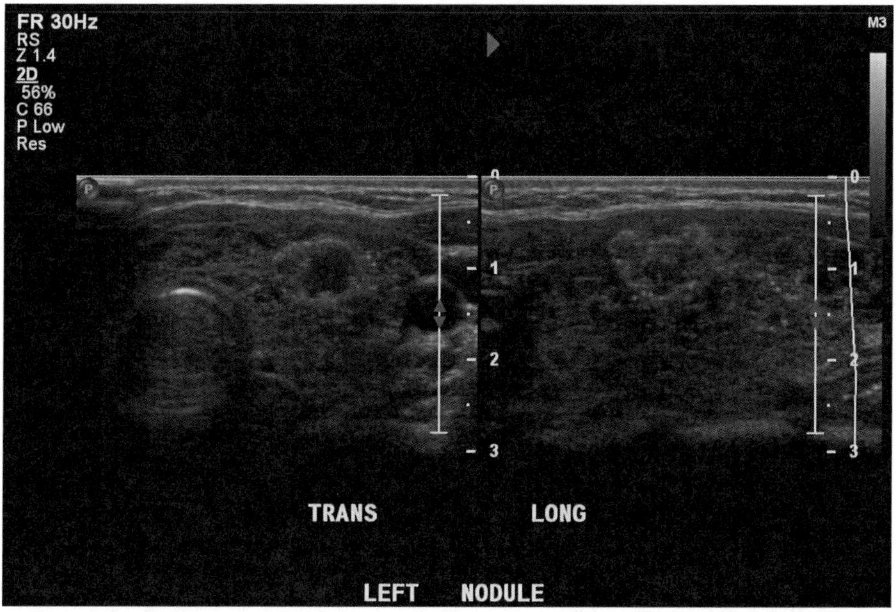

Fig. 2.1 Transverse and longitudinal ultrasound images of a 1.2 cm thyroid nodule with microcalcifications and irregular borders in a 24-year-old woman, which was a papillary thyroid cancer on fine needle aspiration biopsy

is very sensitive for cancer, it is not highly specific. Graves' disease, thyroiditis, and some benign nodules may also have FDG-PET uptake. The literature demonstrates a high incidence of malignancy within FDG-PET avid thyroid incidentalomas, with most studies revealing a malignancy rate of approximately 35% [24–27]. The high sensitivity of PET scan in detecting thyroid cancer underscores the importance of working up FDG-PET avid thyroid lesions, but the low specificity prevents PET scanning from being useful in the routine evaluation of thyroid nodules.

In hyperthyroid patients, a radionuclide thyroid scan should be performed. If there is increased tracer uptake in the nodule compared to the surrounding thyroid parenchyma (i.e., a "hot" nodule) and there are no suspicious features on ultrasound, then the risk of malignancy is extremely low [5–7].

Laboratory Studies

All patients with thyroid nodules should have a serum thyrotropin (thyroid-stimulating hormone, TSH) measurement. Interestingly, several recent studies have found that a higher TSH concentration, even if within the normal range, may be associated with an increased risk of thyroid cancer in a thyroid nodule [18, 28, 29].

The routine use of serum calcitonin measurement to screen all patients with thyroid nodules for medullary thyroid cancer has, thus far, not been advocated in the U.S. Several European studies, and now one study in the U.S., have demonstrated that the routine evaluation of serum calcitonin level in the initial evaluation of all thyroid nodules would be cost-effective [30–33].

Fine Needle Aspiration Biopsy

FNA biopsy should be considered for all patients depending on nodule size, appearance on ultrasound, and patient risk factors for thyroid cancer. FNA biopsy, particularly when done under ultrasound guidance, is the most cost-effective and accurate way to evaluate a thyroid nodule [7]. FNA biopsy has decreased the cost of care of thyroid nodules by 25% [34]. The sensitivity of FNA biopsy is 65–98% with a specificity of 72–100%. Any thyroid nodule in the setting of a suspicious-appearing cervical lymph node, especially when ipsilateral, should undergo FNA biopsy (as should the cervical lymph node) [22].

Consensus guidelines vary regarding clinical thresholds for FNA biopsy. The ATA guidelines recommend FNA biopsy of all nodules >1–1.5 cm [7]. The NCCN and AACE/AME guidelines recommend FNA biopsy of all nodules >1 cm or of those <1 cm with suspicious criteria by ultrasound, with increased tracer uptake on PET scan, or in a patient with risk factors for thyroid cancer [5, 6]. The SRU guidelines recommend FNA biopsy of a ≥1 cm solitary nodule with microcalcifications, of a ≥1.5 cm solitary solid nodule or one containing coarse calcifications, and of a ≥2 cm mixed solid and cystic or almost entirely cystic nodule with a solid mural component [22]. While cystic or mixed solid and cystic thyroid nodules are usually benign, some papillary thyroid cancers may be cystic and therefore warrant FNA biopsy. In the setting of a multinodular goiter, selection of thyroid nodules for FNA biopsy should be based on suspicious ultrasound features rather than on nodule size [6, 7, 22].

Management of Asymptomatic Thyroid Nodules

Management of an asymptomatic thyroid nodule depends, in part, on the findings from the FNA biopsy. The nomenclature used to describe the cytopathologic findings is highly variable between institutions and even individual cytopathologists. At the most basic level, the biopsy results are either diagnostic or nondiagnostic. Nondiagnostic specimens are usually referred to as "unsatisfactory," "inadequate," or "insufficient," because they have an inadequate number of follicular cells to render a diagnosis. This may be due to the nodule being predominantly cystic or highly vascular, or it could be due to poor biopsy technique or slide preparation. Approximately 11–15% of FNA biopsies are nondiagnostic [35, 36], and repeat

FNA biopsy is recommended [5, 7], usually after waiting at least 12 weeks. It is particularly important to repeat the FNA biopsy under ultrasound-guidance, and immediate cytologic review for adequacy should be considered. Surgical excision should be considered for repeatedly nondiagnostic specimens, particularly if the nodule is solid [7]. Large series report a malignancy rate of 5–9% in nodules with nondiagnostic FNA biopsy results that underwent surgical resection [37, 38].

Diagnostic specimens fall into many categories which also frequently vary from institution to institution, as at the present time there is no standardized terminology. The most commonly used categories are "benign," occurring in 68–74% of cases, "malignant," occurring in 4–5% of cases, and "suspicious," occurring in 11–13% of cases [35, 36]. Sometimes an "indeterminate" category is used, which includes diagnoses such as "follicular lesion" or "follicular neoplasm" [7].

In 2006, both the ATA and AACE/AME published proposed diagnostic terminology schemes, which included variations of the above categories [6, 7] (Table 2.1). In 2007, the National Cancer Institute (NCI) convened a Thyroid FNA State of the Science Conference with the goal of further trying to standardize the terminology used to describe FNA biopsies of thyroid nodules [39]. The committee members of this conference proposed the following six diagnostic categories: "non-diagnostic," "benign," "malignant," "suspicious for malignancy," "neoplasm," and "follicular lesion of undetermined significance" [39] (Table 2.1), although these have not yet been adopted into standard practice. These largely overlap with the ATA and AACE/AME categories, and the management of thyroid nodules in each of these categories is described below.

Asymptomatic benign thyroid nodules, smaller than 4 cm, should be followed up, as the false negative rate of FNA biopsies is about 4% [40]. Thyroid nodules ≥4 cm have higher false negative rates of 13–17% [41, 42] and should be considered

Table 2.1 Thyroid fine needle aspiration classification schemes and risk of malignancy

American Thyroid Association 2006 [7]	American Association of Clinical Endocrinologists and Associazione Medici Endocrinologi 2006 [6]	National Cancer Institute 2007 [39]	Risk of malignancy [39]
Benign	Benign	Benign	<5%
Malignant	Malignant or suspicious	Malignant	100% for malignant
Indeterminate – suspect for carcinoma	–	Suspicious for malignancy	50–75%
Indeterminate – suspect for neoplasia	Follicular neoplasia	Neoplasm	20–30%
–	–	Follicular lesion of undetermined significance	5–10%
Inadequate	Nondiagnostic or ultrasound suspicious	Nondiagnostic	–

for diagnostic lobectomy regardless of the biopsy results. The natural history of benign thyroid nodules is poorly understood, as studies examining this issue are often retrospective and contain a substantial number of patients who undergo surgery for various reasons. Nevertheless, these studies have shown that between 13 and 89% of thyroid nodules will increase in size over 5–15 years, and that the risk of thyroid cancer in these nodules is extremely variable from 1 to 26% [43, 44]. Consensus guidelines recommend periodic lifelong follow-up of benign thyroid nodules every 6–24 months, with re-biopsy if there is a significant change in size or appearance [6, 7].

Malignant thyroid nodules are most commonly papillary cancers, although other malignancies such as medullary and anaplastic cancers can be diagnosed by FNA biopsy. Lymphoma and metastatic cancers to the thyroid gland can also be diagnosed or suspected on FNA or core biopsy. Patients with primary malignancies of the thyroid gland should undergo thyroidectomy. The preoperative evaluation, extent of surgical resection, and postoperative therapy and surveillance will depend on the particular histologic type of thyroid cancer, and are described in detail in chapters 3–5.

FNA biopsies interpreted as "suspicious for malignancy" have a cancer rate of 50–75% [39]. The great majority of these cases are suspicious for papillary thyroid cancer, particularly the follicular variant of papillary thyroid cancer, but lymphomas or cancers metastatic to the thyroid might also be placed into this category. Treatment options for lesions suspicious for a differentiated thyroid cancer include diagnostic thyroid lobectomy with or without intraoperative frozen section versus total thyroidectomy at the outset depending on patient risk factors, patient preference, and presence of nodules in the contralateral thyroid lobe.

Thyroid nodule biopsies read as "neoplasm," "follicular neoplasm," "Hürthle cell neoplasm," "suspicious for neoplasm," or "follicular lesion" are indeterminate and have a risk of malignancy up to 20–30% [39]. Because the diagnosis of malignancy in follicular and Hürthle cell carcinoma is made depending on the presence of capsular or vascular invasion, repeat FNA biopsy is not useful for indeterminate nodules, and these patients should undergo diagnostic thyroid lobectomy. Several investigators are studying molecular markers in an attempt to make a diagnosis without surgical resection, but these methods are currently preclinical because of insufficient data [45, 46]. Because in most institutions it is not practical to freeze and section the entire capsule intraoperatively, a final benign or malignant diagnosis is usually rendered several days postoperatively. Reoperation for completion thyroidectomy may be necessary due to these limitations. Alternatively a patient may prefer to undergo total thyroidectomy at the outset on the basis of willingness to undergo completion thyroidectomy, risk factors for complications and cancer, and presence of nodules on the contralateral side.

Finally, thyroid nodule biopsies that are classified as "follicular lesion of undetermined significance," a new category proposed by the 2007 NCI State of the Science Conference, include those FNA biopsies that are not convincingly benign, but whose cellular or architectural features are not sufficiently concerning to place them into a "suspicious for malignancy" or "neoplasm" category [39].

The members of the State of the Science committee advocate minimizing the use of this category, and recommend repeat FNA biopsy in order to make a diagnosis [39].

Management of Symptomatic Thyroid Nodules

Patients with symptomatic thyroid nodules usually either have symptoms of compression or of hyperfunction. Compressive symptoms include pain, dysphagia, dyspnea, or hoarseness. Sometimes patients can have tracheal deviation and compression and be relatively asymptomatic. Figure 2.2 shows the CT scan of a patient with an asymptomatic 6.6 cm left thyroid nodule with substernal extension and rightward tracheal deviation. Patients with compressive symptoms should undergo thyroidectomy.

Patients with autonomously hyperfunctioning thyroid nodules who are symptomatic can be treated surgically or with radioactive iodine ablation. Most patients are treated with radioactive iodine ablation, usually requiring only one dose, with variable rates of postablation hypothyroidism of 0–35% and rates of recurrent hyperthyroidism from 2 to 7% [47–50]. Surgery is usually reserved for patients with larger nodules, younger patients, or those who desire or require immediate control of their hyperthyroidism.

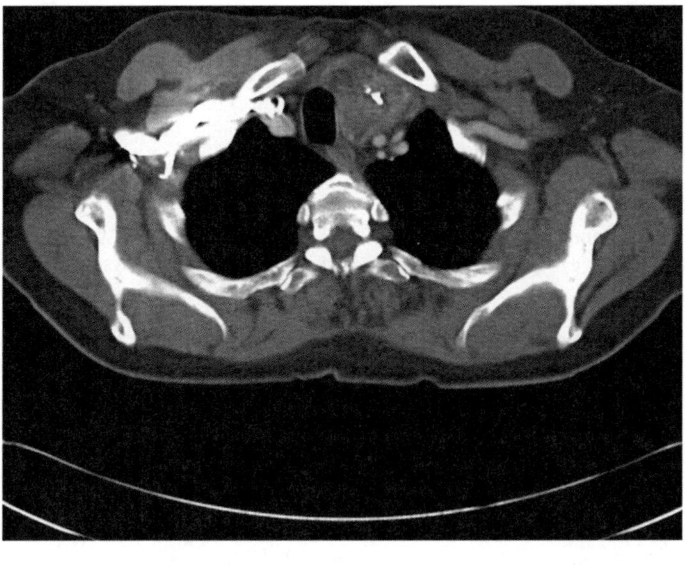

Fig. 2.2 Axial computed tomographic (CT) image of an asymptomatic 69-year-old man with a 6.6 cm left thyroid nodule with coarse calcifications that was causing rightward tracheal deviation. Fine needle aspiration (FNA) biopsy was indeterminate for neoplasm. Final pathologic examination showed a follicular adenoma

Summary

Thyroid nodules are very common in the general population, while thyroid cancer is relatively uncommon. The goal of the evaluation of the thyroid nodule is to identify and surgically treat patients with malignancies, while identifying and avoiding surgery in those with benign, asymptomatic thyroid nodules. The evaluation of the thyroid nodule begins with patient history, risk factor assessment, and physical exam. All patients with a thyroid nodule should undergo cervical ultrasonography and have serum TSH measured. Further diagnostic evaluation is done by FNA biopsy depending on patient risk factors, physical exam findings, nodule size and appearance on ultrasound, and serum TSH. Multiple diagnostic categories for FNA biopsies of thyroid nodules have been developed, each with its own risk of malignancy. Benign asymptomatic thyroid nodules smaller than 4 cm can be observed in low-risk patients. Thyroid nodule size greater than 4 cm, or FNA results classified as "malignant," "suspicious for malignancy," or "indeterminate" should prompt surgical excision. Small, asymptomatic nodules classified as "follicular lesions of undetermined significance" require at least a repeat FNA biopsy. Thyroid nodules that cause compressive symptoms should be treated surgically, while autonomously functioning ("hot") thyroid nodules may be treated with radioactive iodine ablation or surgery depending on the clinical scenario.

References

1. Tan GH, Gharib H (1997) Thyroid incidentalomas: management approaches to nonpalpable nodules discovered incidentally on thyroid imaging. Ann Intern Med 126:226–231
2. Walker J, Findlay D, Amar SS, Small PG, Wastie ML, Pegg CA (1985) A prospective study of thyroid ultrasound scan in the clinically solitary thyroid nodule. Br J Radiol 58:617–619
3. Tan GH, Gharib H, Reading CC (1995) Solitary thyroid nodule. Comparison between palpation and ultrasonography. Arch Intern Med 155:2418–2423
4. Hegedus L (2004) Clinical practice. The thyroid nodule. N Engl J Med 351:1764–1771
5. National Comprehensive Cancer Network (2008) Clinical Practice Guidelines in Oncology: Thyroid Carcinoma V.I.2008. http://www.nccn.org/professionals/physician_gls/PDF/thyroid.pdf Accessed 1 Nov 2008
6. American Association of Clinical Endocrinologists and Associazione Medici Endocrinologi (2006) Medical guidelines for clinical practice for the diagnosis and management of thyroid nodules. Endocr Pract 12:63–102
7. Cooper DS, Doherty GM, Haugen BR et al (2006) Management guidelines for patients with thyroid nodules and differentiated thyroid cancer. Thyroid 16:109–142
8. Jemal A, Siegel R, Ward E et al (2008) Cancer statistics, 2008. CA Cancer J Clin 58:71–96
9. Davies L, Welch HG (2006) Increasing incidence of thyroid cancer in the United States, 1973–2002. JAMA 295:2164–2167
10. Mazzaferri EL, Jhiang SM (1994) Long-term impact of initial surgical and medical therapy on papillary and follicular thyroid cancer. Am J Med 97:418–428
11. Ron E (1998) Ionizing radiation and cancer risk: evidence from epidemiology. Radiat Res 150:S30–S41
12. Shibata Y, Yamashita S, Masyakin VB, Panasyuk GD, Nagataki S (2001) 15 years after Chernobyl: new evidence of thyroid cancer. Lancet 358:1965–1966

13. Imaizumi M, Usa T, Tominaga T et al (2006) Radiation dose–response relationships for thyroid nodules and autoimmune thyroid diseases in Hiroshima and Nagasaki atomic bomb survivors 55–58 years after radiation exposure. JAMA 295:1011–1022
14. Goldgar DE, Easton DF, Cannon-Albright LA, Skolnick MH (1994) Systematic population-based assessment of cancer risk in first-degree relatives of cancer probands. J Natl Cancer Inst 86:1600–1608
15. Hemminki K, Eng C, Chen B (2005) Familial risks for nonmedullary thyroid cancer. J Clin Endocrinol Metab 90:5747–5753
16. Musholt TJ, Musholt PB, Petrich T, Oetting G, Knapp WH, Klempnauer J (2000) Familial papillary thyroid carcinoma: genetics, criteria for diagnosis, clinical features, and surgical treatment. World J Surg 24:1409–1417
17. Evans DB, Shapiro SE, Cote GJ (2007) Invited commentary: medullary thyroid cancer: the importance of RET testing. Surgery 141:96–99
18. Boelaert K, Horacek J, Holder RL, Watkinson JC, Sheppard MC, Franklyn JA (2006) Serum thyrotropin concentration as a novel predictor of malignancy in thyroid nodules investigated by fine-needle aspiration. J Clin Endocrinol Metab 91:4295–4301
19. Schlosser K, Zeuner M, Wagner M, et al (2007) Laryngoscopy in thyroid surgery – essential standard or unnecessary routine? Surgery 142:858–864; discussion 64 e1–e2
20. Randolph GW, Kamani D (2006) The importance of preoperative laryngoscopy in patients undergoing thyroidectomy: voice, vocal cord function, and the preoperative detection of invasive thyroid malignancy. Surgery 139:357–362
21. Jarhult J, Lindestad PA, Nordenstrom J, Perbeck L (1991) Routine examination of the vocal cords before and after thyroid and parathyroid surgery. Br J Surg 78:1116–1117
22. Frates MC, Benson CB, Charboneau JW et al (2005) Management of thyroid nodules detected at US: society of radiologists in ultrasound consensus conference statement. Radiology 237:794–800
23. Papini E, Guglielmi R, Bianchini A et al (2002) Risk of malignancy in nonpalpable thyroid nodules: predictive value of ultrasound and color-Doppler features. J Clin Endocrinol Metab 87:1941–1946
24. Chu QD, Connor MS, Lilien DL, Johnson LW, Turnage RH, Li BD (2006) Positron emission tomography (PET) positive thyroid incidentaloma: the risk of malignancy observed in a tertiary referral center. Am Surg 72:272–275
25. King DL, Stack BC Jr, Spring PM, Walker R, Bodenner DL (2007) Incidence of thyroid carcinoma in fluorodeoxyglucose positron emission tomography-positive thyroid incidentalomas. Otolaryngol Head Neck Surg 137:400–404
26. Are C, Hsu JF, Schoder H, Shah JP, Larson SM, Shaha AR (2007) FDG-PET detected thyroid incidentalomas: need for further investigation? Ann Surg Oncol 14:239–247
27. Kim TY, Kim WB, Ryu JS, Gong G, Hong SJ, Shong YK (2005) 18F-fluorodeoxyglucose uptake in thyroid from positron emission tomogram (PET) for evaluation in cancer patients: high prevalence of malignancy in thyroid PET incidentaloma. Laryngoscope 115:1074–1078
28. Polyzos SA, Kita M, Efstathiadou Z et al (2008) Serum thyrotropin concentration as a biochemical predictor of thyroid malignancy in patients presenting with thyroid nodules. J Cancer Res Clin Oncol 134:953–960
29. Haymart MR, Repplinger DJ, Leverson GE et al (2008) Higher serum thyroid stimulating hormone level in thyroid nodule patients is associated with greater risks of differentiated thyroid cancer and advanced tumor stage. J Clin Endocrinol Metab 93:809–814
30. Cheung K, Roman SA, Wang TS, Walker HD, Sosa JA (2008) Calcitonin measurement in the evaluation of thyroid nodules in the United States: a cost-effectiveness and decision analysis. J Clin Endocrinol Metab 93:2173–2180
31. Elisei R, Bottici V, Luchetti F et al (2004) Impact of routine measurement of serum calcitonin on the diagnosis and outcome of medullary thyroid cancer: experience in 10, 864 patients with nodular thyroid disorders. J Clin Endocrinol Metab 89:163–168
32. Costante G, Meringolo D, Durante C et al (2007) Predictive value of serum calcitonin levels for preoperative diagnosis of medullary thyroid carcinoma in a cohort of 5817 consecutive patients with thyroid nodules. J Clin Endocrinol Metab 92:450–455

33. Vierhapper H, Niederle B, Bieglmayer C, Kaserer K, Baumgartner-Parzer S (2005) Early diagnosis and curative therapy of medullary thyroid carcinoma by routine measurement of serum calcitonin in patients with thyroid disorders. Thyroid 15:1267–1272
34. Gharib H, Goellner JR (1993) Fine-needle aspiration biopsy of the thyroid: an appraisal. Ann Intern Med 118:282–289
35. Grant CS, Hay ID, Gough IR, McCarthy PM, Goellner JR (1989) Long-term follow-up of patients with benign thyroid fine-needle aspiration cytologic diagnoses. Surgery 106:980–985; discussion 5–6
36. Mazzaferri EL (1993) Management of a solitary thyroid nodule. N Engl J Med 328:553–559
37. Alexander EK, Heering JP, Benson CB et al (2002) Assessment of nondiagnostic ultrasound-guided fine needle aspirations of thyroid nodules. J Clin Endocrinol Metab 87:4924–4927
38. McHenry CR, Walfish PG, Rosen IB (1993) Non-diagnostic fine needle aspiration biopsy: a dilemma in management of nodular thyroid disease. Am Surg 59:415–419
39. National Cancer Institute Thyroid Fine Needle Aspiration (FNA) State of the Science Conference (2008) http://thyroidfna.cancer.gov/pages/conclusions/. Accessed 1 Nov 2008
40. Ylagan LR, Farkas T, Dehner LP (2004) Fine needle aspiration of the thyroid: a cytohistologic correlation and study of discrepant cases. Thyroid 14:35–41
41. McCoy KL, Jabbour N, Ogilvie JB, Ohori NP, Carty SE, Yim JH (2007) The incidence of cancer and rate of false-negative cytology in thyroid nodules greater than or equal to 4 cm in size. Surgery 142:837–844; discussion 44 e1–e3
42. Meko JB, Norton JA (1995) Large cystic/solid thyroid nodules: a potential false-negative fine-needle aspiration. Surgery 118:996–1003; discussion 1003–1004
43. Kuma K, Matsuzuka F, Kobayashi A, et al (1992) Outcome of long standing solitary thyroid nodules. World J surg 16:583–587; discussion 7–8
44. Alexander EK, Hurwitz S, Heering JP et al (2003) Natural history of benign solid and cystic thyroid nodules. Ann Intern Med 138:315–318
45. Kebebew E, Peng M, Reiff E, Duh QY, Clark OH, McMillan A (2005) ECM1 and TMPRSS4 are diagnostic markers of malignant thyroid neoplasms and improve the accuracy of fine needle aspiration biopsy. Ann surg 242:353–361; discussion 61–63
46. Bartolazzi A, Orlandi F, Saggiorato E et al (2008) Galectin-3-expression analysis in the surgical selection of follicular thyroid nodules with indeterminate fine-needle aspiration cytology: a prospective multicentre study. Lancet oncol 9:543–549
47. Ross DS, Ridgway EC, Daniels GH (1984) Successful treatment of solitary toxic thyroid nodules with relatively low-dose iodine-131, with low prevalence of hypothyroidism. Ann Intern Med 101:488–490
48. Ratcliffe GE, Cooke S, Fogelman I, Maisey MN (1986) Radioiodine treatment of solitary functioning thyroid nodules. Br J Radiol 59:385–387
49. Huysmans DA, Corstens FH, Kloppenborg PW (1991) Long-term follow-up in toxic solitary autonomous thyroid nodules treated with radioactive iodine. J Nucl Med 32:27–30
50. O'Brien T, Gharib H, Suman VJ, van Heerden JA (1992) Treatment of toxic solitary thyroid nodules: surgery versus radioactive iodine. Surgery 112:1166–1170

Chapter 3
Differentiated Thyroid Cancers of Follicular Cell Origin

Linwah Yip and Sally E. Carty

In the early 1800s, thyroid cancer was one of the first thyroid diseases to be described. Although trends for all other cancers are decreasing, the incidence of thyroid carcinoma is increasing and an estimated 37,340 new cases of thyroid cancer are expected to be diagnosed in 2008. Thyroid cancer (TC) is now the sixth most common malignancy diagnosed in women [1]. The increase in TC incidence can be predominantly attributed to the detection and diagnosis of small (<2 cm) papillary thyroid carcinomas [2]. Although approximately 1 in 127 persons will be diagnosed with TC over their lifetime, TC mortality is low with an estimated 1,590 deaths expected in 2008 [1]. Overall, 5-year TC survival rates have remained stable at 93% from1975 to 1977 and 97% from 1996 to 2003 [1].

Embryologically, both differentiated thyroid carcinoma (DTC) and undifferentiated or anaplastic thyroid carcinoma (ATC) arise from the follicular epithelial cells that produce thyroid hormone and line thyroid follicles. DTC makes up the majority (95%) of TC. DTC histologic subtypes include papillary thyroid carcinoma (PTC; 85%), follicular thyroid carcinoma (FTC; 10%), and oncocytic (Hürthle) cell carcinoma (HCC; 3%) [3]. ATC is rare (1–2%) and patients uniformly have a poor prognosis; its management is addressed in Chap. 5. Medullary thyroid carcinoma accounts for 3–4% of all TC and arises from the calcitonin-producing parafollicular C-cells which are most abundant in the superior thyroid poles. Other rare thyroid neoplasias include primary lymphoma, paraganglioma, and metastases to the thyroid gland [4].

Genetics of Differentiated Thyroid Cancer

More than 70% of PTCs either have a nonoverlapping genetic alteration in *BRAF*, *RAS*, and *NTRK1*, or have a *RET/PTC* genetic rearrangement (Table 3.1). The proto-oncogene *BRAF*, one of the intracellular effectors involved in the MAPK

S.E. Carty (✉)
University of Pittsburgh School of Medicine, Suite 101 Kaufmann Building,
3471 Fifth Avenue, Pittsburgh, PA, 15213, USA
e-mail: cartyse@upmc.edu

C. Sturgeon (ed.), *Endocrine Neoplasia*, Cancer Treatment and Research, vol 153,
DOI 10.1007/978-1-4419-0857-5_3, © Springer Science+Business Media, LLC 2010

Table 3.1 Genetic alterations in differentiated thyroid carcinoma

Histologic subtype	Genetic alteration	Characteristics
Papillary	*BRAF* mutations	Tall-cell, conventional, and oncocytic variants
		Aggressive tumor features
		Poor prognosis
	RET/PTC rearrangements	Classic variant
		Pediatric patients
		Exposure to radiation
	NTRK1 rearrangement	Exposure to radiation
	Ras mutations	Follicular variant
Follicular	*Ras* mutations	Follicular adenomas
	PAX8-PPARγ rearrangement	Exposure to radiation
Oncocytic (Hürthle) cell	*PAX8-PPARγ* rearrangement	
	GRIM-19	Also in oncocytic variant PTC
Medullary	*RET* mutations	Germline mutations seen in multiple endocrine neoplasia types 2A, 2B and familial medullary thyroid carcinoma
Poorly differentiated/ anaplastic	*Ras* or *BRAF* mutations	May predispose to malignant progression
	p53 mutations	Less common in PTC and FTC
	CTNNB1 (β-catenin) mutations	Not seen in DTC

cascade, is located on chromosome 7q24 and encodes a serine/threonine kinase [5]. After activation of membrane tyrosine kinase receptors, RAS is activated, resulting in phosphorylation of BRAF and subsequent activation of extracellular signal-regulated kinase (ERK), leading to transcription of genes regulating cell differentiation, proliferation, and survival [6]. The most common activating point mutation in BRAF results in a valine to glutamate substitution at 600 (V600E). V600E mutations have been identified in 29–69% of PTC, are 100% specific for PTC, and occur predominantly in the classic and tall cell PTC variants [7, 8]. PTCs with BRAF mutations have aggressive characteristics that include lymph node and distant metastases and advanced stage at diagnosis [7–11]. BRAF expression has also been demonstrated to be an independent predictor of tumor recurrence and survival regardless of initial stage at diagnosis [11].

At least 15 *RET/PTC* rearrangements have been identified to date. All are chimeras of the 3′ portion of the *RET* gene fused to the 5′ portion of a variety of other heterologous genes. In vitro studies suggest that the downstream effects of RET/PTC are dependent on an intact BRAF protein and MAPK pathway [12]. These rearrangements have been identified in 13–43% of PTC, 25% of HCC, and 20% of Hürthle cell adenomas [13, 14] with the highest incidence seen in childhood PTC secondary to radiation exposure. PTCs with *RET/PTC* rearrangement usually present at a younger age, have a higher rate of lymph node metastasis, and have better prognosis. *NTRK1* (neurotrophic receptor-tyrosine kinase) rearrangements also result in the downstream activation of a number of signal transduction cascades, including ERK, and are seen in 5–13% of PTC [5].

RAS genes (*HRAS*, *KRAS*, and *NRAS*) encode G-proteins that mediate membrane receptor signaling and downstream signaling pathways. Point mutations in *RAS* that result in a constitutively activated form are less common in PTC (10%), but are seen in FTC (40–50%) and occasionally in follicular adenomas (30%) [15]. *RAS* mutations in vitro promote chromosomal instability which may explain why *RAS*-positive FTC exhibit aggressive characteristics such as extrathyroidal extension, vascular invasion, and distant metastases [16, 17]. Other studies have seen more indolent characteristics associated with *RAS*-positive TCs [18]. *RAS* mutations are also frequently found in ATC and undifferentiated TC.

PAX8-PPARγ rearrangements are identified in up to 50% of FTC and 10% of benign follicular adenomas. PAX8 is a thyroid-specific transcription factor and PPARγ is a nuclear receptor, peroxisome proliferator-activated receptor γ, which is normally expressed in adipose tissue. It is unclear how this fusion protein plays a role in thyroid carcinogenesis [19, 20]. Patients with *PAX8-PPARγ* rearrangements may present at a younger age and be more likely to have vascular invasion [15].

Mitochondrial DNA mutations are possible etiologic factors in the formation of HCC. Mutations in *GRIM-19*, a regulatory gene involved in apoptosis and mitochondrial metabolism, have been identified in ~15% of oncocytic or Hürthle cell variants of follicular and papillary thyroid carcinoma [21]. Two allelic loci have been linked to HCC, TCO and NMTC1, but the corresponding genes have not yet been identified [22].

Even though the field is young, identifying the genetic changes involved in thyroid tumorigenesis has already led to improvements in thyroid cancer diagnosis. Evaluation of cytologic samples for the genetic mutations and rearrangements known to be altered in thyroid cancer cells was initially reported in small series [23]. In larger series, cytologic evaluation of *BRAF* and *RET/PTC* had a high positive predictive value; fine needle aspiration (FNA) samples with *BRAF* mutations or *RET/PTC* rearrangements have up to 100% PPV for PTC, while samples with *RAS* mutations have up to 90% PPV for malignancy [24]. Routine cytologic evaluation of FNA samples even in indeterminate or inadequate categories has shown that identification of *BRAF* is highly specific for PTC [8]. Molecular pathology evaluation of FNA samples may eventually become part of the routine diagnostic evaluation of thyroid nodules and may well influence the extent and conduct of thyroid surgery.

Other molecular techniques have recently been studied to determine their diagnostic utility. Gene expression profiling using microarrays which can determine the expression patterns of up to 20,000 genes with one assay has identified patterns that can differentiate between the DTC histologic subtypes [25]. Among these studies are a number of genes that are expressed in a consistently significant pattern. Using a panel of the most commonly identified genes may also prove to be a useful diagnostic strategy [26].

Allelic loss can also be used to differentiate malignant from benign nodules. Loss of heterozygosity (LOH) at the von Hippel Lindau locus has been associated with follicular carcinomas, but not adenomas [27]. In another study, LOH analysis was performed for a panel of 13 well-established tumor suppressor genes for follicular carcinomas and adenomas. The fractional allelic loss was lower for adenomas (11% vs. 56%, $p<0.001$) and, moreover, correlated with recurrence and survival [28].

Understanding of the molecular pathways involved in thyroid carcinogenesis has also led to therapeutic advances. Clinical trials are ongoing to evaluate the effectiveness and role of targeted therapies such as sunitinib, a tyrosine kinase inhibitor, and motesanib diphosphate (AMG-706), a VEGF and PDGF inhibitor [29, 30]. In vitro studies have demonstrated that the expression of thyroid-specific genes which may play a role in the ability of thyroid cells to concentrate iodine (such as the sodium/iodide symporter (NIS) and thyroperoxidase) are decreased in the presence of the BRAF V600E mutation [31]. Additional investigation is needed to determine if blocking the downstream effectors of BRAF can potentially induce expression of these thyroid-specific genes to result in more effective radioiodine uptake [5, 32].

Biology of Differentiated Thyroid Cancer

Risk factors: Women are 2–4 times more likely to develop DTC with a median age at diagnosis between 40 and 50 years [1]. Radiation exposure is a well-known environmental risk factor for DTC. Radiation-induced TC can develop either from exposure to nuclear fallout or after receiving therapeutic ionizing radiation to the head and neck. PTC is by far the most common TC type associated with radiation exposure, but FTC and HCC are also seen. The risk is higher with women, younger age at exposure, and at increasing doses of exposure [33]. The latency period is between 25 and 30 years, but the effects of exposure can be significant for up to 40 years [34, 35]. The pathogenesis of radiation-associated TC may be the induction of chromosomal breakpoints resulting in gene rearrangements such as *RET/PTC*. A number of other environmental risk factors have also been studied for DTC association. Iodine deficiency is associated with an increased risk of FTC. Diets high in iodine, either by iodine supplementation or by intake of high iodine sources, have no demonstrated association with DTC. Case control studies of hormonal, reproductive, and anthropometric factors have also not demonstrated consistent associations with DTC [36].

Inherited syndromes: Inherited patterns of DTC are usually associated with known genetic syndromes. Between 3 and 10% of patients with **Cowden syndrome** develop FTC; this syndrome is autosomal dominant, arises from germline mutations in the PTEN tumor suppressor gene, and is associated with macrocephaly, characteristic mucocutaneous lesions, and increased risks of breast cancer (20–50%) and both papillary and follicular thyroid cancers [37]. Characteristic manifestations of **Carney complex type 1** include cardiac myxomas, skin and mucosal pigmentations, benign follicular adenomas (6%), and an increased risk of DTC (4%) which can be either FTC or PTC [38]; mutations of the protein kinase A regulatory subunit type 1 alpha gene have been identified in affected patients [39]. PTC is diagnosed in up to 12% of patients with **familial adenomatous polyposis** (FAP) which is a colon cancer syndrome caused by mutations in APC [39]. There is also an increased DTC risk in patients with CHEK-2 mutations which are associated with inherited susceptibility to breast, prostate, and kidney cancer [40]. Genetic linkage analyses of large kindreds affected with DTC have identified possible chromosomal regions associated with both benign thyroid nodules and familial nonmedullary thyroid cancers, including chromosome 1q21 (fPTC/PRN), 2q21 (fNMTC1), 19p13.2 (TCO), and 14q31 (MNG1) [41].

Differences between subtypes: Biologic behavior varies among the TC subtypes. The majority of DTCs are indolent with 10-year survival for PTC, FTC, and HCC of 93%, 85%, and 76%, respectively [3]. Among patients who present with small or moderate-sized FTC or PTC (<4 cm) confined to the thyroid gland, overall survival is >95%. The prognosis for PTC and FTC is slightly better (99–100%) than for HCC (94–95%) and younger patients, especially those <45 years old, also have better prognosis [3]. Five-year survival for FTC with capsular invasion alone is excellent (98–99%) while FTC with vascular invasion is associated with a poorer prognosis (80%) [42, 43].

Even among PTCs, there is a range of tumor aggressiveness. Multifocality is common among PTCs, representing multiple primary tumors in an estimated 40–50% and likely locally metastatic disease in the remainder [44, 45]. Histologic PTC subtypes include follicular variant (FVPTC), tall cell variant (TCV-PTC), and other less common insular, oncocytic, clear cell, and sclerosing variants. FVPTC is the most common PTC variant. FVPTC tumors tend to be smaller with a lower risk of lymph node metastasis [46]. FVPTC can be mistakenly classified as FTC and even among expert pathologists, the degree of concordance in differentiating between FTC, FA, and FVPTC is <50% [47]. Immunohistochemical markers such as CK-19, HBME-1, and Galectin-2 are more strongly expressed in FVPTC than in FTC and can be an important diagnostic adjunct [48]. TCV is seen in ~1% of PTC and is associated with more aggressive features such as local metastases, persistent disease after surgery, and persistence after radioactive iodine ablation [49, 50].

HCC is usually considered to be a variant of FTC. Some studies have not found a significant difference in biological behavior between the two [51, 52] but in other studies HCC has demonstrated an older age at presentation, a more aggressive clinical course, a higher rate of locoregional and distant metastatic disease, and worse 10-year overall survival [3, 53]. Similar to PTC, HCC can be multifocal – whereas FTC is often unifocal. Unlike both FTC and PTC, HCC does not often concentrate iodine well, limiting its use in salvage therapy.

Staging systems: A number of DTC staging systems exist including metastases, age, completeness of resection, invasion, and size (MACIS); age, grade, extent, and size (AGES); age, metastases, extent, and size (AMES); and the European Organization for Research and Treatment of Cancer (EORTC) system. The most commonly used staging system is that of the American Joint Committee on Cancer, sixth edition which utilizes tumor size, nodal status, and metastases [54] (TNM; Table 3.2). All clinical scoring systems are still somewhat imprecise and even patients in low-risk groups can still die of thyroid cancer [3, 55].

Dedifferentiation: It is speculated that approximately 1–2% of DTC can undergo additional genetic alterations that lead to dedifferentiation into ATC. Pathologic examinations of ATC can show areas of papillary or follicular structures interspersed with poorly differentiated regions. *p53* mutations in a background of DTC are thought to be the initiating genetic alteration [56]. DTC with BRAF and RAS mutations has also been associated with ATC, suggesting that both close surveillance of these patients and aggressive treatment of recurrent disease may be indicated [57, 58].

Table 3.2 American Joint Committee on Cancer (AJCC) 6th Edition, TNM staging for papillary or follicular thyroid cancer [54]

Primary Tumor (T):

Tx	Primary tumor cannot be assessed
T0	No evidence of primary tumor
T1	Tumor 2 cm or less in greatest dimension limited to the thyroid
T2	Tumor more than 2 cm but not more than 4 cm in greatest dimension limited to the thyroid
T3	Tumor more than 4 cm in greatest dimension limited to the thyroid or any tumor with minimal extrathyroid extension (e.g., extension to sternothyroid muscle or perithyroid soft tissues)
T4a	Tumor of any size extending beyond the thyroid capsule to invade subcutaneous soft tissues, larynx, trachea, esophagus, or recurrent laryngeal nerve
T4b	Tumor invades prevertebral fascia or encases carotid artery or mediastinal vessels

Regional Lymph Nodes (N):

Regional lymph nodes are the central compartment, lateral cervical, and upper mediastinal lymph nodes.

Nx	Regional lymph nodes cannot be assessed
N0	No regional lymph node metastasis
N1	Regional lymph node metastasis
N1a	Metastasis to Level VI (pretracheal, paratracheal, prelaryngeal/ Delphian lymph nodes)
N1b	Metastasis to unilateral, bilateral, or contralateral cervical or superior mediastinal lymph nodes

Distant Metastasis (M):

Mx	Distant metastasis cannot be assessed
M0	No distant metastasis
M1	Distant metastasis

Staging Grouping:	**Under 45 years**	**45 years and older**		
I	Any T Any N M0	T1	N0	M0
II	Any T Any N M1	T2	N0	M0
III		T3	N0	M0
		T1	N1a	M0
		T2	N1a	M0
		T3	N1a	M0
IVa		T4a	N0	M0
		T4a	N1a	M0
		T1	N1b	M0
		T2	N1b	M0
		T3	N1b	M0
		T4a	N1b	M0
IVb		T4b	Any N	M0
IVc		Any	T Any	N M1

Treatment of Differentiated Thyroid Cancer

In general, aspects of the treatment of DTC are still actively debated. Because of the indolent course of disease, the number of patients needed to conduct prospective randomized clinical trials with a cause-specific mortality endpoint has been estimated to be prohibitively high and trials would also require decades of follow-up and significant expense [59]. As a result, treatment recommendations are largely based on retrospective, single-institution studies from high volume centers. The principles of DTC treatment include adequate staging, complete tumor resection, adjuvant therapy, and surveillance. Unique to DTC is the relationship of each treatment modality to the next.

The initial treatment of DTC is thyroidectomy. The extent and conduct of thyroidectomy depends on whether the diagnosis of DTC is reached by preoperative FNA biopsy, or by postoperative histologic examination. The classic modern paradigm in DTC is patient presentation with a thyroid nodule noted or suspected on physical examination, and further evaluated with ultrasound and FNA biopsy. The details and algorithms of thyroid nodule evaluation are addressed in Chap. 2. It is important to keep in mind that although PTC can often be readily diagnosed on FNA cytology, the diagnoses of FV-PTC, FTC, and HCC require, in each case, histologic examination of the entire nodule and its capsule in relation to the adjacent thyroid lobe tissue.

Thyroidectomy for DTC Diagnosed by FNA biopsy: When FNA cytology shows PTC, thyroidectomy is recommended. The false negative rate of FNA cytology that is positive for DTC is quite low (1–2%), but patients should be counseled preoperatively about the possibility of false positive results. As recently stated, the specific goals of thyroidectomy for DTC are to remove the primary tumor and lymphadenopathy, if present; to minimize treatment-related morbidity; to permit accurate staging; to facilitate treatment with radioiodine when appropriate; to permit accurate long-term surveillance for recurrence as appropriate; and to minimize the risk of recurrence and spread [60]. The minimum operation for DTC is ipsilateral complete lobectomy and isthmusectomy. The thyroid isthmus is an important anatomic and surgical margin intraoperatively. Total thyroidectomy or near-total thyroidectomy (which leaves approximately 50 mg of tissue at the ligament of Berry) is considered the procedure of choice for DTC >1 cm in size [60].

Diagnostic Thyroidectomy: Often, DTC is first diagnosed on postoperative histology. For FNA biopsy results in the indeterminate, persistently nondiagnostic, or suspicious categories, diagnostic thyroid lobectomy with isthmusectomy is indicated and is associated with histologic TC in 20%, 5–10%, and 50% of cases respectively. Partial thyroid lobectomy is an outmoded operation that puts the ipsilateral recurrent laryngeal nerve at unnecessary risk should reoperation be required. Because lobectomy with isthmusectomy is associated with a 25–40% chance of surgical hypothyroidism requiring chronic replacement l-thyroxine therapy, patients should be counseled about this possibility preoperatively.

Extent of Initial Thyroidectomy: The extent of initial thyroidectomy is influenced by several clinical factors. For patients with FNA-proven DTC <1 cm in size or who have FNA biopsy results in the indeterminate, suspicious, or persistently nondiagnostic categories, the evidence to date supports initial total thyroidectomy for patients who have a history of radiation exposure, diagnosed hypothyroidism, a family history of DTC, toxic nodular goiter, a contralateral macronodule (>1 cm), or regional or distant metastases. Older age (>45 years) may also be an indication for initial total thyroidectomy [60]. In addition, with increasing nodule size, a number of studies have demonstrated an increased risk of thyroid malignancy. In one report of 639 patients with indeterminate or suspicious FNA results, nodules that were >2.5 cm had a significant association between malignancy and size; for every 1 cm increase in nodule size, there was a 40% increased risk of malignancy [61]. Nodule size >4 cm has been recently reported to be associated with increased malignant risk in Hürthle cell neoplasms [62, 63], in follicular neoplasms [64], and even in 13% of thyroid masses ≥4 cm that are cytologically benign on ultrasound-directed FNA [64]. In the future, the results of tumor mutation profiling such as *BRAF* positivity may also be an indication for initial total thyroidectomy [8].

Completion Total Thyroidectomy: The extent of surgery for papillary microcarcinoma (<1 cm) remains controversial. Microcarcinomas can be seen in up to 50% of thyroidectomies [65, 66]. Although most studies suggest that PTC <1 cm is generally associated with an excellent long-term survival regardless of surgical procedure [67, 68], there is a small but real percentage of patients who develop lymph node metastases (up to 40%) and distant metastases (<1%). In one meta-analysis, recurrent disease from papillary microcarcinomas was associated with multifocality, "nonincidental" disease, age <45 years, and the presence of lymph node disease at presentation [69]. In the absence of these factors, thyroid lobectomy is usually considered adequate treatment for unifocal papillary microcarcinoma.

Among low-risk DTC patients who undergo lobectomy only, studies suggest a higher rate of local (up to 30%) and contralateral lobe (5–10%) recurrence; however, effects on long-term survival are less clear [70, 71]. For any DTC patient >45 years who also has extrathyroidal extension and/or palpable lymph node metastases (i.e., TNM stage III disease), total thyroidectomy compared to lobectomy improves cause-specific mortality at 30 years (20% vs. 39%) [72]. A recent retrospective study of >50,000 PTC patients from the National Cancer Data Base, demonstrated a statistically significant improvement in 10-year local recurrence rates (7.7% vs. 9.8%) and 10-year survival (98.4% vs. 97.1%) among patients who undergo total thyroidectomy compared to lobectomy; for PTC <1 cm, the type of surgery made no difference in recurrence or survival, but the findings of this study are limited by heterogeneity in PTC pathologic subtypes, radioactive iodine ablation, and management with TSH-suppression [73]. Among FTCs and HCCs that are <1 cm in size, risk factors also determine the extent of thyroidectomy. FTC with minimal vascular invasion or wide invasion is associated with a worse prognosis [55] and such patients should undergo total thyroidectomy. Because HCC can be multifocal and does not take up radioactive iodine as effectively, many support an aggressive surgical approach with total thyroidectomy for all HCC regardless of size.

Completion total thyroidectomy (also termed reoperative contralateral lobectomy) is performed to facilitate the use of radioiodine in staging and therapy, and is also performed for tumors at high risk of multifocality. Its benefits must be balanced against the risks. Among experienced thyroid surgeons initial total thyroidectomy is usually associated with a <1% risk of recurrent laryngeal nerve injury and a <1% risk of permanent hypoparathyroidism [74]. The risks of reoperative thyroid surgery vary but range from 0 to 22% for permanent hypocalcemia and 0–13% for permanent recurrent laryngeal nerve injury [75]. Overall, the recently revised American Thyroid Association Guidelines [60] recommend completion total thyroidectomy for DTC (to a thyroid remnant ≤1 gm) if total thyroidectomy would have been recommended had the diagnosis been known preoperatively, i.e., unless the tumor is <1cm, low-risk, unifocal, intrathyroidal, with no prior irradiation, and with no apparent nodal involvement on preoperative staging.

Nodal clearance: Although cervical lymph node involvement is the rule in DTC, ranging from 20 to 90% depending on the sensitivity and/or tenacity of the detection method [60, 76, 77], the prognostic significance of lymph node metastasis is controversial. Nodal disease is clinically apparent in <10% of patients with PTC or HCC. The clinical relevance of occult micrometastases is likely minimal and has little to no prognostic significance for most patients. Micrometastatic disease responds especially well to radioiodine therapy. Metastatic PTC documented in cervical nodes is associated with a higher risk of local recurrence. Whether there is also an association with long-term PTC survival has not been clearly demonstrable although many studies have examined the issue [67, 78, 79]. In large SEER database studies evaluating patient outcomes, lymph node metastases have recently been shown to be a poor prognostic indicator among FTC and older (>45 years) PTC patients [80]. Resection of involved lymph nodes by prophylactic neck dissection has not consistently been shown to improve long-term survival or to reduce local recurrence [81].

In the preoperative staging of DTC, ultrasound (lymph node mapping) is the best test currently used to identify nodal metastases. Suspicious sonographic lymph node characteristics include microcalcifications, peripheral vascularization, loss of fatty hilum, rounded shape, and cystic appearance [82]. FNA biopsy, with or without thyroglobulin measurement on the aspirate, is recommended when clinical or sonographic evidence is present. When cervical metastasis is confirmed, functional compartment-oriented or selective therapeutic lymphadenectomy is advocated to decrease local recurrence [60, 83] and may in fact do so compared to berry-picking, but again this has not yet been studied prospectively.

DTC usually metastasizes first to the central compartment (Level VI) bilaterally [84]. As discussed above, routine prophylactic lateral neck dissection is not indicated for DTC. Although still controversial, routine prophylactic central neck dissection is performed often for T3 and T4 tumors because it is relatively simple and because the level VI compartments are necessarily dissected during total thyroidectomy. The incidence of permanent hypoparathyroidism and recurrent laryngeal nerve injury may increase with central compartment dissection, but conversely these complications may also be higher with cervical reoperation [85]. For small and apparently node-negative DTC, intraoperative inspection of the central compartment may prompt central compartment dissection only as needed, yet it is important to keep in mind that central compartment dissection may upstage some patients >45 years from AJCC stage I to III (clinical N0 to pathologic N1a) [60]. Routine clearance of central compartment nodal tissue has been demonstrated to lower postoperative thyroglobulin levels at 6 months [86]. No studies have yet demonstrated any advantage in long-term survival or locoregional recurrence.

Whether synchronous or metachronous, the presence of clinically apparent lymph node disease prompts surgical local control to prevent complications related to airway and venous obstruction. Metachronous lymph node metastasis is associated with a higher rate of recurrence and disease-specific mortality and develops in <5% of patients with PTC after thyroidectomy and RAI ablation [87–89]. In contrast, metachronous nodal disease develops in approximately 25% of patients after thyroidectomy for HCC; however, not all patients received radioiodine postoperatively [53]. Synchronous and metachronous lymph node metastases are rare in FTC and are an indicator of poor prognosis [90, 91]. Prophylactic central neck dissection has been proposed for all HCC patients, but has not been prospectively studied.

Radioiodine Staging and Ablation: Because normal thyroid tissue takes up radioiodine better than does DTC tissue, it is important to keep in mind that implicit in several DTC staging schema is the information provided by the use of radioiodine, which in turn depends upon either total thyroidectomy or on lobectomy with subsequent two-stage ablation of the contralateral lobe.

The observed results of radioiodine ablation on survival and local recurrence in retrospective studies have been variable [92]. Among DTC patients with low-risk thyroid cancers, the risk of mortality at 10 years is <2% and no improvement in survival or local regional recurrence has been consistently demonstrated with RAI ablation [67, 68]. RAI ablation in high-risk DTC patients, e.g., patients with tumors >1.5 cm, incomplete tumor resection, stage III or IV disease, or residual disease, may be associated with improved disease-specific survival and local recurrence [67, 71]. Among patients with HCC, RAI ablation may be associated with a longer interval to disease progression and disease-specific mortality [93]. Two-stage ablation, i.e., nonoperative destruction of the contralateral lobe after diagnostic lobectomy and isthmusectomy, is occasionally used instead of completion total thyroidectomy if there is a major contraindication to reoperation such as vocal cord paralysis.

Few would disagree that RAI remnant ablation facilitates long-term surveillance. Thyroglobulin levels in the absence of thyroglobulin antibodies are a sensitive indicator of recurrent or persistent disease. RAI ablation is generally recommended for all PTC patients with stage III or IV disease, all patients with stage II disease who are <45 years, most patients with stage II disease who are >45 years, and patients with stage I disease who have aggressive pathologic findings such as multifocality, extrathyroidal (either gross or microscopic), or vascular invasion [60]. The presence of histologic subtypes such as tall cell, columnar cell, insular, or poorly differentiated should also be considered. RAI remnant ablation is recommended for almost all HCC and FTC patients. Small (<1 cm) FTC without vascular invasion and FVPTC generally have an excellent overall prognosis and may not need postoperative RAI.

Optimal radioactive iodine uptake is achieved through TSH stimulation either by T4 withdrawal or recombinant human TSH (rhTSH). Recombinant human TSH has been shown to have equivalent efficacy at remnant ablation compared to T4 withdrawal when using a standard ^{131}I ablative dose of either 50 or 100 mci. In short-term follow-up, recurrent and persistent disease, as measured by whole-body scans and TSH-stimulated thyroglobulin levels after ablation, were similar [94, 95].

Quality of life indicators also suggest an advantage for use of rhTSH compared to T4 withdrawal [94, 96]. A stimulated TSH of >30 mU/L has been associated with increased tumor radioiodine uptake; however, no controlled studies have been performed. A low iodine diet (<50 μg/day) for 2 weeks prior to RAI ablation has been recommended to increase thyrocyte iodine uptake [60]. The diet restricts intake of iodized or sea salt, dairy products, and seafoods.

Prior to giving the therapeutic ^{131}I dose, a pretherapy scan can be performed using 1–3 mCi ^{131}I in order to determine the amount of thyroid tissue remaining following thyroidectomy. Decreased RAI uptake following the pretherapy scan, or thyroid stunning, is theorized to occur by a mechanism that may be related to down regulation of the sodium-iodide symporter [97]. Although decreased ^{131}I uptake may occur, the issue is controversial and not all studies have demonstrated an associated decrease in thyroid remnant ablation [98]. Limiting the pretherapy scan to the lowest dose of ^{131}I may reduce this effect. Studies evaluating the effects of using ^{123}I instead for pretherapy scans are ongoing.

^{131}I can be administered in an empiric fixed low (30 mCi) or high (100 mCi) dose, by quantitative tumor dosimetry, or by quantitative whole-body dosimetry. Whole-body dosimetry is usually reserved for widespread metastatic disease. Empiric fixed doses are most commonly utilized; however, the optimal dose is under ongoing study. While lower doses are associated with both lower costs and reduced exposure to radioactivity, they are also somewhat less successful in ablating residual thyroid tissue [99, 100]. Retrospective studies are confounded by the variability in completeness of thyroidectomy, method of TSH stimulation, and endpoint determination. While two large randomized trials are ongoing in Europe and will be valuable in guiding future recommendations, current recommendations suggest using the minimum activity needed for remnant ablation while taking into account the patient's risk of recurrent disease [60].

A posttherapy whole-body scan is often obtained 5–8 days after administration of therapeutic ^{131}I to evaluate for metastatic disease. In ~10% of patients, the posttherapy scan demonstrates clinically relevant disease, most often in the neck, chest, and mediastinum, which is not seen on the pretherapy scan and this justifies its routine use [101].

RAI has been associated with salivary gland dysfunction (sialadenitis, dry mouth, alterations in taste, or salivary duct stones) and premature menopause [68]. Large thyroid remnants may develop thyroiditis sometimes requiring corticosteroids for symptomatic treatment. Transient testicular failure may develop if large (>300 mCi) doses of ^{131}I are administered. No differences in infertility, miscarriage, or premature births are seen in large long-term studies of women who became pregnant after receiving ^{131}I [102]. In an earlier study, an observed low but increased frequency of second malignancies in DTC patients who received RAI led to the estimation that 100 mCi ^{131}I induces 53 solid malignant tumors and three leukemias in 10,000 patients over a 10-year follow-up [103]. A causative RAI effect has been difficult to determine and the increased risk for secondary cancers may also be due to an inherent epidemiologic or genetic predisposition to malignancy in DTC patients [104, 105].

TSH Suppression

In vitro studies demonstrated that thyroid cells are dependent on TSH for differentiation and growth [106] and this together with the clinical observation that levothyroxine can prevent tumor growth has led to the routine use of levothyroxine to suppress TSH in DTC patients. Retrospective studies have shown that patients treated with TSH suppression may experience a 25% reduction in disease recurrence and a 50% improvement in survival [87]. A more recent meta-analysis also suggested that TSH suppression is likely favorable towards preventing disease progression and mortality [107]. The benefits of TSH suppression on overall survival and disease-specific survival appear to be more significant for high-risk patients [68].

The amount of TSH suppression has been difficult to determine and must now be balanced against its risks. TSH suppression, even to subclinical levels, is associated with a two- to threefold increase in risk of developing atrial fibrillation, impaired cardiac reserve, and postmenopausal osteoporosis [108, 109]. Surgical treatment and RAI ablation are confounding factors; TSH in patients who undergo total or near total thyroidectomy followed by RAI ablation can be suppressed to a greater degree than in those who do not. However, studies have demonstrated that maintaining a higher degree of TSH suppression (<0.1 mU/L) may be associated with improved rates of disease progression, particularly in higher risk patients [110, 111]. Treating low-risk patients with this amount of TSH suppression has not been beneficial. Currently, recommendations support maintaining TSH suppression to <0.1 mU/L for high-risk patients while a TSH of 0.1–0.5 mU/L is considered adequate for low-risk patients [60]. For most adults, 2.2–2.5 μg levothyroxine per kg lean body weight per day is required to achieve TSH suppression.

Surveillance

Long-term surveillance strategies can also be stratified according to recurrence risk (Table 3.3). Low-risk patients are those who do not have nodal or distant metastasis, residual disease, or aggressive histologic features. Intermediate risk patients have microscopic extrathyroidal extension, or aggressive histologic features such as angiolymphatic invasion or tall cell, insular, or columnar cell carcinomas. High-risk patients include those with distant metastases, evidence of extrathyroidal ^{131}I uptake, incomplete resection, or macroscopic tumor invasion [60]. Surveillance methods include whole-body radioiodine scanning, simultaneous measurement of serum TSH, thyroglobulin (Tg), and anti thyroglobulin antibodies, physical exam, and neck ultrasound.

Whole-body iodine scanning (WBS) is often obtained following the administration of therapeutic ^{131}I and can be used to identify iodine-avid metastatic disease. Among patients with negative posttherapy WBS, the routine use of surveillance WBS is not a sensitive method to detect recurrent disease. Distant metastases do

Table 3.3 Patient stratification according to recurrence risk

	Primary tumor	Extrathyroidal disease
Low	• Complete resection • No tumor invasion of local tissues/ structures • Not an aggressive histologic subtype[a]	• None • No ^{131}I uptake outside the thyroid bed on initial WBS
Intermediate	• Microscopic tumor invasion into perithyroidal soft tissues • Aggressive histologic subtype[a] • Vascular invasion	• Cervical lymph node metastasis • ^{131}I uptake outside the thyroid bed on WBS after remnant ablation
High	• Macroscopic tumor invasion • Incomplete resection	• Distant metastasis • Significantly elevated Tg not consistent with WBS results

[a]Aggressive histologic subtype: tall cell, columnar cell, or insular
WBS Whole-body scan; *Tg* Thyroglobulin. Ref. [60]

not always concentrate iodine well, which may explain why only 4–10% of patients with distant metastases have a positive surveillance WBS [112]. Once there is suspicion of recurrent disease, WBS is helpful in determining if ^{131}I will be a useful treatment adjunct.

In a euthyroid patient, it has been estimated that a Tg of 1 μg/L corresponds to 1 g of normal thyroid tissue [113]. Approximately 25% of DTC patients have circulating antithyroglobulin antibodies which interfere with the assay for Tg. Therefore, Tg and antithyroglobulin antibodies should always be obtained simultaneously when conducting DTC surveillance. Persistently elevated antithyroglobulin antibodies may be indicative of persistent or recurrent disease [60]. Assay variability in Tg levels between laboratories can make comparisons between Tg levels from different laboratories difficult [113].

Elevated Tg obtained with TSH stimulation and in the absence of anti thyroglobulin antibodies has been shown to be highly sensitive in identifying recurrent or persistent DTC. A Tg >2 μg/L can identify metastatic disease with a sensitivity of 89% and a specificity of 96% [114]. Mildly elevated Tg levels (between 0.5 and 2 μg/L) can be seen immediately after thyroidectomy and RAI; however, the majority (>90%) of these patients have a spontaneous decline of Tg to undetectable levels within 3 years [114]. A rising Tg can be an indicator of persistent or recurrent disease.

Cervical ultrasound is considered the surveillance imaging modality of choice and can detect local thyroid bed or nodal recurrence with up to 94% sensitivity [115]. US can detect cervical disease that is not palpable and can also facilitate pathologic confirmation with FNA biopsy [116]. Metastatic disease can be diagnosed either by the presence of malignant cells seen on cytopathology or by an elevated aspirate thyroglobulin level [117]. The clinical significance of recurrent disease diagnosed by US in patients with undetectable Tg levels is still unclear.

The majority of patients with DTC are low-risk with expected prolonged survival. As a result, a strategy utilizing sensitive testing that is also cost-effective is important. Among patients with no clinical evidence of recurrent disease who have an undetectable (<0.5 μg/L) TSH-stimulated Tg with negative Tg-antibodies, an annual TSH-stimulated Tg along with physical exam is considered adequate follow-up. If the initial TSH-stimulated Tg is mildly elevated (0.5–2 μg/L), it should be monitored closely until it either decreases to <0.5 μg/L or increases to >2 μg/L. If the initial TSH-stimulated Tg is elevated (>2 μg/L), a cervical US and CXR should be obtained [60]. The long-term surveillance of intermediate or high-risk patients is less defined, but annual Tg and Tg-Ab testing with periodic cervical US is recommended [118].

Long-Term Outcomes

Patients with AJCC TNM stage I or II PTC or FTC have almost equivalent 5-year survivals; 99–100% [3]. For patients with early stage HCC, 5-year survival is also excellent; 94–95%. Overall survival at 10 years is 9% lower for HCC patients compared to PTC and FTC patients. Approximately 5% of DTC patients present with distant metastases and have a 5-year survival of 50% [3].

Prognosis is also affected by age at diagnosis. Patients over 60 years old have a significantly higher disease-related mortality rate compared to younger patients (31% vs. 1.2%) [119]. Older patients present with more aggressive disease with an increased likelihood of extrathyroidal extension, lymph node and distant metastases. DTC in elderly patients is also less iodine-avid [120].

Recurrent/Persistent Disease

Recurrent or persistent disease is often heralded by elevated Tg levels. At the time of remnant ablation, a Tg >30 ng/mL has a 70% positive predictive value for recurrent disease [121]. A Tg level obtained at least 6 months after treatment also has independent prognostic value [122]. Elevated Tg levels following thyroidectomy and RAI ablation should prompt further evaluation with cervical ultrasound. WBS identifies cervical recurrence with a significantly lower (45%) sensitivity [115] but can also be helpful if distant disease is present. Patients with persistent disease should have levothyroxine adjusted to maintain the serum TSH <0.1 mU/L.

Suspicious cervical disease should be FNA biopsied and recurrent or persistent cervical disease confirmed by cytology and/or elevated Tg levels in the aspirate. Treatment is surgical resection which may be associated with a higher likelihood of lowering Tg levels [123]. Compartment-oriented lymph node dissection is often utilized because of the possibility of more extensive microscopic disease not visualized radiographically [124]. In patients with recurrent or persistent disease in a previously operated field, ultrasound guidance can greatly facilitate focused resection with negligible morbidity and with an observed subsequent decrease in postoperative Tg level [125]. Subsequent therapeutic I131 is also considered after reoperative cervical exploration.

Persistent DTC has been associated with a 60% reduction in median life expectancy [126] and recurrent disease has been demonstrated to be a predictor of cancer-specific mortality [127]. Up to 40% of persistent and recurrent disease can be attributed to incomplete surgical resection [83] emphasizing the importance of accurate preoperative imaging prior to initial surgical treatment.

^{18}F-FDG PET is useful in patients with elevations in Tg, but no evidence of disease on US or WBS. This is thought to be due to the inverse relationship between loss of iodine-avidity and gain of glucose utilization that occurs with tumor dedifferentiation [116]. PET has a sensitivity of 50–70% with an increase in sensitivity as the Tg level increases. No significant differences appear to occur when the study is obtained with or without TSH-stimulation [128]. HCC, in particular, has high avidity for ^{18}F-FDG and the avidity may also have prognostic significance; metastatic HCC lesions with a higher maximum SUV (>10) have been associated with a poorer outcome compared to those with a lower maximum SUV (5-year mortality of 64% vs. 92%) [129].

Although external beam radiation (EBRT) can be used for locoregional control and palliation of recurrent or persistent disease that is not surgically resectable, it has no proven benefit to date. There may be some benefit for patients with microscopic noniodine avid residual disease secondary to extrathyroidal extension or positive surgical margins, associated with locoregional control rates at 4 years of 70% [130]. Acute toxicities can include mucositis, dysphagia, and/or dermatitis requiring placement of a gastrostomy (30%), fatigue, dry mouth, and/or hoarseness requiring placement of a tracheostomy (10%), and the difficulties of reoperation in an irradiated field should it be required subsequently [130].

Distant Metastasis

Among patients with synchronous metastases, age is a strong prognostic indicator; pediatric patients with DTC who present with metastatic disease have a reported 10-year survival of 100% [131] while older patients have a 5-year survival of 35–50% [132]. Pulmonary metastases are the most common, especially in PTC and HCC, while bone metastases are more common among FTC patients. Treatment should still include total thyroidectomy and resection of gross cervical disease for local control, prevention of airway and vascular complications, and optimization of ^{131}I treatment. In a study of 169 patients with locoregional and distant metastases, Tg levels obtained with a suppressed TSH correlated to site of metastasis. Tg >100 ng/mL correlates with lung and/or bone metastasis although lung metastasis can be found in patients with TSH-suppressed Tg levels as low as 2.5 ng/mL. Tg levels >300 ng/mL are associated with patients who have at least 3 metastatic sites [133]. Tg levels in patients with FTC are higher than those of patients with comparably sized PTC [134].

Metachronous metastatic PTC lesions that are iodine-avid have a better prognosis compared to FTC or HCC metastases [132]. These are usually treated with ^{131}I with response and long-term survival related to disease volume [135] and a maximum cumulative dose of 600 mCi ^{131}I is usually recommended. Above this, the risk of leukemia significantly increases. If pulmonary lesions are present, RAI should be administered to limit whole-body retention at 48 h to <80 mCi to prevent pulmonary fibrosis. Surgical metastasectomy of bone lesions has been associated with improved long-term survival [136].

Radioiodine resistant lesions have a poor prognosis with 10-year survival <15%. Conventional cytotoxic chemotherapies have not been effective in treating progressive metastatic disease with response rates ranging from 5 to 25% for doxorubicin alone or in combination therapy [137, 138]. Other studies have attempted to induce iodine uptake by the redifferentiation of thyroid cancer cells with 13-cis-retinoic acid. Despite promising in vitro studies, translation into clinical use has shown disappointing results. Partial responses have been achieved with newer molecular targeted chemotherapies. In a phase II study, the multikinase inhibitor motesanib diphosphate has demonstrated a 12% partial or complete response rate and a 69% stable disease rate [29]. A partial response has been reported in 30% of patients treated with the tyrosine kinase inhibitor sorafenib [139]. Further studies are needed to determine if these partial responses translate into improvements in recurrence and overall survival.

References

1. Ries LAG, Melbert D, Krapcho M et al (eds). SEER Cancer Statistics Review, 1975–2005, National Cancer Institute. Bethesda, MD, http://seer.cancer.gov/csr/1975_2005/, based on November 2007 SEER data submission, posted to the SEER web site, 2008
2. Davies L, Welch HG (2006) Increasing incidence of thyroid cancer in the United States, 1973–2002. JAMA 295:2164–2167
3. Hundahl SA, Fleming ID, Fremgen AM, Menck HR (1998) A National Cancer Data Base report on 53, 856 cases of thyroid carcinoma treated in the US, 1985–1995. Cancer 83:2638–2648
4. Baloch ZW, Cibas ES, Clark DP, Layfield LJ, Ljung BM, Pitman MB et al (2008) The National Cancer Institute thyroid fine-needle aspiration state of the science conference: a summation. Cytojournal 5:6
5. Nikiforov YE (2008) Thyroid carcinoma: molecular pathways and therapeutic targets. Mod Pathol 21(Suppl 2):S37–S43
6. Motti ML, DeMarco C, Califano D et al (2007) Loss of p27 expression through RAS ->BRAF ->MAP kinase-dependent pathway in human thyroid carcinomas. Cell Cycle 15:2817–2825
7. Lupi C, Giannini R, Ugolini C et al (2007) Association of BRAF V600E mutation with poor clinicopathological outcomes in 500 consecutive cases of papillary thyroid carcinoma. J Clin Endocrinol Metab 92:4085–4090
8. Yip L, Nikiforova MN, Carty SE et al (2009) Optimizing surgical treatment of papillary thyroid carcinoma associated with BRAF mutation. Under review
9. Kebebew E, Weng J, Bauer J et al (2007) The prevalence and prognostic value of BRAF mutation in thyroid cancer. Ann Surg 246:466–471

10. Xing M, Westra WH, Tufano RP et al (2005) BRAF mutation predicts a poorer clinicl prognosis for papillary thyroid cancer. J Clin Endocrinol Metab 90:6373–6379
11. Elisei R, Ugolini C, Viola D et al (2008) BRAF V600E mutation and outcome of patients with papillary thyroid carcinoma: a 15-year median follow-up study. J Clin Endocrinol Metab 93:3943–3949
12. Kimura ET, Nikiforova MD, Zhu Z et al (2003) High prevalence of BRAF mutations in thyroid cancer: genetic evidence for constitutive activation of the RET/PTC-RAS-BRAF signaling pathway in papillary thyroid carcinoma. Cancer Res 63:1454–1457
13. Jhiang SM (2000) The RET proto-oncogene in human cancers. Oncogene 19:5590–5597
14. Cheung CC, Ezzat S, Ramyar L, Freeman JL, Asa SL (2000) Molecular basis of Hurthle cell papillary thyroid carcinoma. J Clin Endocrinol Metab 85:878–882
15. Nikiforova MN, Lynch RA, Biddinger PW et al (2003) RAS point mutations and PAX8-PPAR gamma rearrangement in thyroid tumors: evidence for distinct molecular pathways in thyroid follicular carcinoma. J Clin Endocrinol Metab 88:2318–2326
16. Garcia-Rostan G, Zhao H, Camp RL et al (2003) ras mutations are associated with aggressive tumor phenotypes and poor prognosis in thyroid cancer. J Clin Oncol 21:3226–3235
17. Basolo F, Pisaturo F, Pollina LE et al (2000) N-ras mutation in poorly differentiated thyroid carcinomas: correlation with bone metastases and inverse correlation to thyroglobulin expression. Thyroid 10:19–23
18. Zhu Z, Gandhi M, Nikiforova MN, Fischer AH, Nikiforov YE (2003) Molecular profile and clinical-pathologic features of the follicular variant of papillary thyroid carcinoma, an unusually high prevalence of RAS mutations. Am J Clin Pathol 120:71–77
19. Dwight T, Thoppe SR, Foukakis T et al (2003) Involvement of the PAX8/peroxisome proliferator-activated receptor gamma rearrangement in follicular thyroid tumors. J Clin Endocrinol Metab 88:4440–4445
20. Cheung L, Messina M, Gill A et al (2003) Detection of the PAX8-PPAR gamma fusion oncogene in both follicular thyroid carcinomas and adenomas. J Clin Endocrinol Metab 88:354–357
21. Máximo V, Botelho T, Capela J, Soares P, Lima J, Taveira A et al (2005) Somatic and germline mutation in GRIM-19, a dual function gene involved in mitochondrial metabolism and cell death, is linked to mitochondrion-rich (Hürthle cell) tumours of the thyroid. Br J Cancer 92:1892–1898
22. Fusco A, Viglietto G, Santoro M (2005) Point mutation in GRIM-19: a new genetic lesion in Hurthle cell thyroid carcinomas. Br J Cancer 92:1817–1818
23. Cohen Y, Rosenbaum E, Clark DP et al (2004) Mutational analysis of BRAF in fine needle aspiration biopsies of the thyroid: a potential application for the preoperative assessment of thyroid nodules. Clin Cancer Res 10:2761–2765
24. Nikiforov YE, Ohori NP, Kuffner HA, Carty SE, LeBeau SO, Hodak SP et al (2008) Introduction of molecular testing of thyroid fine needle aspiration (FNA) samples into routine clinical practice: one year experience at the University of Pittsburgh Medical Center. American Thyroid Association.
25. Chevillard S, Ugolin N, Vielh P et al (2004) Gene expression profiling of differentiated thyroid neoplasms: diagnostic and clinical implications. Clin Cancer Res 10:6586–6597
26. Griffith OL, Melck A, Jones SJ, Wiseman SM (2006) Meta-analysis and meta-review of thyroid cancer gene expression profiling studies identifies important diagnostic biomarkers. J Clin Oncol 24:5043–5051
27. Hunt JL, Livolsi VA, Baloch ZW et al (2003) A novel microdissection and genotyping of follicular-derived thyroid tumors to predict aggressiveness. Hum Pathol 34:375–380
28. Hunt JL, Yim JH, Carty SE (2006) Fractional allelic loss of tumor suppressor genes identifies malignancy and predicts clinical outcome in follicular thyroid tumors. Thyroid 16:643–649
29. Sherman SI, Wirth LJ, Droz JP et al (2008) Motesanib diphosphate in progressive differentiated thyroid cancer. N Engl J Med 359:31–42
30. Dawson SJ, Conus NM, Toner GC et al (2008) Sustained clinical responses to tyrosine kinase inhibitor sunitinib in thyroid carcinoma. Anticancer Drugs 19:547–552

31. Durante C, Puxeddu E, Ferretti E et al (2007) BRAF mutations in papillary thyroid carcinomas inhibit genes involved in iodine metabolism. J Clin Endocrinol Metab 92:2840–2843
32. Liu D, Hu S, Hou P, Jiang D, Condouris S, Xing M (2007) Suppression of BRAF/MEK/MAP kinase pathway restores expression of iodide-metabolizing genes in thyroid cells expressing the V600E BRAF mutant. Clin Cancer Res 15:1341–1349
33. Zablotska LB, Bogdanova TI, Ron E et al (2008) A cohort study of thyroid cancer and other thyroid diseases after the Chornobyl accident: dose–response analysis of thyroid follicular adenomas detected during first screening in Ukraine (1998–2000). Am J Epidemiol 167:305–312
34. Schneider AB, Ron E, Lubin J, Stovall M, Gierlowski TC (1993) Dose–response relationships for radiation-induced thyroid cancer and thyroid nodules: evidence for the prolonged effects of radiation on the thyroid. J Clin Endocrinol Metab 77:362–369
35. Kikuchi S, Perrier ND, Ituarte P, Siperstein AE, Duh QY, Clark OH (2004) Latency period of thyroid neoplasia after radiation exposure. Ann Surg 239:536–543
36. Dal Maso L, Bosetti C, La Vecchia C, Franceschi S (2009) Risk factors for thyroid cancer: an epidemiological review focused on nutritional factors. Cancer Causes Control 20:75–86
37. Malchoff CD, Malchoff DM (2002) The genetics of hereditary nonmedullary thyroid carcinoma. J Clin Endocrinol Metab 87:2455–2459
38. Stratakis CA, Courcoutsakis NA, Abati A et al (1997) Thyroid gland abnormalities in patients with the syndrome of spotty skin pigmentation, myxomas, endocrine overactivity and schwannomas (Carney Complex). J Clin Endocrinol Metab 82:2037–2043
39. Bertherat J, Horvath A, Groussin L et al (2009) Mutations in regulatory subunit type 1A of cyclic AMP-dependent protein kinase (PRKAR1A): phenotype analysis in 353 patients and 80 different genotypes. J Clin Endocrinol Metab 94(6):2085–2091
40. Cybulski C, Górski B, Huzarski T et al (2004) CHEK2 is a multiorgan cancer susceptibility gene. Am J Hum Genet 75:1131–1135
41. Moore FD Jr (2006) Inherited aspects of papillary thyroid carcinoma. J Surg Oncol 94:719–724
42. van Heerden JA, Hay ID, Goellner JR, Salomao D, Ebersold JR, Bergstralh EJ et al (1992) Follicular thyroid carcinoma with capsular invasion alone: a nonthreatening malignancy. Surgery 112:1130–1136
43. D'Avanzo A, Treseler P, Ituarte PHG, Wong M, Streja L, Greenspan FS et al (2004) Follicular thyroid carcinoma: histology and prognosis. Cancer 100:1123–1129
44. McCarthy RP, Wang M, Jones TD, Strate RW, Cheng L (2006) Molecular evidence for the same clonal origin of multifocal papillary thyroid carcinomas. Clin Cancer Res 112:2414–2418
45. Shattuck TM, Westra WH, Ladenson PW, Arnold A (2005) Independent clonal origins of distinct tumor foci in multifocal papillary thyroid carcinoma. N Engl J Med 352:2406–2412
46. Tielens ET, Sherman ST, Hruban RH, Ladenson PW (1994) Follicular variant of papillary thyroid carcinoma: a clinicopathologic study. Cancer 73:424–431
47. Elsheikh TM, Asa SL, Chan JK, DeLellis RA, Heffess CS, LiVolsi VA et al (2008) Interobserver and intraobserver variation among experts in the diagnosis of thyroid follicular lesions with borderline nuclear features of papillary carcinoma. Am J Clin Pathol 130:736–744
48. Park YJ, Kwak SH, Kim DC et al (2007) Diagnostic value of galectin-3, HBME-1, cytokeratin 19, high molecular weight cytokeratin, cyclin D1 and p27 (kip1) in the differential diagnosis of thyroid nodules. J Korean Med Sci 22:621–628
49. Johnson TL, Lloyd RV, Thompson NW, Beierwaltes WH, Sisson JC (1988) Prognostic implications of the tall cell variant of papillary thyroid carcinoma. Am J Surg Pathol 12:22–27
50. Ghossein RA, Leboeuf R, Patel KN et al (2007) Tall cell variant of papillary thyroid carcinoma without extrathyroid extension: biologic behavior and clinical implications. Thyroid 17:655–661
51. Haigh PI, Urbach DR (2005) The treatment and prognosis of Hürthle cell follicular thyroid carcinoma compared with its non-Hürthle cell counterpart. Surgery 138:1152–1158
52. Evans HL, Vassilopoulou-Sellin R (1998) Follicular and Hürthle cell carcinomas of the thyroid: a comparative study. Am J Surg Pathol 22:1512–1520

53. Kushchayeva Y, Duh QY, Kebebew E, Clark OH (2004) Prognostic indications for Hürthle cell cancer. World J Surg 28:1266–1270
54. American Joint Committee on Cancer (2003) AJCC cancer staging manual, 6th edn. Springer, New York
55. D'Avanzo A, Ituarte PHG, Treseler P et al (2004) Prognostic scoring systems in patients with follicular thyroid cancer: a comparison of different staging systems in predicting the patient outcome. Thyroid 14:453–458
56. Nikiforov YE (2004) Genetic alterations involved in the transition from well-differentiated to poorly differentiated and anaplastic thyroid carcinomas. Endocr Pathol 15:319–327
57. Wang HM, Huang YW, Huang JS et al (2007) Anaplastic carcinoma of the thyroid arising more often from follicular carcinoma than papillary carcinoma. Ann Surg Oncol 14:3011–3018
58. Quiros RM, Ding HG, Gattuso P, Prinz RA, Xu X (2005) Evidence that one subset of anaplastic thyroid carcinomas are derived from papillary carcinomas due to BRAF and p53 mutations. Cancer 103:2261–2268
59. Udelsman R, Lakatos E, Ladenson P (1996) Optimal surgery for papillary thyroid carcinoma. World J Surg 20:88–93
60. American Thyroid Association Guidelines Taskforce (2009) Revised management guidelines for patients with thyroid nodules and differentiated thyroid cancer. Thyroid, in press
61. Banks ND, Kowalski J, Tsai HL et al (2008) A diagnostic predictor model for indeterminate or suspicious thyroid FNA samples. Thyroid 18:933–941
62. Sippel RS, Elaraj DM, Khanafshar E, Zarnegar R, Kebebew E, Duh QY et al (2008) Tumor size predicts malignant potential in Hürthle cell neoplasms of the thyroid. World J Surg 32:702–707
63. Chen H, Nicol TL, Zeiger MA, Dooley WC, Ladenson PW, Cooper DS et al (1998) Hürthle cell neoplasms of the thyroid: are there factors predictive of malignancy. Ann Surg 227:542–546
64. McCoy KL, Jabbour N, Ogilvie JB, Ohori NP, Carty SE, Yim JH (2007) The incidence of cancer and rate of false-negative cytology in thyroid nodules greater than or equal to 4 cm in size. Surgery 142:837–844
65. Mercante G, Frasoldati A, Pefroni C et al (2009) Prognostic factors affecting neck lymph node recurrence and distant metastasis in papillary microcarcinoma of the thyroid: results of a study in 445 patients. Thyroid 19(7):707–716
66. Chow SM, Law SC, Chan JK, Yau S, Lau WH (2003) Papillary microcarcinoma of the thyroid – prognostic significance of lymph node metastasis and multifocality. Cancer 98:31–40
67. Lundgren CI, Hall P, Dickman PW, Zedenius J (2007) Influence of surgical and postoperative treatment on survival in differentiated thyroid cancer. Br J Surg 94:571–577
68. Jonklaas J, Sarlis NJ, Litofsky D et al (2006) Outcomes of patients with differentiated thyroid carcinoma following initial therapy. Thyroid 16:1229–1242
69. Roti E, Degli Uberti EC, Bondanelli M, Braverman LE (2008) Thyroid papillary microcarcinoma: a descriptive and meta-analysis study. Eur J Endocrinol 159:659–673
70. Mazzaferri EL, Kloos RT (2001) Clinical review 128: current approaches to primary therapy for papillary and follicular thyroid cancer. J Clin Endocrinol Metab 86:1447–1463
71. Tsang RW, Brierley SWJ, Panzarella T, Gospodarowicz MK, Sutcliffe SB (1998) The effects of surgery, radioiodine, and external radiation therapy on the clinical outcome of patients with differentiated thyroid carcinoma. Cancer 82:375–388
72. Hay ID, Bergstralh EJ, Grant CS et al (1999) Impact of primary surgery on outcome in 300 patients with pathologic tumor-node-metastasis stage III papillary thyroid carcinoma treated at one institution from 1940 through 1989. Surgery 126:1173–1181
73. Bilimoria KY, Bentrem DJ, Linn JG et al (2007) Utilization of total thyroidectomy for papillary thyroid cancer in the United States. Surgery 142:906–913
74. Sosa JA, Bowman HM, Tielsch JM, Powe NR, Gordon TA, Udelsman R (1998) The importance of surgeon experience for clinical and economic outcomes from thyroidectomy. Ann Surg 228:320–330

75. Moalem J, Suh I, Duh QY (2008) Treatment and prevention of recurrence of multinodular goiter: an evidence-based review of the literature. World J Surg 32:1301–1312
76. Qubain SW, Nakano S, Baba M, Takao S, Aikou T (2002) Distribution of lymph node micrometastasis in pN0 well-differentiated thyroid carcinoma. Surgery 131:249–256
77. Arturi F, Russo D, Giuffrida D, Ippolito A, Perrotti N, Vigneri R et al (1997) Early diagnosis by genetic analysis of differentiated thyroid cancer metastases in small lymph nodes. J Clin Endocrinol Metab 82:1638–1641
78. Grebe SK, Hay ID (1996) Thyroid cancer nodal meatastases: biologic significance and therapeutic considerations. Surg Oncol Clin N Am 5:43–63
79. Loh KC, Greenspan FS, Gee L, Miller TR, Yeo PP (1997) Pathological tumor-node-metastasis (pTNM) staging for papillary and follicular thyroid carcinomas: a retrospective analysis of 700 patients. J Clin Endocrinol Metab 82:3553–3562
80. Zavdfudim V, Feurer ID, Griffin MR, Phay JE (2008) The impact of lymph node involvement on survival in patients with papillary and follicular thyroid carcinoma. Surgery 144:1070–1077
81. Gemsenjäger E, Perren A, Seifert B, Schüler G, Schweizer I, Heitz PU (2003) Lymph node surgery in papillary thyroid carcinoma. J Am Coll Surg 197:182–190
82. Leboulleux S, Girard E, Rose M et al (2007) Ultrasound criteria of malignancy for cervical lymph nodes in patients followed up for differentiated thyroid cancer. J Clin Endocrinol Metab 92:3590–3594
83. Kouvaraki MA, Lee JE, Shapiro SE, Sherman SI, Evans DB (2004) Preventable reoperations for persistent and recurrent papillary thyroid carcinoma. Surgery 136:1183–1191
84. Gimm O, Rath FW, Dralle H (1998) Pattern of lymph node metastases in papillary thyroid carcinoma. Br J Surg 85:252–254
85. White ML, Gauger PG, Doherty GM (2007) Central lymph node dissectionin differentiated thyroid cancer. World J Surg 31:895–904
86. Sywak M, Cornford L, Roach P, Stalberg P, Sidhu S, Delbridge L (2006) Routine ipsilateral level VI lymphadenectomy reduces postoperative thyroglobulin levels in papillary thyrdoi cancer. Surgery 140:1000–1005
87. Mazzaferri EL, Jhiang SM (1994) Long-term impact of initial surgical and medical therapy on papillary and follicular thyroid cancer. Am J Med 97:418–428
88. Palazzo FF, Gosnell J, Savio R et al (2006) Lympadenectomy for papillary thyroid cancer: changes in practice over four decades. Eur J Surg Oncol 32:340–344
89. Ito Y, Higashiyama T, Takamura Y et al (2007) Risk factors for recurrence to the lymph node in papillary thyroid carcinoma patients without preoperatively detectable lateral node metastasis: validity of prophylactic modified radical neck dissection. World J Surg 31:2085–2091
90. Grebe SK, Hay ID (1995) Follicular thyroid cancer. Endocrinol Metab Clin North Am 24:761–801
91. Witte J, Goretzki PE, Dieken J, Simon D, Röher HD (2002) Importance of lymph node metastases in follicular thyroid cancer. World J Surg 26:1017–1022
92. Sawka AM, Brierley JD, Tsang RW et al (2008) An updated systematic review and commentary examining the effectiveness of radioactive iodine remnant ablation in well-differentiated thyroid cancer. Endocrinol Metab Clin North Am 37:457–480
93. Lopez-Penabad L, Chiu AC et al (2003) Prognostic factors in patients with Hürthle cell neoplasms of the thyroid. Cancer 97:1186–1194
94. Pacini F, Ladenson PW, Schlumberger M et al (2006) Radioiodine ablation of thyroid remnants after preparation with recombinant human thyrotropin in differentiated thyroid carcinoma: results of an international, randomized, controlled study. J Clin Endocrinol Metab 91:926–932
95. Tuttle RM, Brokhin M, Omry G et al (2008) Recombinant human TSH-assisted radioactive iodine remnant ablation achieves short-term clinical recurrence rates similar to those of traditional thyroid hormone withdrawal. J Nucl Med 49:767–770
96. Taïeb D, Sebag F, Cherenko M et al (2008) Quality of life changes and clinical outcomes in thyroid cancer patients undergoing radioiodine remnant ablation with recombinant human thyrotropin: a randomized controlled study. Clin Endocrinol Sep 17, epub
97. Nordén MM, Larsson F, Tedelind S et al (2007) Down-regulation of the sodium/iodide symporter explains 131I-induced thyroid stunning. Cancer Res 67:7512–7517

98. Sisson JC, Avram AM, Lawson SA, Gauger PG, Doherty GM (2006) The so-called stunning of thyroid tissue. J Nucl Med 47:1406–1412
99. Doi SA, Woodhouse NJ (2000) Ablation of the thyroid remnant and 131I dose in differentiated thyroid cancer. Clin Endocrinol (Oxf) 52:765–773
100. Hackshaw A, Harmer C, Mallick U, Haq M, Franklyn JA (2007) 131I activity for remnant ablation in patients with differentiated thyroid cancer: a systematic review. J Clin Endocrinol Metab 92:28–38
101. Souza Rosario PW, Barroso AL, Rezende LL, Padrao EL, Fagundes TA, Penna GC, Purisch S (2004) Post I-131 therapy scanning in patients with thyroid carcinoma metastases: an unnecessary cost or a relevant contribution? Clin Nucl Med 29:795–798
102. Garsi JP, Schlumberger M, Rubino C, Ricard M, Labbé M, Ceccarelli C et al (2008) Therapeutic administration of ^{131}I for differentiated thyroid cancer: radiation dose to ovaries and outcome of pregnancies. J Nucl Med 49:845–852
103. Rubino C, de Vathaire F, Dottorini ME, Hall P, Schvartz C, Couette JE et al (2003) Second primary malignancies in thyroid cancer patients. Br J Cancer 89:1638–1644
104. Sandeep TC, Strachan MW, Reynolds RM, Brewster DH, Scélo G, Pukkala E et al (2006) Second primary cancers in thyroid cancer patients: a multinational record linkage study. J Clin Endocrinol Metab 91:1819–1825
105. Verkooijen RB, Smit JW, Romijn JA, Stokkel MP (2006) The incidence of second primary tumors in thyroid cancer patients is increased, but not related to treatment of thyroid cancer. Eur J Endocrinol 155:801–806
106. Brabant G (2008) Thyrotropin suppressive therapy in thyroid carcinoma: what are the targets? J Clin Endocrinol Metab 93:1167–1169
107. McGriff NJ, Csako G, Gourgiotis L, Lori CG, Pucino F, Sarlis NJ (2002) Effects of thyroid hormone suppression therapy on adverse clinical outcomes in thyroid cancer. Ann Med 34:554–564
108. Cappola AR, Fried LP, Arnold AM et al (2006) Thyroid status, cardiovascular risk, and mortality in older adults. JAMA 295:1033–1041
109. Toft AD (2001) Clinical practice: subclinical hyperthyroidism. N Engl J Med 34:512–516
110. Pujol P, Daures JP, Nsakala N, Baldet L, Bringer J, Jaffiol C (1996) Degree of thyrotropin suppression as a prognostic determinant in differentiated thyroid cancer. J Clin Endocrinol Metab 81:4318–4323
111. Cooper DS, Speckler B, Ho M et al (1998) Thyrotropin suppression and disease progression in patients with differentiated thyroid cancer: results from the National Thyroid Cancer Treatment Cooperative Registry. Thyroid 8:737–744
112. Mazzaferri EL, Robbins RJ, Spencer CA et al (2003) A consensus report of the role of serum thyroglobulin as a monitoring method for low-risk patients with papillary thyroid carcinoma. J Clin Endocrinol Metab 88:1433–1441
113. SpencerCA LoPresti JS, Fatemi S, Nicoloff JT (1999) Detection of residual and recurrent differentiated thyroid carcinoma by serum thyroglobulin measurement. Thyroid 9:435–441
114. Kloos RT, Mazzaferri EL (2005) A single recombinant human thyrotropin-stimulated serum thyroglobulin measurement predicts differentiated thyroid carcinoma metastases three to five years later. J Clin Endocrinol Metab 90:5047–5057
115. Frasoldati A, Pesenti M, Gallo M, Caroggio A, Salvo D, Valcavi R (2003) Diagnosis of neck recurrences in patients with differentiated thyroid carcinoma. Cancer 97:90–96
116. Johnson NA, Tublin ME (2008) Postoperative surveillance of differentiated thyroid carcinoma: rationale, techniques, and controversies. Radiology 249:429–444
117. Boi F, Baghino G, Atzeni F, Lai ML, Faa G, Mariotti S (2006) The diagnostic value for differentiated thyroid carcinoma metastases of thyroblogulin (Tg) measurement in washout fluid from fine-needle aspiration biopsy of neck lymph nodes is maintained in the presence of circulating anti-Tg antibodies. J Clin Endocrinol Metab 91:1364–1369
118. The NCCN Clinical Practice Guidelines in Oncology(TM) Thyroid Carcinoma (Version 1.2009). 2009 National Comprehensive Cancer Network, Inc. Available at: NCCN.org. Accessed [10/19/2009]

119. Cady B (1998) Papillary carcinoma of the thyroid gland: treatment based on risk group definition. Surg Oncol Clin N Am 7:633–644
120. Biliotti GC, Martini F, Vezzosi V et al (2006) Specific features of differentiated thyroid carcinoma in patients over 70 years of age. J Surg Oncol 93:194–198
121. Kim TY, Kim WB, Kim ES et al (2005) Serum thyroglobulin levels at the time of 131I remnant ablation just after thyroidectomy are useful for early prediction of clinical recurrence in low-risk patients with differentiated thyroid carcinoma. J Clin Endocrinol Metab 90:1440–1445
122. Heemstra KA, Liu YY, Stokkel M et al (2007) Serum thyroglobulin concentrations predict disease-free remission and death in differentiated thyroid carcinoma. Clin Endocrinol 66:58–64
123. Kloos RT (2008) Approach to the patient with a positive serum thyroglobulin and a negative radioiodine scan after initial therapy for differentiated thyroid cancer. J Clin Endocrinol Metab 93:1519–1525
124. Elaraj DM, Clark OH (2007) Changing management in patients with papillary thyroid cancer. Curr Treat Options in Oncol 8:305–313
125. McCoy KL, Yim JH, Tublin ME, Burmeister LA, Ogilvie JB, Carty SE (2007) Same-day ultrasound guidance in reoperation for locally recurrent papillary thyroid cancer. Surgery 142:965–972
126. Links TP, van Tol KM, Jager PL et al (2005) Life expectancy in diffentiated thyroid cancer: a novel approach to survival analysis. Endocr Relat Cancer 12:273–280
127. Grant CS, Hay ID, Gough IR, Bergstralh EJ, Goellner JR, McConahey WM (1988) Local recurrence in papillary thyroid carcinoma: is extent of surgical resection important? Surgery 104:954–962
128. Shammas A, Degirmenci B, Mountz JM, McCook BM, Branstetter B, Bencherif B et al (2007) ^{18}F-FDG PET/CT in patients with suspected recurrent or metastatic well-differentiated thyroid cancer. J Nucl Med 48:221–226
129. Pryma DA, Schöder H, Gönen M, Robbins RJ, Larson SM, Yeung HW (2006) Diagnostic accuracy and prognostic value of ^{18}F-FDG PET in Hürthle cell thyroid cancer patients. J Nucl Med 47:1260–1266
130. Terezakis SA, Lee KS, Ghossein RA et al (2009) Role of external beam radiotherapy in patients with advanced or recurrent nonanaplastic thyroid cancer: Memorial Sloan-Kettering Cancer Center experience. Int J Radiat Oncol Biol Phys 73:795–801
131. La Quaglia MP, Black T, Holcomb GW III et al (2000) Differentiated thyroid cancer: clinical characteristics, treatment, and outcome in patients under 21 years of age who present with distant metastases. J Pediatr Surg 35:955–959
132. Sampson E, Brierley JD, Le LW, Rotstein L, Tsang RW (2007) Clinical management and outcome of papillary and follicular (differentiated) thyroid cancer presenting with distant metastsis at diagnosis. Cancer 110:1451–1456
133. Robbins RJ, Srivastava S, Shaha A et al (2004) Factors influencing the basal and recombinant human thyrotropin-stimulated serum thyroglobulin in patients with metastatic thyroid carcinoma. J Clin Endocrinol Metab 89:6010–6016
134. Dralle H, Schwarzrock R, Lang W et al (1985) Comparison of histology and immunohistochemistry with thyroglobulin serum levels and radioiodine uptake in recurrences and metastases of differentiated thyroid carcinomas. Acta Endocrinol 108:504–510
135. Zanotti-Fregonara P, Hindie E, Faugeron I et al (2008) Update on the diagnosis and therapy of distant metastases of differentiated thyroid carcinoma. Minerva Endocrinol 33:313–327
136. Zettinig G, Fueger BJ, Passler C, Kaserer K, Pirich C, Dudczak R et al (2002) Long-term follow-up of patients with bone metastases from differentiated thyroid carcinoma – surgery or conventional therapy? Clin Endocrinol 56:377–382
137. Argiris A, Agarwala SS, Karamouzis MV, Burmeister LA, Carty SE (2008) A phase II trial of doxorubisin and interferon alpha 2b in advanced non-medullary thyroid cancer. Invest New Drugs 26:183–188
138. Shimaoka K, Schoenfield DA, DeWys WD, Creech RH, DeConti R (1985) A randomized trial of doxorubicin versus doxorubicin plus cisplatin in patients with advanced thyroid carcinoma. Cancer 59:2155–2160
139. Gupta-Abramson V, Troxel AB, Nellore A et al (2008) Phase II trial of sorafenib in advanced thyroid cancer. J Clin Oncol 26:4714–4719

Chapter 4
Sporadic Medullary Thyroid Cancer

Adrian Harvey and Janice L. Pasieka

Introduction

Medullary thyroid cancer (MTC), is a tumor of the parafollicular / c-cells of the thyroid gland. These cells are derived from the embryonic neural crests and make up 1% of the thyroid cells. C-cells can be found anywhere in the gland but are concentrated in the upper poles of the thyroid lobes. Among other substances, these cells produce calcitonin which contributes to the regulation of serum calcium. This tumor, first described in 1959, is characterized by early spread to regional lymph nodes, and long-term survival even with disseminated disease [1]. Common sites of distant metastases include lung, liver, brain, bone, and soft tissue [2].

MTC accounts for 5–10% of thyroid cancers. Overall 70–75% of MTC appear to be sporadic, while 25–30% have been linked to a hereditary form. Several hereditary forms exist, including those tumors associated with MEN-2A and 2B, as well as familial medullary thyroid cancer (FMTC). In MEN-2A, MTC is associated with pheochromocytoma, hyperparathyroidism, cutaneous lichen amyloidosis, and occasionally Hirschsprung's disease [3–5]. Patients with MEN-2B also have an elevated risk of developing pheochromocytoma; in addition, they have marfanoid habitus and typically develop multiple neural ganglioma (most commonly of the digestive tract mucosa) [6]. Familial forms are inherited in an autosomal dominant fashion because of a germline mutation in the RET proto-oncogene found on chromosome 10 [7–9]. While in familial forms, MTC tends to be multifocal and bilateral, and arises in a background of C-cell hyperplasia, sporadic tumors are commonly solitary and unilateral, and may arise in an otherwise normal gland [10, 11].

J.L. Pasieka (✉)
Department of Surgery, University of Calgary, North Tower Floor 10, 1403 29th Street NW, Calgary, AB, Canada, T2N 2T9
e-mail: janice.pasieka@albertahealthservices.ca

C. Sturgeon (ed.), *Endocrine Neoplasia*, Cancer Treatment and Research, vol 153,
DOI 10.1007/978-1-4419-0857-5_4, © Springer Science+Business Media, LLC 2010

Diagnosis

While patients with familial disease may present with positive genetic screening or surveillance, sporadic MTC most commonly presents with a palpable thyroid nodule and 50% of these patients present with palpable lymph node metastases or signs of local compression. In addition, high levels of calcitonin can result in systemic symptoms including flushing and diarrhea. The work up of patients with MTC begins with a thorough history and physical examination. In particular, evidence of familial disease should be elucidated through family history of MTC or associated endocrinopathies. Symptoms associated with local compression or invasion including change in voice, dysphagia, cough, and shortness of breath are present in up to 15% of patients with MTC [12]. Ultrasound and fine needle aspiration biopsy have become mainstays in the work-up and diagnosis of nodular thyroid disease. In MTC, ultrasound can be used to assess the size, extent, and potential multifocality of the tumor as well as the regional lymph node basins. Ultrasound may also be used to guide fine needle aspiration biopsies. Fine needle aspiration cytology is highly sensitive for the diagnosis of MTC. Specimens are stained for calcitonin as well as amyloid and carcinoembryonic antigen (CEA) in some cases. In the setting of nodular thyroid disease the sensitivity of fine needle aspiration cytology approaches 100% in the evaluation of nodules larger than 10 mm [13].

Biochemical Markers in Medullary Thyroid Cancer

A number of substances are released by MTC cells. These include, but are not limited to, calcitonin, CEA, chromogranin A, serotonin, neuron specific enolase, somatostatin, gastrin related peptide, and substance P. Prior to genetic testing, calcitonin was used for screening asymptomatic members of families affected with MEN-2. More recently, a number of authors have argued for routine measurement of calcitonin in the work-up of nodular thyroid disease [13–15]. Elisei et al. published the results of routine calcitonin screening in 10,864 patients with nodular thyroid disease [14]. MTC was found in 44 patients (0.4%). Screening serum calcitonin demonstrated a higher sensitivity than fine needle aspiration for the detection of MTC in these patients. Complete biochemical remission in these 44 patients was significantly higher than in a historical comparison group diagnosed before routine screening. In a similar series, 1,167 patients with nodular thyroid disease were screened with basal calcitonin and in some cases stimulated levels [15]. Elevated basal calcitonin was seen in 34 patients. On histological examination of surgical specimens, the prevalence of MTC was found to be 1.37% (16 patients). Of these 16 patients, 14 had elevated basal calcitonin levels. The authors therefore recommended that calcitonin levels should become part of the routine workup of nodular thyroid disease arguing that "occult" MTC could be detected preoperatively and more extensive primary surgery performed. Although this approach is commonly used in Europe, North American centers have not yet utilized calcitonin in the routine screening of a multinodular goiter because of the poor positive predicted value. Calcitonin is however useful in the screening and diagnosis of persistent or recurrent MTC following surgical therapy.

A number of the other substances released by MTC cells have been evaluated as biochemical markers for clinical use. In a study of 46 patients with histologically proven MTC, de Groot et al. examined the neuroendocrine profile of these tumors [16]. In addition to calcitonin, other potential serum markers (CEA, chromogranin A, catecholamines, tryptase, and platelet serotonin), and urinary markers (catecholamines, histamine, and serotonin metabolites) were evaluated. Patients were divided into three groups. Group 1 consisted of those with no clinical evidence of disease, group 2 were those with clinically apparent but stable disease, and group 3 consisted of patients with progressive disease. The results demonstrated that of these markers, only CEA and chromogranin A were able to distinguish stable from progressive disease. The authors concluded that the most useful biochemical markers in the follow-up of MTC were calcitonin and CEA [16].

Biochemical markers may also provide prognostic information in MTC. In one series, Laure Giraudet et al. performed repeat imaging in 55 patients with MTC and persistent elevations in calcitonin [17]. Serum levels of CEA and calcitonin were measured in an attempt to define a relationship between serum markers and disease progression. On repeat imaging, 10 patients had no evidence of disease. In the remaining 45 patients a significant relationship was found between serum marker doubling time and disease progression. Doubling times of greater than 24 months were strongly associated with stable disease. In contrast, serum marker doubling times of shorter than 24 months were more commonly seen in those with progressive MTC.

Preoperative CEA has also been shown to correlate with progression of disease. In a retrospective review of 150 patients with histological proven MTC, 54 of these patients were found to have elevated preoperative levels of CEA [18]. On multivariate analysis, CEA level was found to be associated with increased tumor size, lymph node involvement and distant metastases. An analysis of those 54 patients with elevated CEA levels demonstrated that surgical cure was rare in patients with levels greater than 30 ng/ml as this was associated with lymph node involvement in the central and ipsilateral lateral neck compartments. CEA levels above 100 ng/ml were associated with lymph node spread to the contralateral neck and distant metastases.

Screening for Familial Disease

Identification of the RET proto-oncogene and delineation of its role in hereditary forms of MTC have allowed for genetic screening in patients with suspected familial disease. As a result, prophylactic thyroidectomy can be performed on patients potentially before the development of MTC and those without a germline mutation can forego continued screening of calcitonin. More recently however, evidence has supported genetic testing even in those with suspected sporadic disease. Elisei et al. retrospectively analyzed a 13 year experience with RET genetic testing in 807 subjects [19]. Four-hundred and eighty-one of these tests were performed in patients with presumed sporadic MTC. In this group, 35 patients (7.3%) were found to have a germline RET mutation, with the majority falling under the category of FMTC.

Unfortunately, genetic testing may take some time to complete. As such, patients may come to surgery for MTC prior to the identification or exclusion of a germline RET mutation. Thus, all patients should still undergo biochemical screening for associated endocrine tumors. In particular, pheochromocytoma should be ruled out by measurement of 24-h urinary, or plasma catecholamines and metanephrines, and serum calcium and parathyroid hormone to rule out hyperparathyroidism. Surgical strategies should include appropriate blockade of a pheochromocytoma and its removal prior to dealing with the MTC. The surgical strategies of hyperparathyroidism depend on the genotype and the surgical findings which will be covered in Chap. 6.

Staging

Staging of MTC is generally by the American Joint Committee on Cancer (AJCC) and International Union against Cancer (UICC) TNM classification systems [20]. The stage of disease is determined by the size of the primary tumor, the involvement of regional lymph nodes, and the presence or absence of distant metastases (Fig. 4.1). As expected, stage of disease has proven to be a significant prognostic indicator in MTC. Survival data on 899 patients with MTC from the French Calcitonin Tumour Study Group were analyzed by Modigliani et al. [21]. This cohort of patients included 57% with sporadic disease. On multivariate analysis the only independent predictors of survival were tumor stage and age. Similar data were seen in a series of 104 patients reported on by Kebebew et al. [22]. In this series 56% had sporadic disease. Cause specific mortality at 10 years was found to be 13.5%. Again, on multivariate analysis, only tumor stage and age were independent predictors of survival.

Treatment

Surgical Treatment of Primary Tumors

MTC is distinct from other forms of differentiated thyroid cancer in that its cells do not organify and concentrate radioactive iodine. Thus surgery represents the best chance for cure. Appropriate surgical therapy, in particular the treatment of the lymph node basins, for MTC has recently been the subject of debate in the literature.

AJCC Stage Grouping			
Medullary Thyroid Cancer			
Stage I	T1	N0	M0
Stage II	T2	N0	M0
Stage III	T3	N0	M0
	T1	N1a	M0
	T2	N1a	M0
	T3	N1a	M0
Stage IVa	T4a	N0	M0
	T4a	N1a	M0
	T1	N1b	M0
	T2	N1b	M0
	T3	N1b	M0
	T4a	N1b	M0
Stage IVb	T4b	Any N	M0
Stage IVc	Any T	Any N	M1

Fig. 4.1 TNM stage grouping: medullary thyroid cancer. Reproduced with permission from *Greene F.L., Page D.L., Fleming I.D., et al. AJCC Cancer Staging Manual, Sixth Edition, pp. 78–79. New York: Springer, 2002*

Total thyroidectomy has generally been considered appropriate in all patients with MTC. In fact, the use of total thyroidectomy has increased over the last three or four decades [23]. However, on the basis of the assumption that sporadic tumors are always solitary and unilateral, Miyauchi et al. recently proposed that hemithyroidectomy with appropriate lymph node dissection may be a reasonable strategy in these patients [24, 25]. In a small prospective series of patients with sporadic disease confirmed by genetic testing, 15 patients were treated with unilateral thyroid surgery with bilateral central and ipsilateral modified radical neck dissection [25]. Using this strategy, 12 of 15 patients (80%) achieved biochemical cure. Two patients however required completion operations (13%). In addition, other reports have cast doubt on the notion that sporadic tumors are always solitary [10, 26]. In fact, on histopathological examination, bilateral gland involvement has been reported in 5–9% of sporadic MTC [10, 26] Therefore, total thyroidectomy remains the best surgical option for sporadic MTC at this time.

The more contentious issue in the treatment of MTC is the extent of lymph node dissection. Metastases to regional lymph nodes are common in MTC. A recent study from the Netherlands evaluated 64 patients undergoing surgery for MTC [27]. Thirty-five of these patients presented with a palpable nodule alone and 29 had suspicious lymph nodes. Of these, 45 patients were classified as having sporadic MTC on the basis of negative family history and in most cases, genetic testing. Central lymph node compartments were dissected in all patients. Unilateral or bilateral lateral compartment neck dissections (level II–V) were performed at the initial operation or at reoperation when clinical or radiological evidence pointed to involvement. Lymph node metastasis was noted in the central compartment in 63%, in the ipsilateral lateral compartment in 55%, and in both lateral compartments in 27%. In addition, 31% of patients had mediastinal lymph node metastases. In a similar series, Moley and colleagues evaluated 73 patients (35 sporadic) who had undergone total thyroidectomy with central and bilateral lateral neck dissection for MTC [28]. All of these patients presented with a palpable thyroid nodule. Overall, 32 patients had unilateral tumors and 41 had bilateral tumors on pathological examination. In those patients with unilateral tumors, 81% had positive nodes in the central and in the ipsilateral lateral neck compartments and 41% had positive nodes in the contralateral neck dissection. In those patients with bilateral tumors, lymph node metastases were noted in 78% of central compartment dissections and lateral neck dissections ipsilateral to the largest tumor and in 44% of lateral neck dissections contralateral to the largest tumor.

Despite the high incidence of lymph node involvement in MTC, total thyroidectomy without a lymph node dissection continues to be performed. Hundahl et al. examined cohort data on 5,583 patients with thyroid cancer from the National Cancer Data Base [29]. Of these, 150 patients were found to have sporadic MTC. Total thyroidectomy without lymph node dissection was performed in 31.1% of patients. The next most common procedure was a total thyroidectomy with limited or selective lymph node dissection.

The concept of compartment oriented lymph node dissection in MTC was introduced by Dralle and colleagues [30, 31]. In a retrospective study these authors reviewed 82 patients with MTC (57 sporadic, 25 hereditary). In total, 142 operations were performed. Selective lymphadenectomies were performed in 63 with systematic compartment-oriented surgery in 35. In those patients with positive lymph nodes, compartment oriented surgery resulted in a significantly higher rate of biochemical cure, defined by normalization of pentagastrin stimulated calcitonin, when compared to selective lymph node surgery (29.2% vs. 8.5%). In addition, a higher portion of those undergoing selective lymphadenectomy required reoperation for recurrent disease. Finally, survival was significantly better in those undergoing compartment oriented microdissection of cervical lymph nodes. In 24 patients undergoing an initial compartment oriented dissection and an additional 11 patients with delayed compartment dissection after a selective lymph node dissection, overall survival was 100% at last follow-up, (4.1 and 12 years respectively). In comparison, in 35 patients undergoing a selective lymphadenectomy only, overall survival was less than 30% at a maximum follow-up of 12 years.

Since this recommendation, other authors have added their support for compartment oriented lymph node dissection in the primary treatment of MTC [32–34]. Kallinowski et al. examined a series of 40 patients with MTC operated on over a period of 15 years [33]. In this series lymph node dissection consisted mostly of the selective removal of clinically enlarged nodes. Six patients received a unilateral neck dissection. The authors reported the mean survival to be 68 months with the primary prognostic factor being involvement of regional lymph nodes. On the basis of these data, the authors recommended that all patients received a total thyroidectomy with bilateral central neck lymph node dissections. In those patients with involved nodes, or persistently elevated postoperative calcitonin, the authors recommended lateral compartment dissections. In a similar series, Weber et al. reviewed their experience with 36 patients (16 sporadic, 20 familial) presenting with clinically evident MTC [34]. All patients had a total thyroidectomy with central and lateral (bilateral in 13) neck lymph node dissections either as primary surgery or within 5 months of the initial operation. Overall biochemical cure, defined as normal basal and pentagastrin stimulated calcitonin levels, at a median follow-up of almost 4 years was 44%. Biochemical cure was achieved in 89% of node negative patients and 30% of those with positive lymph nodes.

More recently published data have supported the growing consensus that more extensive primary surgical therapy is appropriate in patients with nonoccult MTC. In a series published in 2003, Yen et al. reviewed a series of 80 patients operated on for MTC at the MD Anderson Cancer Center [35]. Of these, 70 patients were operated on with the intent of cure in the setting of primary ($n=23$), or recurrent ($n=47$) disease. Forty-five of these patients were classified as having sporadic disease. The standard procedure for sporadic disease was to perform a bilateral central neck dissection and unilateral lateral dissection in those without clinical or radiographic evidence of lymph node involvement. Bilateral lateral compartment procedures were performed in those with clinical or radiographic evidence of disease in the lymph nodes. Recurrence in this study was found in 18 (26%) patients at a median 35 month follow-up. In just 10 (14%) of these patients the recurrence was found in the neck. This rate of cervical recurrence was lower than the 20–60% rate previously published in the literature.

In a similar study from the Netherlands, de Groot et al. looked at 64 patients (45 sporadic) with MTC presenting clinically as either a palpable thyroid nodule ($n=35$) or palpable lymph nodes ($n=29$) [27]. Standard surgical therapy in this center at that time consisted of a total thyroidectomy with bilateral central compartment lymph node dissections. Management of the lateral or mediastinal compartments was on the basis of clinical or radiological evidence of disease. Interestingly, 64% of patients in this series received postoperative external beam radiation therapy. In those patients presenting with a palpable nodule, lymph node involvement was found in the central compartment in 31%, the ipsilateral, lateral compartment in 23%, and in the contralateral and mediastinal compartments in 14%. However, it should be noted that compartments not dissected were considered free of disease if no clinical or radiographic evidence was found. Thus the actual rate of involved lymph nodes may have been underestimated. In those patients who presented with palpable lymph nodes 100% had central compartment involvement, 93% had ipsilateral, and 45% had contralateral lateral lymph node spread. Mediastinal lymph nodes were involved in 52%. In the group with a palpable thyroid nodule, 13 patients had "less than standard" operations at other centers prior to referral. In this subgroup of patients locoregional recurrence was significantly higher. Overall, loco-regional recurrence in this series was 46%. In a similar, but smaller series reported on by Greenblatt et al., [36] cure rates were significantly higher in those patients who underwent a lymph node dissection.

In general, most authors have supported compartment oriented lymph node dissection at the primary surgery. In fact, delayed dissection of the central lymph nodes has been associated with higher complication rates. Fleming et al. reported on 40 patients (23 sporadic, 17 familial) with MTC operated on at a single center [37]. Of these patients, 11 were undergoing primary surgery, 13 had previous thyroidectomy but had postoperative elevations in calcitonin without clinical/radiological evidence of lymph node involvement, and the remaining 16 had previous thyroidectomy with radiological evidence of lymph node metastases. In this series, a 17% rate of permanent postoperative hypoparathyroidism was observed. Interestingly, most of these cases (5/7) occurred in the third group in which normalization of postoperative calcitonin was seen in only one patient.

In summary, the general consensus for primary surgical therapy of MTC is a total thyroidectomy and compartment oriented lymph node dissection. However, the number of compartments that should be dissected has remained a focus of some controversy. In a 2002 article, Dralle et al. published revised recommendations regarding the extent of lymph node dissection [38]. Citing a significant rate of involvement of both the ipsilateral (35%) and contralateral (20%) lateral neck compartments at primary surgery, the authors recommended total thyroidectomy with central and bilateral lateral compartment dissection for most patients with MTC at primary or completion surgery. Mediastinal lymph node dissection was recommended for cases of known nodal spread. In cases of distant micrometastases the authors proposed that the local-regional disease is of paramount importance and recommended a bilateral central and ipsilateral lateral compartment dissection. Finally, in cases of distant macrometastases the authors recommended total thyroidectomy with only selective removal of symptomatic lymph nodes. Similarly, Moley and DeBenedetti recommended total thyroidectomy with bilateral central and lateral compartment neck dissections for all patients with palpable MTC. Their recommendations were on the basis of a series of 73 patients operated on, (either primary or reoperative surgery) at a single center. In this series, lymph node metastases were found in 78% of central compartment, 71% of ipsilateral, and 49% of contralateral lateral compartment dissections. This rate of positive lymph nodes was higher than that previously published in the literature. The authors explained this by the fact that all patients in the series had full neck dissections, whereas many previous studies had assumed that compartments not dissected were free of disease. However the authors did acknowledge that a potential referral bias may have artificially inflated these numbers.

Scollo et al. following a retrospective review of 101 patients with MTC also recommended total thyroidectomy with bilateral central and lateral neck compartment dissections in all patients with MTC [39]. This recommendation was on the basis of a significant rate of positive nodes in the contralateral lateral compartment (19%) and the inability to predict lymph node involvement by tumor size. The authors did propose that contralateral lateral compartment dissection could be left out in patients with unilateral, sporadic tumors and no clinical evidence of lymph nodes metastases in the central or ipsilateral lateral compartments on preoperative imaging. In 2000, Kebebew recommended that a standard surgical procedure for patients with MTC should consist of total thyroidectomy with bilateral central compartment as well as an ipsilateral lateral neck compartment dissection [40]. Contralateral lateral neck dissection was recommended for bilateral primary tumors and those with extensive lymph node involvement on the ipsilateral side. Mediastinal dissection was also recommended in the presence of extensive involvement of cervical lymph nodes but not prophylactically [40]. Some authors do include mediastinal lymph node dissection in their recommendations for standard surgical therapy [27, 38]. The ability to adequately remove Level VII requires a sternal split; therefore, many centers do not prophylactically remove this level unless gross disease is found.

One potential caveat to the strong recommendation for compartment oriented lymph node dissection may be in cases of sporadic "micro" MTC found incidentally during or prior to procedures for nodular thyroid disease. Lymph node dissection may be unnecessary in these subcentimeter lesions. Hamy et al. examined specimens from 43 patients with sporadic micro MTC [41]. Clinically apparent cervical adenopathy was noted in two patients. Of these, 36 underwent a formal bilateral central compartment lymph node dissection, with the remainder having "node picking" procedures. A total of 601 lymph nodes from the 41 subclinical patients were examined and no metastatic involvement was found. As well, normalization of postoperative calcitonin levels was seen in all of the 41 subclinical patients at a mean follow-up of 32 months, including those having undergone lesser procedures.

The search for consensus in the surgical treatment of MTC has been elusive. In a survey among members of the International Association of Endocrine Surgeons (IAES) Dotzenrath et al. examined pattern of diagnostic and therapeutic management in MTC [42]. Of the 263 surveys distributed, 75 responses, representing 73 international endocrine units were received. For the purpose of this study, the authors defined "standard surgical therapy" according to the German guidelines calling for total thyroidectomy and central compartment lymph node dissection combined with ipsilateral (in sporadic MTC) or bilateral (in hereditary MTC) modified functional neck dissection. Overall, only 25–40% of respondents utilized this standard procedure. In addition, Kebebew et al. retrospectively examined 1,070 patients with MTC entered in the Surveillance, Epidemiology, and End-Results (SEER) database [23]. The authors concluded that a significant portion of patients were receiving initial surgical treatment that was "less than optimal." Even over the last 7 years of the study (1994–2000), 15% of patients received less than a total or near total thyroidectomy and 41% did not undergo any formal lymph node dissection at their primary surgery.

Persistent or Recurrent Medullary Thyroid Cancer

Despite more aggressive primary surgical therapy, a significant percentage of patients will have persistent disease or develop locoregional recurrence. Persistent or recurrent elevations in basal or stimulated calcitonin are seen in at least 50% of patients [12, 43, 44]. The concept of cervical reoperation for persistently elevated calcitonin was introduced by Tisell et al. in 1986 [45]. In this series, 11 patients with persistently elevated postoperative calcitonin underwent microdissection of central and lateral neck compartments. Four of these patients experienced normalization of calcitonin levels. Overall, cervical reoperation based on persistently elevated calcitonin levels results in normalization of calcitonin in approximately 33% of patients [45–47]. In addition, another 50% will experience a fall in postoperative calcitonin levels. Unfortunately, up to 30–50% of patients will have no significant change in calcitonin levels following cervical reoperation [46, 47].

Reoperative neck surgery is technically difficult with the possibility of significant complications, including permanent hypoparathyroidism, injury to the recurrent laryngeal nerve (RLN), and/or the thoracic duct [2]. In fact, the rate of RLN injury ranges from 2% to 15% [2, 46, 47]. Given this, the avoidance of reoperative neck surgery in patients unlikely to experience benefit is desirable. As a result, a more extensive search for metastatic disease generally precedes a return visit to the operating room. Patients presenting with persistent or recurrent elevations in calcitonin should first have their operative notes reviewed to determine if they have undergone adequate initial surgical therapy. Given the ongoing changes in recommendations regarding primary surgical treatment, this will be center-dependent and, for the time being, somewhat of a "moving target." In addition, patients should undergo a physical exam and radiologic studies to search for evidence of disease. Imaging studies may include CT, MRI, or ultrasound of the neck, and CT or MRI of the chest/mediastinum and abdomen [48–51]. In addition, bone scans, nuclear medicine studies, and selective venous sampling have been used to localize the sites of disease [48–51]. In a recent study examining the metastatic work-up of MTC patients with elevated calcitonin, bone metastases were demonstrated in 40% by bone scan and 40% by MRI [52]. Both bone scan and MRI were needed as these modalities were found to be complimentary for lesions of the axial skeleton. Recently, FDG-PET scanning has been utilized and examined as part of the metastatic work-up in patients with MTC. Initial results have been mixed, but this modality shows promise in the work-up of patients with persistent or recurrent MTC [52–54]. As well, in patients proceeding to surgical re-exploration of the neck, laparoscopy is recommended as up to 25% of patients will have liver metastases not detected on preoperative imaging [55].

In patients with elevated levels of calcitonin after adequate primary surgery, but no clinical or radiological evidence of disease, close follow-up is a reasonable approach. Van Heerden et al. followed 31 patients, (11 sporadic, 20 hereditary), with persistently elevated levels of calcitonin on either basal or stimulated testing [12, 56]. All 31 patients had their initial operation at the Mayo clinic and were deemed to have "adequate" primary surgery with removal of all disease. No clinical or radiological evidence of disease was noted at the initiation of the study. Median follow-up was 11.9 years. Eleven patients developed radiological or clinical evidence of disease during follow-up and underwent reoperation. Overall 5 and 10 year survivals were 90 and 86%, respectively.

More recent series have suggested improved results with respect to normalization or reduction in postoperative calcitonin levels [37, 50, 57]. Moley et al. reported a series of 62 patients operated on for persistent or recurrent MTC [50]. Of these patients, seven were known to have distant metastases and underwent palliative debulking to alleviate symptoms. In addition, 10 patients were found to have liver metastases on laparoscopy that were not evident on preoperative imaging. These 10 patients did not subsequently undergo a cervical reoperation. Thus, a cervical reoperation, with curative intent was undertaken in 45 patients. Of these patients, only 38% experienced normalization of postoperative calcitonin, with only 13% not experiencing a significant decrease. Ten-year follow-up on 54 of these patients found that 26% had normal, stimulated calcitonin levels and an additional 20% had levels less than 100 pg/ml. [48]. All the patients, with levels less than 100 pg/ml had no radiological evidence of recurrent disease.

In summary, reoperation for persistent or recurrent MTC appears to be beneficial in properly selected patients. Biochemical cure can be achieved in 35–40% with the majority of patients demonstrating at least a reduction in basal and/or stimulated calcitonin levels postoperatively [50]. In general, cervical reoperation should be reserved for those having undergone inadequate primary surgical therapy and those with radiological evidence of loco-regional disease without distant metastases [2]. All patients should have a laparoscopy prior to reoperation in order to rule out liver metastases that might have been missed on imaging studies [55]. Palliative reoperation may also be beneficial to prevent local invasion or compression and reduce systemic symptoms, when present [2].

Adjuvant Treatment for Medullary Thyroid Cancer

In general, primary surgical therapy represents the best chance for cure in MTC. To date, the results of adjuvant therapy have been disappointing. Unlike thyroid cancers of follicular cell origin, the cells of MTC do not take up and concentrate iodine. As such, radioactive iodine is considered largely ineffective for the elimination of residual disease except however, in a small series of seven patients that demonstrated a decrease in calcitonin in three patients following such therapy. [58]. This is likely due to the "bystander" effect from poor initial surgical clearance of all thyroid tissue and therefore, radioiodine is not recommended.

Traditional systemic chemotherapy regimes have also been investigated for the treatment of MTC [59–62]. Overall the results have been disappointing. Nocera et al. gave alternating combinations of doxorubicin/streptozocin and 5-FU/dacarbazine to 20 patients with advanced MTC [59]. No complete responses and just three partial responses were seen. However long-term stabilization was seen in ten patients.

Targeted molecular therapy with tyrosine kinase inhibition has shown some early promise in the treatment of metastatic MTC [63–68]. Imatinib mesylate (STI571, Gleevec) has been the most common agent utilized. In one open-label clinical trial six of nine patients showed stabilization of disease, with a median progression free survival of 6 months [66]. As well, the use of the multi-kinase inhibitor Sorafenib has recently been reported with a promising response [67].

The known production of CEA by MTC cells has served as a target for a number of newer systemic therapies under investigation [69, 70]. Radiolabeled anti-CEA antibodies appear promising, especially in those with advanced, progressive disease. Chatal et al. reported a series of 29 patients with advanced medullary thyroid cancer who received treatment with I^{131} labeled antiCEA antibodies [69]. All patients had progressive disease as defined by a calcitonin doubling time of less than 2 years. Comparisons were made to a nonrandomized group of 39 controls with similar prognostic indicators. Overall survival was significantly higher in the treated group. As well, the traditional radiosensitizer, paclitaxel has been shown to improve the efficacy of this targeted, radio-immunotherapy in animal models [71]. Finally, a humanized, monoclonal antibody to CEA (labetuzumab) has also shown direct anti-tumor effects and enhancement of dacarbazine toxicity against MTC in animal models [72].

The observation that metastatic neuroendocrine tumors, including MTC, show uptake on somatostatin receptor scintigraphy and MIBG scans in some patients has led to the use or radiolabeled octreotide and MIBG in the treatment of advanced metastatic disease [73–75]. Overall, an objective tumor response is seen in 12–33%, stability of disease in 46–66%, and progression in 0–41% over the course of treatment. However, in one series, progression was seen in 75% of patients at 18 months following the last treatment [73]. Symptomatic improvement was reported in 75% of patients in one series, particularly relief of bone pain from distant metastases [75].

The use of external beam radiation for the treatment of MTC is unclear. An early study by Samaan et al. reported worse survival in those treated with external beam radiation after surgery for MTC [76]. However, despite being matched for extent of disease, the groups were not randomized and only patients suspected of having residual MTC after primary surgical therapy were referred for therapy. Thus a significant referral bias is likely responsible for this result. In contrast, more recent reports have not shown a difference in either survival or locoregional control with external beam radiation [27, 77].

In summary, while several promising therapies are on the horizon, surgical therapy is currently the best hope for cure in patients with MTC. The role of adjuvant therapies is currently poorly defined. Many centers use external beam radiation in an attempt to improve local control in patients with residual disease after appropriate surgical therapy, but the effectiveness of this is unclear. Newer targeted therapies require more extensive testing on larger number of patients and should be the subject of clinical trials.

Prognosis

MTC is a disease characterized by early spread to loco-regional lymph nodes. Even after adequate surgical therapy, more than 50% of patients can expect to have persistent or recurrent disease. Fortunately, even in cases of disseminated disease, long-term survival is common. Overall survival rates are approximately 80–85% and 70–80% at 5 and 10 years, respectively [12]. Survival rates are however heavily dependent on stage. Five-year overall survival rates are 98% in stages 1 and 2, 73% for stage 3, and 40% for stage 4 [12].

Adequate primary surgery provides the best chance for long-term survival. In the series from the French Calcitonin Tumors study Group, biochemical cure, achieved in 43% of patients following surgery, predicted a 10-year survival of 97.7% [21]. In those patients in whom biochemical cure was achieved, 4.9% experienced a recurrence indicated by an elevation of calcitonin. However, survival in those patients not achieving biochemical cure, was still 80% and 70% at 5 and 10 years, respectively. Thus long-term survival is common in MTC, but a significant portion of these patients will be living with recurrent or persistent disease.

Conclusion

MTC is a tumor arising from the parafollicular / C-cells of the thyroid, and occurs in a hereditary form in 25% and a sporadic form in 75%. Sporadic MTC most commonly presents as a thyroid nodule. As with most thyroid tumors, the work up typically involves a history, physical exam, ultrasound, and fine needle aspiration biopsy. More recently, it has been suggested that all patients being worked up for nodular thyroid disease have a serum calcitonin level done, as 0.4–1.3% will have an unanticipated MTC [14]. In addition, genetic screening should be considered for all MTC patients, even for those with apparently sporadic disease as recent evidence indicates that 7–8% will have a germline mutation in the RET proto-oncogene [19]. Preoperative calcitonin and CEA are useful biochemical markers of disease. It is important to rule out MEN syndromes prior to surgical intervention.

In general, surgical therapy represents the best chance for cure. Lymph node metastases are common. As a result, recommendations for standard surgical therapy at the initial operation have progressively become more aggressive [27, 28, 38–40]. Currently, there appears to be consensus (with a few caveats) that the initial operation should involve a total thyroidectomy with bilateral central lymph node dissection. In addition, given the relatively high rate of lymph node metastases in both the ipsilateral and contralateral lateral neck compartments, many authors are currently recommending ipsilateral and possibly bilateral lateral neck dissections at primary surgery [28, 38, 39]. While no randomized control trials exist, series of patients treated with this more aggressive approach seem to have improved rates of biochemical cure and lower rates of reoperation [27, 36].

Reoperation for persistently elevated calcitonin can achieve biochemical cure in a third of properly selected patients. In general, reoperation should be reserved for patients with radiographic evidence of disease in the neck and no sign of distant metastases as well as those who underwent "less than adequate" primary surgery [2, 50]. Reoperative neck surgery may be performed in those with distant disease to alleviate local compressive or systemic symptoms. Overall, survival rates for MTC are approximately 70–80% at 10 years [12, 40]. With biochemical cure following primary surgery, 10-year survival rates as high as 98–99% have been reported [12]. However, even in those with distant disease, long-term survival is not uncommon. The role of traditional cytotoxic chemotherapy and external beam radiation in the treatment of MTC are unclear as no survival benefits have been clearly demonstrated. Newer targeted therapies have shown promise in animal and early clinical trials, but further studies including larger numbers of patients are required to define their role.

References

1. Hazard JB, Hawk WA, Crile G Jr (1959) Medullary (solid) carcinoma of the thyroid; a clinicopathologic entity. J Clin Endocrinol Metab 19(1):152–161
2. Moley JF, Fialkowski EA (2007) Evidence-based approach to the management of sporadic medullary thyroid carcinoma. World J Surg 31(5):946–956
3. Edery P, Lyonnet S, Mulligan LM, Pelet A, Dow E, Abel L et al (1994) Mutations of the RET proto-oncogene in Hirschsprung's disease. Nature 367(6461):378–380
4. Gagel RF, Levy ML, Donovan DT, Alford BR, Wheeler T, Tschen JA (1989) Multiple endocrine neoplasia type 2a associated with cutaneous lichen amyloidosis. Ann Intern Med 111(10):802–806
5. Howe JR, Norton JA, Wells SA Jr (1993) Prevalence of pheochromocytoma and hyperparathyroidism in multiple endocrine neoplasia type 2A: results of long-term follow-up. Surgery 114(6):1070–1077
6. O'Riordain DS, O'Brien T, Crotty TB, Gharib H, Grant CS, van Heerden JA (1995) Multiple endocrine neoplasia type 2B: more than an endocrine disorder. Surgery 118(6):936–942
7. Hofstra RM, Landsvater RM, Ceccherini I, Stulp RP, Stelwagen T, Luo Y et al (1994) A mutation in the RET proto-oncogene associated with multiple endocrine neoplasia type 2B and sporadic medullary thyroid carcinoma. Nature 367(6461):375–376
8. Mulligan LM, Kwok JB, Healey CS, Elsdon MJ, Eng C, Gardner E et al (1993) Germ-line mutations of the RET proto-oncogene in multiple endocrine neoplasia type 2A. Nature 363(6428):458–460
9. Mulligan LM, Eng C, Healey CS, Clayton D, Kwok JB, Gardner E et al (1994) Specific mutations of the RET proto-oncogene are related to disease phenotype in MEN 2A and FMTC. Nat Genet 6(1):70–74
10. Kaserer K, Scheuba C, Neuhold N, Weinhausel A, Haas OA, Vierhapper H et al (2001) Sporadic versus familial medullary thyroid microcarcinoma: a histopathologic study of 50 consecutive patients. Am J Surg Pathol 25(10):1245–1251
11. Machens A, Niccoli-Sire P, Hoegel J, Frank-Raue K, van Vroonhoven TJ, Roeher HD et al (2003) Early malignant progression of hereditary medullary thyroid cancer. N Engl J Med 349(16):1517–1525
12. Fialkowski EA, Moley JF (2006) Current approaches to medullary thyroid carcinoma, sporadic and familial. J Surg Oncol 94(8):737–747

13. Papi G, Corsello SM, Cioni K, Pizzini AM, Corrado S, Carapezzi C et al (2006) Value of routine measurement of serum calcitonin concentrations in patients with nodular thyroid disease: a multicenter study. J Endocrinol Invest 29(5):427–437
14. Elisei R, Bottici V, Luchetti F, Di Coscio G, Romei C, Grasso L et al (2004) Impact of routine measurement of serum calcitonin on the diagnosis and outcome of medullary thyroid cancer: experience in 10, 864 patients with nodular thyroid disorders. J Clin Endocrinol Metab 89(1):163–168
15. Niccoli P, Wion-Barbot N, Caron P, Henry JF, de Micco C, Saint Andre JP et al (1997) Interest of routine measurement of serum calcitonin: study in a large series of thyroidectomized patients. The French Medullary Study Group. J Clin Endocrinol Metab 82(2):338–341
16. de Groot JW, Kema IP, Breukelman H, van der Veer E, Wiggers T, Plukker JT et al (2006) Biochemical markers in the follow-up of medullary thyroid cancer. Thyroid 16(11):1163–1170
17. Laure GA, Al Ghulzan A, Auperin A, Leboulleux S, Chehboun A, Troalen F et al (2008) Progression of medullary thyroid carcinoma: assessment with calcitonin and carcinoembryonic antigen doubling times. Eur J Endocrinol 158(2):239–246
18. Machens A, Ukkat J, Hauptmann S, Dralle H (2007) Abnormal carcinoembryonic antigen levels and medullary thyroid cancer progression: a multivariate analysis. Arch Surg 142(3):289–293
19. Elisei R, Romei C, Cosci B, Agate L, Bottici V, Molinaro E et al (2007) RET genetic screening in patients with medullary thyroid cancer and their relatives: experience with 807 individuals at one center. J Clin Endocrinol Metab 92(12):4725–4729
20. Sobin LH, Wittekind C (2002) TNM classification of malignant tumours, 6th edn. Wiley-Liss, New York
21. Modigliani E, Cohen R, Campos JM, Conte-Devolx B, Maes B, Boneu A et al (1998) Prognostic factors for survival and for biochemical cure in medullary thyroid carcinoma: results in 899 patients. The GETC Study Group. Groupe d'etude des tumeurs a calcitonine. Clin Endocrinol (Oxf) 48(3):265–273
22. Kebebew E, Ituarte PH, Siperstein AE, Duh QY, Clark OH (2000) Medullary thyroid carcinoma: clinical characteristics, treatment, prognostic factors, and a comparison of staging systems. Cancer 88(5):1139–1148
23. Kebebew E, Greenspan FS, Clark OH, Woeber KA, Grunwell J (2005) Extent of disease and practice patterns for medullary thyroid cancer. J Am Coll Surg 200(6):890–896
24. Miyauchi A, Matsuzuka F, Hirai K, Yokozawa T, Kobayashi K, Kuma S et al (2000) Unilateral surgery supported by germline RET oncogene mutation analysis in patients with sporadic medullary thyroid carcinoma. World J Surg 24(11):1367–1372
25. Miyauchi A, Matsuzuka F, Hirai K, Yokozawa T, Kobayashi K, Ito Y et al (2002) Prospective trial of unilateral surgery for nonhereditary medullary thyroid carcinoma in patients without germline RET mutations. World J Surg 26(8):1023–1028
26. Machens A, Hauptmann S, Dralle H (2007) Increased risk of lymph node metastasis in multifocal hereditary and sporadic medullary thyroid cancer. World J Surg 31(10):1960–1965
27. de Groot JW, Links TP, Sluiter WJ, Wolffenbuttel BH, Wiggers T, Plukker JT (2007) Locoregional control in patients with palpable medullary thyroid cancer: results of standardized compartment-oriented surgery. Head Neck 29(9):857–863
28. Moley JF, DeBenedetti MK (1999) Patterns of nodal metastases in palpable medullary thyroid carcinoma: recommendations for extent of node dissection. Ann Surg 229(6):880–887
29. Hundahl SA, Cady B, Cunningham MP, Mazzaferri E, McKee RF, Rosai J et al (2000) Initial results from a prospective cohort study of 5583 cases of thyroid carcinoma treated in the united states during 1996. U.S. and German Thyroid Cancer Study Group. An American College of Surgeons Commission on Cancer Patient Care Evaluation study. Cancer 89(1):202–217
30. Dralle H, Damm I, Scheumann GF, Kotzerke J, Kupsch E (1992) Frequency and significance of cervicomediastinal lymph node metastases in medullary thyroid carcinoma: results of a compartment-oriented microdissection method. Henry Ford Hosp Med J 40(3–4):264–267
31. Dralle H, Damm I, Scheumann GF, Kotzerke J, Kupsch E, Geerlings H et al (1994) Compartment-oriented microdissection of regional lymph nodes in medullary thyroid carcinoma. Surg Today 24(2):112–121

32. Ellenhorn JD, Shah JP, Brennan MF (1993) Impact of therapeutic regional lymph node dissection for medullary carcinoma of the thyroid gland. Surgery 114(6):1078–1081
33. Kallinowski F, Buhr HJ, Meybier H, Eberhardt M, Herfarth C (1993) Medullary carcinoma of the thyroid – therapeutic strategy derived from fifteen years of experience. Surgery 114(3):491–496
34. Weber T, Schilling T, Frank-Raue K, Colombo-Benkmann M, Hinz U, Ziegler R et al (2001) Impact of modified radical neck dissection on biochemical cure in medullary thyroid carcinomas. Surgery 130(6):1044–1049
35. Yen TW, Shapiro SE, Gagel RF, Sherman SI, Lee JE, Evans DB (2003) Medullary thyroid carcinoma: results of a standardized surgical approach in a contemporary series of 80 consecutive patients. Surgery 134(6):890–899
36. Greenblatt DY, Elson D, Mack E, Chen H (2007) Initial lymph node dissection increases cure rates in patients with medullary thyroid cancer. Asian J Surg 30(2):108–112
37. Fleming JB, Lee JE, Bouvet M, Schultz PN, Sherman SI, Sellin RV et al (1999) Surgical strategy for the treatment of medullary thyroid carcinoma. Ann Surg 230(5):697–707
38. Dralle H (2002) Lymph node dissection and medullary thyroid carcinoma. Br J Surg 89(9):1073–1075
39. Scollo C, Baudin E, Travagli JP, Caillou B, Bellon N, Leboulleux S et al (2003) Rationale for central and bilateral lymph node dissection in sporadic and hereditary medullary thyroid cancer. J Clin Endocrinol Metab 88(5):2070–2075
40. Kebebew E, Clark OH (2000) Medullary thyroid cancer. Curr Treat Options Oncol 1(4):359–367
41. Hamy A, Pessaux P, Mirallie E, Mucci-Hennekinne S, Gibelin H, Mor-Martinez C et al (2005) Central neck dissection in the management of sporadic medullary thyroid microcarcinoma. Eur J Surg Oncol 31(7):774–777
42. Dotzenrath C, Goretzki PE, Cupisti K, Simon D, Witte J, Yang Q et al (2001) Is there any consensus in diagnostic and operative strategy with respect to medullary thyroid cancer? A questionnaire answered by 73 endocrine surgical units. Langenbecks Arch Surg 386(1):47–52
43. Pellegriti G, Leboulleux S, Baudin E, Bellon N, Scollo C, Travagli JP et al (2003) Long-term outcome of medullary thyroid carcinoma in patients with normal postoperative medical imaging. Br J Cancer 88(10):1537–1542
44. Quayle FJ, Moley JF (2005) Medullary thyroid carcinoma: including MEN 2A and MEN 2B syndromes. J Surg Oncol 89(3):122–129
45. Tisell LE, Hansson G, Jansson S, Salander H (1986) Reoperation in the treatment of asymptomatic metastasizing medullary thyroid carcinoma. Surgery 99(1):60–66
46. Kebebew E, Kikuchi S, Duh QY, Clark OH (2000) Long-term results of reoperation and localizing studies in patients with persistent or recurrent medullary thyroid cancer. Arch Surg 135(8):895–901
47. Moley JF, Wells SA, Dilley WG, Tisell LE (1993) Reoperation for recurrent or persistent medullary thyroid cancer. Surgery 114(6):1090–1095
48. Fialkowski E, Debenedetti M, Moley J (2008) Long-term outcome of reoperations for medullary thyroid carcinoma. World J Surg 32(5):754–765
49. Juweid M, Sharkey RM, Swayne LC, Goldenberg DM (1997) Improved selection of patients for reoperation for medullary thyroid cancer by imaging with radiolabeled anticarcinoembryonic antigen antibodies. Surgery 122(6):1156–1165
50. Moley JF, Dilley WG, DeBenedetti MK (1997) Improved results of cervical reoperation for medullary thyroid carcinoma. Ann Surg 225(6):734–740
51. Vriens B, Van Hee R (2007) Re-operation for recurrent lymph node metastasis of medullary thyroid cancer – is it useful? Acta Chir Belg 107(3):331–335
52. Giraudet AL, Vanel D, Leboulleux S, Auperin A, Dromain C, Chami L et al (2007) Imaging medullary thyroid carcinoma with persistent elevated calcitonin levels. J Clin Endocrinol Metab 92(11):4185–4190
53. de Groot JW, Links TP, Jager PL, Kahraman T, Plukker JT (2004) Impact of 18F-fluoro-2-deoxy-D-glucose positron emission tomography (FDG-PET) in patients with biochemical evidence of recurrent or residual medullary thyroid cancer. Ann Surg Oncol 11(8):786–794

54. Oudoux A, Salaun PY, Bournaud C, Campion L, Ansquer C, Rousseau C et al (2007) Sensitivity and prognostic value of positron emission tomography with F-18-fluorodeoxyglucose and sensitivity of immunoscintigraphy in patients with medullary thyroid carcinoma treated with anticarcinoembryonic antigen-targeted radioimmunotherapy. J Clin Endocrinol Metab 92(12):4590–4597
55. Tung WS, Vesely TM, Moley JF (1995) Laparoscopic detection of hepatic metastases in patients with residual or recurrent medullary thyroid cancer. Surgery 118(6):1024–1029
56. van Heerden JA, Grant CS, Gharib H, Hay ID, Ilstrup DM (1990) Long-term course of patients with persistent hypercalcitoninemia after apparent curative primary surgery for medullary thyroid carcinoma. Ann Surg 212(4):395–400
57. Fernandez Vila JM, Peix JL, Mandry AC, Mezzadri NA, Lifante JC (2007) Biochemical results of reoperations for medullary thyroid carcinoma. Laryngoscope 117(5):886–889
58. Faik EM, Gursoy A, Erdogan G, Kamel N (2006) Radioactive iodine treatment in medullary thyroid carcinoma. Nucl Med Commun 27(4):359–362
59. Nocera M, Baudin E, Pellegriti G, Cailleux AF, Mechelany-Corone C, Schlumberger M (2000) Treatment of advanced medullary thyroid cancer with an alternating combination of doxorubicin-streptozocin and 5 FU-dacarbazine. Groupe d'Etude des Tumeurs a Calcitonine (GETC). Br J Cancer 83(6):715–718
60. Orlandi F, Caraci P, Berruti A, Puligheddu B, Pivano G, Dogliotti L et al (1994) Chemotherapy with dacarbazine and 5-fluorouracil in advanced medullary thyroid cancer. Ann Oncol 5(8):763–765
61. Scherubl H, Raue F, Ziegler R (1990) Combination chemotherapy of advanced medullary and differentiated thyroid cancer. Phase II study. J Cancer Res Clin Oncol 116(1):21–23
62. Schlumberger M, Abdelmoumene N, Delisle MJ, Couette JE (1995) Treatment of advanced medullary thyroid cancer with an alternating combination of 5 FU-streptozocin and 5 FU-dacarbazine. The Groupe d'Etude des Tumeurs a Calcitonine (GETC). Br J Cancer 71(2):363–365
63. de Groot JW, Plaza MI, Schepers H, Drenth-Diephuis LJ, Osinga J, Plukker JT et al (2006) Cellular effects of imatinib on medullary thyroid cancer cells harboring multiple endocrine neoplasia Type 2A and 2B associated RET mutations. Surgery 139(6):806–814
64. de Groot JW, Zonnenberg BA, Ufford-Mannesse PQ, de Vries MM, Links TP, Lips CJ et al (2007) A phase II trial of imatinib therapy for metastatic medullary thyroid carcinoma. J Clin Endocrinol Metab 92(9):3466–3469
65. Ezzat S, Huang P, Dackiw A, Asa SL (2005) Dual inhibition of RET and FGFR4 restrains medullary thyroid cancer cell growth. Clin Cancer Res 11(3):1336–1341
66. Frank-Raue K, Fabel M, Delorme S, Haberkorn U, Raue F (2007) Efficacy of imatinib mesylate in advanced medullary thyroid carcinoma. Eur J Endocrinol 157(2):215–220
67. Hong D, Ye L, Gagel R, Chintala L, El Naggar AK, Wright J et al (2008) Medullary thyroid cancer: targeting the RET kinase pathway with sorafenib/tipifarnib. Mol Cancer Ther 7(5):1001–1006
68. Strock CJ, Park JI, Rosen DM, Ruggeri B, Denmeade SR, Ball DW et al (2006) Activity of irinotecan and the tyrosine kinase inhibitor CEP-751 in medullary thyroid cancer. J Clin Endocrinol Metab 91(1):79–84
69. Chatal JF, Campion L, Kraeber-Bodere F, Bardet S, Vuillez JP, Charbonnel B et al (2006) Survival improvement in patients with medullary thyroid carcinoma who undergo pretargeted anti-carcinoembryonic-antigen radioimmunotherapy: a collaborative study with the French Endocrine Tumor Group. J Clin Oncol 24(11):1705–1711
70. Juweid ME, Hajjar G, Stein R, Sharkey RM, Herskovic T, Swayne LC et al (2000) Initial experience with high-dose radioimmunotherapy of metastatic medullary thyroid cancer using 131I-MN-14 F(ab)2 anti-carcinoembryonic antigen MAb and AHSCR. J Nucl Med 41(1):93–103
71. Kraeber-Bodere F, Sai-Maurel C, Campion L, Faivre-Chauvet A, Mirallie E, Cherel M et al (2002) Enhanced antitumor activity of combined pretargeted radioimmunotherapy and paclitaxel in medullary thyroid cancer xenograft. Mol Cancer Ther 1(4):267–274

72. Stein R, Goldenberg DM (2004) A humanized monoclonal antibody to carcinoembryonic antigen, labetuzumab, inhibits tumor growth and sensitizes human medullary thyroid cancer xenografts to dacarbazine chemotherapy. Mol Cancer Ther 3(12):1559–1564
73. Buscombe JR, Cwikla JB, Caplin ME, Hilson AJ (2005) Long-term efficacy of low activity meta-[131I]iodobenzylguanidine therapy in patients with disseminated neuroendocrine tumours depends on initial response. Nucl Med Commun 26(11):969–976
74. Gao ZR, An R, Zhang YX, Biersack HJ (2006) Targeted radionuclide therapy for patients with metastatic medullary thyroid carcinoma. Zhonghua Zhong Liu Za Zhi 28(8):621–624
75. Pasieka JL, McEwan AJ, Rorstad O (2004) The palliative role of 131I-MIBG and 111In-octreotide therapy in patients with metastatic progressive neuroendocrine neoplasms. Surgery 136(6):1218–1226
76. Samaan NA, Schultz PN, Hickey RC (1989) Medullary thyroid carcinoma: prognosis of familial versus nonfamilial disease and the role of radiotherapy. Horm Metab Res Suppl 21:21–25
77. Brierley J, Tsang R, Simpson WJ, Gospodarowicz M, Sutcliffe S, Panzarella T (1996) Medullary thyroid cancer: analyses of survival and prognostic factors and the role of radiation therapy in local control. Thyroid 6(4):305–310

Chapter 5
Anaplastic Thyroid Cancer

Alan P.B. Dackiw

Dedication

This chapter is dedicated to the memory of my patients I have cared for, who have suffered anaplastic thyroid cancer and also their families and to the hope that we will soon have more effective treatments strategies for their therapy.

Recent Patient Presentation

Although the majority of thyroid cancer patients presenting to our surgical endocrinology clinics present with resectable and often curable disease, patients may rarely present with a history and physical findings suggestive of an anaplastic thyroid cancer. The endocrine surgeon should recognize, diagnose, and treat this patient urgently and promptly. The clinical course and findings from two patients who presented to our endocrine surgery clinic recently are summarized below from the patients' clinical notes.

Patient 1

A 69-year-old male noted swelling in his neck approximately a month and a half prior to presentation. The patient initially noted swelling more so on the left side of his neck but then noted that the swelling began to enlarge, encompassing all of his left neck and crossing over toward the midline to involve the right neck.

A.P.B. Dackiw (✉)
Department of Surgery, Division of Endocrine and Oncologic Surgery, Section of Endocrine Surgery, Johns Hopkins Hospital, Johns Hopkins University School of Medicine, Baltimore, MD, USA
e-mail: adackiw1@jhmi.edu

C. Sturgeon (ed.), *Endocrine Neoplasia*, Cancer Treatment and Research, vol 153,
DOI 10.1007/978-1-4419-0857-5_5, © Springer Science+Business Media, LLC 2010

Associated with the swelling was discomfort and difficulty with swallowing. Mild shortness of breath ensued and he noted increasing hoarseness of his voice. A CT scan was subsequently ordered of the patient's neck and chest along with needle biopsy of the thyroid mass and biopsy of a supraclavicular lymph node. The results of the CT scan (Fig. 5.1) were as follows: (1) Large mass in the region of the left thyroid lobe extending into the mediastinum and left supraclavicular region with mediastinal lymphadenopathy and multiple pulmonary nodules concerning for malignancy with metastatic disease. (2) Possible left mainstem endobronchial lesion. Specifically, the CT demonstrated a prominent mass arising from the left thyroid plane and extending inferiorly to the level of the aortic arch and extending superiorly to the level of the tonsillar fossa with invasion into the left hypopharynx and the left paraglottic space. The mass surrounded the distal common carotid artery and the proximal left internal carotid artery. Given the lack of definition and the prominent necrosis of this lesion, this was felt to be representative of a highly malignant thyroid mass. Mediastinal lymphadenopathy was also noted. Lymphadenopathy was also noted in the pretracheal, right hilar, and subcarinal regions, with lymph nodes measuring 1.5 × 1.5 cm. Multiple pulmonary nodules were also noted. Biopsies revealed partially necrotic carcinoma with a mixed component of well-differentiated papillary thyroid carcinoma and anaplastic thyroid carcinoma. The mass was assessed as not surgically resectable. Radiation therapy was begun and percutaneous gastrostomy (PEG) tube placed for nutrition. The patient returned with increasing shortness of breath, airway narrowing, and dysphagia. Intravenous dexamethasone and albuterol nebulizers were given.

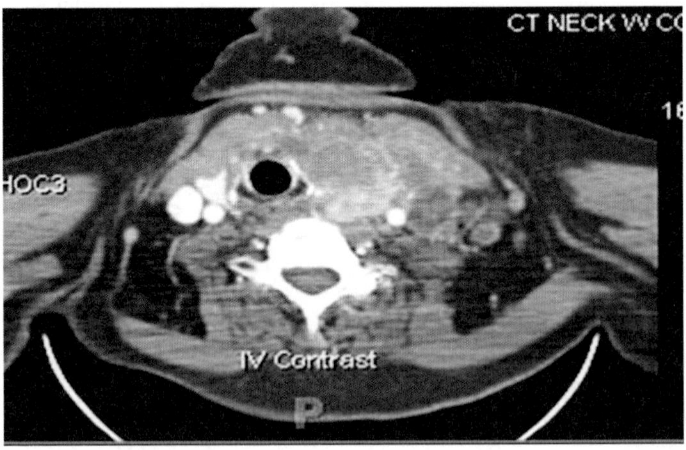

Fig. 5.1 CT scan of *Patient 1* demonstrates a prominent mass arising from the left thyroid and extending inferiorly to the level of the aortic arch and extending superiorly to the level of the tonsillar fossa with invasion into the left hypopharynx and the left paraglottic space. The mass surrounds the distal common carotid artery and the proximal left internal carotid artery. Given the lack of definition and the prominent necrosis of this lesion, this is representative of a highly malignant thyroid mass

Unfortunately, despite radiation his condition continued to deteriorate and after discussion with family it was decided to institute comfort measures. He died of his disease 1 month after his initial presentation.

Patient 2

A 72-year-old female noticed left neck fullness, hoarseness, and voice changes for 1 month with additional symptoms of dyspnea and dysphagia. There was no family history of thyroid cancer and no personal history of head or neck irradiation. FNA of the left thyroid lobe and isthmic masses suggested poorly differentiated/anaplastic malignancy. CT scan revealed a 6.5 cm mass replacing the left lobe of the thyroid and isthmus with tracheal infiltration, deviation and narrowing, and involvement of the cricoid cartilage with possible infiltration of the esophagus/prevertebral fascia and abutment of the carotid sheath extending inferiorly into the superior mediastinum (Fig. 5.2). An abnormal 1.2 cm left upper jugular chain node, suggestive of metastasis and posterior cervical triangle node, measuring 0.8 cm, as well as bilateral lower lung nodules, are seen. The mass was felt to be unresectable without significant patient morbidity and combined chemoradiation therapy was begun. The patient succumbed to her disease 4 months following her initial presentation.

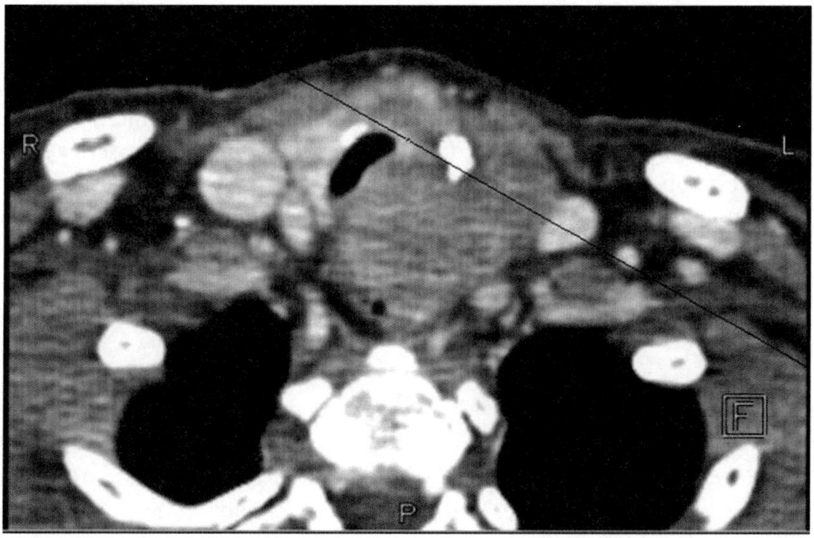

Fig. 5.2 CT scan of *Patient 2* demonstrates a 6.5 cm mass replacing the left lobe of the thyroid and isthmus with tracheal infiltration, deviation and narrowing and involvement of the cricoid cartilage with probable infiltration of the esophagus/prevertebral fascia and abutment of the carotid sheath extending inferiorly into the superior mediastinum A left upper jugular chain node measuring 1.2 cm suggestive of metastasis and posterior cervical triangle node 0.8 cm are seen as well as bilateral lower lung nodules

Definition/Introduction

Anaplastic thyroid cancer is an uncommon malignancy of the thyroid but unfortunately is almost always fatal as it is usually unresectable and systemic therapies have proven largely ineffective. The mean survival time is often less than 6 months [1]. The incidence of anaplastic thyroid cancer appears to be decreasing. The annual incidence is approximately one to two cases per million, but the overall incidence of this disease is highest in areas of endemic goiter [2]. In this review of the National Cancer Data Base, 893 patients were reported to have anaplastic thyroid cancer in a total series of 53,856 thyroid cancer patients representing 2% of the thyroid cancer population.

Pathology/Etiology

Grossly, ATC's are unencapsulated tumors with direct extension into the surrounding tissues of the neck. Microscopically three histologic patterns of anaplastic thyroid cancer (spindle, giant cell and squamoid) are described, all with the same prognosis. It is however important to distinguish anaplastic thyroid cancers from thyroid lymphoma and poorly differentiated medullary thyroid cancer with the latter staining for NSE, chromogranin or calcitonin and the former being more uniform small cell carcinomas.

It remains controversial as to whether ATC arises de novo or from dedifferentiation of a previously well-differentiated thyroid cancer. Similar to *Patient 1* presented above, whose pathology specimen demonstrated areas of tumor consisting of both papillary and anaplastic thyroid cancer, a review of the case series suggests that at least a subset of these undifferentiated tumors arise in patients with previously differentiated thyroid tumors [2, 3]. As noted, the incidence of thyroid cancer is also higher in areas of endemic goiter and in patients with previously incompletely treated papillary or follicular thyroid cancer.

Molecular Biology

Mutations of the p53 tumor suppressor gene, a transcription factor that controls both apoptosis and the cell cycle, leads to the production of an inactive p53 protein and occurs in the majority of anaplastic thyroid carcinomas. On the basis of the suggestion that differentiated thyroid carcinomas may degenerate into anaplastic thyroid carcinomas, it has been hypothesized that gene mutations may provide an early growth advantage and that p53 mutations are the final hit in the development of an anaplastic carcinoma. There is evidence to support and as well as refute this hypothesis. A recent study found that approximately 10% of anaplastic thyroid carcinomas contained a mutation of the BRAF gene [4]. Similar to *Patient 1* presented as an introduction to this chapter, these anaplastic thyroid carcinomas had well-differentiated regions suggesting papillary thyroid carcinoma, which also contained the same mutation. It thus seems possible that in some cases papillary thyroid carcinoma may dedifferentiate into anaplastic thyroid carcinoma. This finding has been corroborated in another study where immunohistochemical (IHC) analysis of RET/PTC rearrangements revealed no positive staining of RET in any of eight ATCs, suggesting that these ATCs are not derived from RET/PTC- rearranged PTC [5]. In contrast, IHC analysis of p53 mutation revealed that p53 was detected in the nuclei of 5 of 5 BRAF-mutated ATCs and 2 of 3 ATCs with wild-type BRAF. p53 staining was present only in anaplastic thyroid tumor cells but not in the neighboring papillary thyroid tumor cells suggesting that many ATCs with papillary components are derived from BRAF-mutated PTC, because of the addition of p53 mutation. This is consistent with another published study where no RET gene rearrangements were detected in 17 anaplastic carcinomas [6].

Clinical Presentation

Anaplastic thyroid cancer is usually seen in elderly patients typically presenting in the seventh decade of life or later. The most common clinical presentation is that of a rapidly enlarging, fixed mass in the central and lateral neck often with associated lymphadenopathy. Locally invasive symptoms such as hoarseness, dysphagia, cervical pain and shortness of breath as are often reported. Some patients may have reported a pre-existing differentiated thyroid cancer or goiter [7].

Physical examination often reveals a firm fixed mass in the central and lateral neck. Laryngoscopy may document vocal cord paralysis due to direct extension of the disease into the larynx or recurrent laryngeal nerve. Coexistent lymphadenopathy on physical exam is a common finding.

Diagnosis

As noted earlier, there must be a strong clinical suspicion of the diagnosis of anaplastic thyroid cancer in a patient who presents with a central neck mass that has been rapidly enlarging with local symptoms, in order that a prompt diagnosis be made and treatment initiated as soon as possible. Fine needle aspiration biopsy can diagnose ATC with the demonstration of spindle or giant cells, atypical multinucleated neoplastic cells with high mitotic activity although core biopsy or open biopsy may sometimes be necessary [8]. Patients may also present themselves with an airway emergency necessitating urgent tracheostomy, which may prove a technical challenge secondary to tumor burden. Tracheostomy may also prove necessary for impending airway obstruction to secure the airway preceding further treatment in these patients with chemotherapy and radiation. Neck and Chest CT define the extent of local cervical disease and lymph node metastases, the position of the trachea and the presence of lung metastases.

Treatment

Surgery

The role of surgery in patients with anaplastic thyroid cancer is both controversial and limited depending on the extent of disease at presentation. Unfortunately the majority of patients with this tumor have unresectable disease. Some authors, however, have concluded that surgery may be indicated and may prolong survival in selected patients with localized disease [9, 10]. It is, however, important to note that there may be potential selection bias in these studies where patients with less aggressive disease underwent more complete resections. Others have reported that neither the extent nor completeness of resection had any effect on long-term survival [7].

When possible, surgical resection is reasonable if complete resection is possible and all gross cervical and mediastinal disease can be removed with limited morbidity (i.e., avoid resection of vital structures: larynx, carotid, esophagus).

Previously, prophylactic tracheostomy was often advocated prior to initiation of chemoradiation therapy in order to protect the airway. However, prophylactic tracheostomies are often difficult to perform in the presence of a large cervical mass and may be associated with significant immediate morbidity and wound problems that may delay chemoradiation [1]. It appears that the number of patients requiring prophylactic tracheostomy has declined with the proper use of radiation therapy [11].

Radiotherapy

A small improvement in survival (3 months vs. 5 months) has been observed in patients receiving radiotherapy compared with those who did not [7]. Hyperfractionated accelerated radiation therapy, a strategy that enables high doses of radiation (>40 Gy) to be delivered over a short time with acceptable toxicity, appears to be associated with improved local disease control. In a retrospective study of 47 patients with anaplastic thyroid cancer who underwent radiotherapy, the 6 month progression-free rate was significantly higher with radical compared with palliative (defined as ≤40 Gy) radiotherapy (94 and 65%, respectively) [12]. There was also a trend toward improved survival with twice-daily fractionation as compared with once-daily fractionation. The radiation fields in patients with anaplastic thyroid cancer include the thyroid bed and the adjacent lymph nodes. No attempt is made to treat the entire neck or mediastinum unless disease is documented in these sites.

Chemotherapy

The most commonly used drugs for anaplastic thyroid cancer are paclitaxel and doxorubicin [13–15]. Response rates as high as 50% are reported in distant metastatic sites, although response duration is unfortunately short and long-term survival not significantly improved.

Combination Therapy

For patients who present themselves with locally advanced inoperable disease, combined radiotherapy and chemotherapy for local control of disease is recommended. Surgical resection for residual tumor may be considered if the disease is responsive. Given the overall poor prognosis of current treatment modalities, consideration should always be given to referring a patient with anaplastic carcinoma for participation in a clinical trial.

Clinical Trials and Novel Therapies

Clinical Trials

Several clinical trials are open and investigating novel treatments for anaplastic thyroid cancer continue. New therapies are obviously needed, since standard treatments, as discussed above, have had limited to no effect on patient mortality. A relatively new agent in recent use is combrestatin A4, a vascular disrupting agent. A current NIH sponsored study is examining the effects of the triple combination of combretastatin, paclitaxel, and carboplatin compared with the triple treatment of paclitaxel and carboplatin. Other open trials include the study of an Experimental New Drug CS7017, an oral PPARγ agonist taken by mouth twice daily in combination with paclitaxel chemotherapy and a Phase II study of sorafenib in patients with advanced anaplastic thyroid cancer (http://www.cancer.gov).

Novel Therapies

Failure of standard treatment regimens demands preclinical investigation of novel treatment strategies. For example, studies have demonstrated that inhibition of the enzyme farnesyltransferase with manumycin in xenograft models of human anaplastic thyroid carcinoma tumors grown in nude mice has a beneficial effect and also potentiates the effect of paclitaxel [16]. Inhibition of tumor angiogenesis by manumycin or an effect on PTHrP levels may be a mechanism for the inhibitory activity [17, 18].

As discussed above, loss of expression of the p53 tumor suppressor may be an important step in the transformation of differentiated thyroid cancers to anaplastic tumors. Interestingly, preclinical gene therapy experiments have demonstrated that restoration of p53 expression decreases the malignant potential of anaplastic carcinoma cell lines, and may restore responsiveness to chemotherapeutic agents [19, 20]. As noted, mutations of BRAF (a member of the RAF family of serine/threonine kinases) may occur in anaplastic thyroid carcinomas suggesting that agents targeting this pathway may also be beneficial. Sorafenib a tyrosine kinase inhibitor that inhibits Raf-1 is being studied for anaplastic thyroid cancers as noted in the clinical trials section above. Preclinical evaluation of RS5444, a high-affinity PPARγ agonist, both alone and in combination with paclitaxel, demonstrated additive antiproliferative activity in cell culture and minimal anaplastic thyroid cancer tumor growth in vivo. RS5444 did not induce apoptosis but combined with paclitaxel, doubled the apoptotic index compared to that of paclitaxel. The authors concluded that functional PPARγ is a molecular target for therapy in and that alone, or in combination with paclitaxel, may provide therapeutic benefit to patients diagnosed with anaplastic thyroid cancer [21, 22]. As noted above, an oral PPARγ agonist is currently being examined in a clinical trial.

Treatment Recommendations

In summary, patients with local disease that is potentially completely resectable, which is a rare clinical presentation, should undergo surgery. If the tumor is completely resected in the absence of distant metastases, adjuvant chemoradiotherapy may be considered but is not necessarily indicated. If after initial staging, the tumor is deemed unresectable, chemoradiation therapy is indicated which may be doxorubicin or paclitaxel based [8, 13]. PEG tube placement and/or tracheostomy may be required during the course of therapy as well as palliative care support and counseling.

Summary

Anaplastic thyroid cancer is a rare but, unfortunately, nearly always a lethal tumor due to local disease extent or metastatic spread. Surgical resection should only be attempted when complete resection of cervical and mediastinal disease is judged to be possible without the sacrifice of major structures resulting in significant patient morbidity. Tracheostomy is best performed for pending airway obstruction rather than for airway prophylaxis. Radiation therapy may be administered postoperatively in a surgically resected patient, preoperatively in a neo-adjuvant setting in a patient who may become resectable or as the primary form of treatment in a patient judged to be unresectable as a therapeutic or palliative strategy. Doxorubicin or paclitaxel based chemotherapy may be considered as a combination therapy. End of life and palliative care issues should be addressed urgently in all patients. Enrollment in the clinical trials discussed above or of others to become available as well as the development of new therapeutic agents is to be encouraged due to the ineffectiveness of these current therapies.

References

1. Are C, Shaha AR (2006) Anaplastic thyroid carcinoma: biology, pathogenesis, prognostic factors, and treatment approaches. Ann Surg Oncol 13:453–464
2. Hundahl SA, Fleming ID, Fremgen AM, Menck HR (1998) A National Cancer Data Base report on 53, 856 cases of thyroid carcinoma treated in the U.S., 1985–1995 [see comments]. Cancer 83:2638–2648
3. Demeter JG, De Jong SA, Lawrence AM, Paloyan E (1991) Anaplastic thyroid carcinoma: risk factors and outcome. Surgery 110:956–961; discussion 961–963
4. Nikiforova MN, Kimura ET, Gandhi M et al (2003) BRAF mutations in thyroid tumors are restricted to papillary carcinomas and anaplastic or poorly differentiated carcinomas arising from papillary carcinomas. J Clin Endocrinol Metab 88:5399–5404
5. Quiros RM, Ding HG, Gattuso P, Prinz RA, Xu X (2005) Evidence that one subset of anaplastic thyroid carcinomas are derived from papillary carcinomas due to BRAF and p53 mutations. Cancer 103:2261–2268
6. Tallini G, Santoro M, Helie M et al (1998) RET/PTC oncogene activation defines a subset of papillary thyroid carcinomas lacking evidence of progression to poorly differentiated or undifferentiated tumor phenotypes. Clin Cancer Res 4:287–294
7. McIver B, Hay ID, Giuffrida DF et al (2001) Anaplastic thyroid carcinoma: a 50-year experience at a single institution. Surgery 130:1028–1034
8. Tennvall J, Lundell G, Wahlberg P et al (2002) Anaplastic thyroid carcinoma: three protocols combining doxorubicin, hyperfractionated radiotherapy and surgery. Br J Cancer 86:1848–1853
9. Haigh PI, Ituarte PH, Wu HS et al (2001) Completely resected anaplastic thyroid carcinoma combined with adjuvant chemotherapy and irradiation is associated with prolonged survival. Cancer 91:2335–2342
10. Venkatesh YS, Ordonez NG, Schultz PN, Hickey RC, Goepfert H, Samaan NA (1990) Anaplastic carcinoma of the thyroid. A clinicopathologic study of 121 cases. Cancer 66:321–330
11. Nilsson O, Lindeberg J, Zedenius J et al (1998) Anaplastic giant cell carcinoma of the thyroid gland: treatment and survival over a 25-year period. World J Surg 22:725–730
12. Wang Y, Tsang R, Asa S, Dickson B, Arenovich T, Brierley J (2006) Clinical outcome of anaplastic thyroid carcinoma treated with radiotherapy of once- and twice-daily fractionation regimens. Cancer 107:1786–1792
13. Ain KB, Egorin MJ, DeSimone PA (2000) Treatment of anaplastic thyroid carcinoma with paclitaxel: phase 2 trial using ninety-six-hour infusion. Collaborative Anaplastic Thyroid Cancer Health Intervention Trials (CATCHIT) Group. Thyroid 10:587–594
14. Ain KB, Tofiq S, Taylor KD (1996) Antineoplastic activity of taxol against human anaplastic thyroid carcinoma cell lines in vitro and in vivo. J Clin Endocrinol Metab 81:3650–3653
15. Voigt W, Kegel T, Weiss M, Mueller T, Simon H, Schmoll HJ (2005) Potential activity of paclitaxel, vinorelbine and gemcitabine in anaplastic thyroid carcinoma. J Cancer Res Clin Oncol 131:585–590

16. Yeung SC, Xu G, Pan J, Christgen M, Bamiagis A (2000) Manumycin enhances the cytotoxic effect of paclitaxel on anaplastic thyroid carcinoma cells. Cancer Res 60:650–656
17. Xu G, Pan J, Martin C, Yeung SC (2001) Angiogenesis inhibition in the in vivo antineoplastic effect of manumycin and paclitaxel against anaplastic thyroid carcinoma. J Clin Endocrinol Metab 86:1769–1777
18. Dackiw A, Pan J, Xu G, Yeung SC (2005) Modulation of parathyroid hormone-related protein levels (PTHrP) in anaplastic thyroid cancer. Surgery 138:456–463
19. Nagayama Y, Yokoi H, Takeda K et al (2000) Adenovirus-mediated tumor suppressor p53 gene therapy for anaplastic thyroid carcinoma in vitro and in vivo. J Clin Endocrinol Metab 85:4081–4086
20. Narimatsu M, Nagayama Y, Akino K et al (1998) Therapeutic usefulness of wild-type p53 gene introduction in a p53-null anaplastic thyroid carcinoma cell line. J Clin Endocrinol Metab 83:3668–3672
21. Copland JA, Marlow LA, Kurakata S et al (2006) Novel high-affinity PPARgamma agonist alone and in combination with paclitaxel inhibits human anaplastic thyroid carcinoma tumor growth via p21WAF1/CIP1. Oncogene 25:2304–2317
22. Smallridge RC, Marlow LA, Copland JA (2009) Anaplastic thyroid cancer: molecular pathogenesis and emerging therapies. Endocr Relat Cancer 16:17–44

Part II
Parathyroid

Chapter 6
Primary Hyperparathyroidism

Kaitlyn J. Kelly, Herbert Chen, and Rebecca S. Sippel

Introduction

Calcium plays an essential role in a variety of body functions, including muscle contraction, nerve conduction, intracellular signaling, bone remodeling and maintenance, and blood clotting. Parathyroid hormone (PTH), which is produced by four small parathyroid glands located just posterior to the thyroid gland, is the key regulator of calcium homeostasis. PTH is an 84-amino acid peptide with a very short half-life (2–4 min) that allows tight, moment-to-moment regulation of the serum calcium level. The parathyroid glands sense when serum calcium concentrations fall and respond by releasing PTH, which in turn directly stimulates calcium reabsorption in the distal nephron of the kidney and the release of calcium from bone, and indirectly stimulates increased absorption of calcium from the GI tract via calcitriol. Under normal circumstances, elevations in serum calcium result in decreased PTH secretion. Primary hyperparathyroidism (PHPT) is defined as autonomous overproduction of PTH from a hyperfunctioning parathyroid gland or glands.

Epidemiology

PHPT is the most common cause of hypercalcemia in the outpatient setting. It is due to a hyperfunctioning single gland, or adenoma, in approximately 85% of cases. The remaining 15% of cases are caused by hyperplasia affecting all glands (10%), double adenomas (4%), or in rare cases, parathyroid carcinoma (1%). The overall prevalence of PHPT is 1% of the adult population. The incidence is approximately 4 cases per 100,000 people per year. PHPT occurs primarily in patients over the age of 55 and is approximately 2–3 times more common in women than in men [1].

R.S. Sippel (✉)
University of Wisconsin Hospital and Clinics, Madison, WI, USA
e-mail: sippel@surgery.wisc.edu

C. Sturgeon (ed.), *Endocrine Neoplasia*, Cancer Treatment and Research, vol 153,
DOI 10.1007/978-1-4419-0857-5_6, © Springer Science+Business Media, LLC 2010

Differential Diagnosis and Clinical Presentation

Differential Diagnosis

The classical diagnosis of PHPT is an abnormally elevated serum calcium level in the setting of a high or high-normal PTH level. Also frequently elevated is 24-h urine calcium excretion (>250 mg/24 h or calcium creatinine clearance ratio (Ca/Cr) >0.02). In addition, about 50% of patients with PHPT have hypophosphatemia because PTH increases excretion of phosphate by the kidneys in a patient with normal kidney function. It is important to note, however, that milder forms of PHPT exist where either the serum calcium level or PTH level is not "elevated" by laboratory definition but the two values are still biochemically abnormal when considered together. For example, a serum calcium level in the high-normal range in the setting of an elevated PTH (ePTH) is biochemically abnormal as this amount of calcium in the blood should suppress PTH secretion. This clinical scenario is termed "normocalcemic hyperparathyroidism" (NCHPT) [2]. Similarly, a normal or high-normal PTH level in the setting of hypercalcemia is biochemically abnormal and has been termed "inappropriate secretion of PTH" (ISP) [2].

Important differentials in the diagnosis of PHPT include familial hypocalciuric hypercalcemia (FHH), vitamin-D deficiency, and secondary hyperparathyroidism. These conditions must be ruled out before a diagnosis of PHPT can be made.

FHH is an autosomal dominant, inherited condition. It results from a heterozygous mutation in the calcium sensing receptor (CaSR) on parathyroid cells. Because of this mutation, the CaSR is not sufficiently activated by normal serum calcium levels. The result is that PTH continues to be secreted when the serum calcium concentration is normal, leading to a normal or ePTH with a high normal or mildly elevated serum calcium. This is similar to the laboratory profile of ISP, a mild form of PHPT. The difference is that in FHH, CaSR in the nephron of the kidney is also mutated and so it reabsorbs calcium from the urine. In FHH, as opposed to PHPT, urinary calcium excretion is low (<200 mg/24 h or calcium-creatinine clearance (Ca/Cr) ratio <0.01). It is important to distinguish between FHH and PHPT because the former is a benign condition and cannot be cured by parathyroidectomy.

Vitamin D deficiency must be ruled out in patients undergoing evaluation for PHPT. Vitamin D deficiency can result from insufficient dietary intake or from lack of exposure to the sun. One function of PTH is to stimulate hydroxylation of 25-hydroxyvitamin D to 1,25-dihydroxyvitamin D, the active form. In vitamin D deficiency, PTH secretion increases as a compensatory mechanism. Patients with ePTH in the setting of vitamin D deficiency should receive vitamin D replacement therapy and then be reevaluated to see if PTH levels normalize.

Secondary hyperparathyroidism develops in patients with chronic kidney disease or malabsorption where reabsorption of calcium at the kidney or GI tract, respectively, is abnormal. Hypocalcemia results and PTH secretion increases as a compensatory mechanism. Secondary hyperparathyroidism is therefore characterized by hypocalcemia and should not be part of the differential diagnosis of PHPT.

Tertiary hyperparathyroidism, however, can develop in patients with secondary hyperparathyroidism when the hyperfunctioning parathyroid glands develop autonomy and continue secreting PTH even after normalization of serum calcium levels. Secondary hyperparathyroidism is best treated by treating the underlying disorder. Patients with chronic kidney disease benefit from kidney transplantation. Tertiary hyperparathyroidism, however, is treated with parathyroidectomy as is PHPT.

Clinical Presentation

Historically, patients with PHPT presented with kidney stones, bone pain or multiple fractures, or neuropsychiatric problems. The most common clinical presentation of the disease today, however, is the finding of a persistently elevated serum calcium level on routine laboratory evaluation in a patient with no complaints. Symptoms of this disease commonly include fatigue, weakness, nausea, constipation, polyuria and nocturia, depression, and memory loss, among others (Table 6.1). Because these symptoms can be vague and because they develop gradually over time, patients often do not notice them enough to report them as a complaint. They attribute these symptoms to lack of sleep or normal aging. Because these symptoms are frequently not recognized as being related to PHPT or are difficult to quantify, many patients are inappropriately labeled as being "asymptomatic" from their disease. PHPT, whether symptomatic or not, can lead to associated conditions including osteoporosis, nephrolithiasis, cardiovascular disease, weight loss, gout, hypertension, and even pancreatitis. Historically, it is the PHPT patients with these associated morbidities that are considered to be "symptomatic." Lastly, all PHPT patients have increased mortality from ischemic heart disease, cerebrovascular disease, and cancer relative to age- and sex-matched controls [3–5]. Whether the degree of hypercalcemia correlates with survival in PHTP patients is a subject of debate. In 1987, Palmér et al. followed 441 PHPT patients and demonstrated that the increased mortality was independent of initial serum calcium level [6]. More recently, however, Wermers et al. followed 435 patients with PHPT and found that higher maximal serum calcium level was an independent predictor of mortality [7].

Table 6.1 Frequently overlooked symptoms of PHPT

Easy fatigue	Abdominal pain
Weakness	Headache
Ataxia	Inability to concentrate
Hyporeflexia	Hearing loss
Myalgia	Memory loss
Dyspepsia	Vision changes
Nausea	Depression
Weight loss	Polyuria
Constipation	Nocturia
Incontinence	Polydypsia
Anorexia	Pruritus

Parathyroid Localization Studies

The diagnosis of PHPT is a based on clinical and laboratory findings. Parathyroid imaging is used to help identify patients with single gland disease and allow appropriate operative planning. Negative imaging should not be used to exclude a diagnosis of PHPT. The purpose of imaging is to distinguish between single adenomas and multiglandular disease, and to detect and localize ectopic glands. Parathyroid imaging has developed considerably over the past decade. Ultrasound, nuclear medicine scanning, computed tomography (CT), and magnetic resonance imaging (MRI) are among the techniques currently in use for noninvasive assessment of parathyroid glands.

Nuclear Imaging

A variety of nuclear imaging techniques are currently available for the identification of parathyroid adenomas, but technetium-99m (^{99m}Tc) sestamibi is the most thoroughly investigated and most frequently used technique to date. Sestamibi is a lipophilic compound that is sequestered by mitochondria within cells. The larger number of mitochondria in parathyroid adenoma cells versus normal thyroid cells results in a differential in clearance of sestamibi from these two tissues. Labeling of sestamibi with ^{99m}Tc allows for both planar and tomographic imaging. In practice, early and delayed imaging of the neck at 10–15 min and 1–3 h after intravenous administration of ^{99m}Tc-sestamibi, respectively, is performed. The delayed images are generally the most informative in terms of localization of abnormal parathyroid tissue as the differential between thyroid and parathyroid uptake of sestamibi is more pronounced at the later time point (Fig. 6.1). ^{99m}Tc-sestamibi has been shown to be up to 88% specific for the detection of solitary parathyroid adenomas [8–10]. Moure and colleagues demonstrated that ^{99m}Tc-sestamibi as a sole localization technique had an overall PPV of 98.4% for detection of a solitary parathyroid adenoma in patients with one solitary uptake on the study [11]. In general, ^{99m}Tc-sestamibi imaging is considered to be the best preoperative imaging modality available for localization of parathyroid adenomas.

Ultrasound

Ultrasound is a noninvasive and relatively inexpensive imaging modality for localization of abnormal parathyroid glands that does not involve radioactivity. It is highly operator-dependent and is generally not considered to be as specific as ^{99m}Tc-sestamibi, but it does provide important adjunctive information that compliments

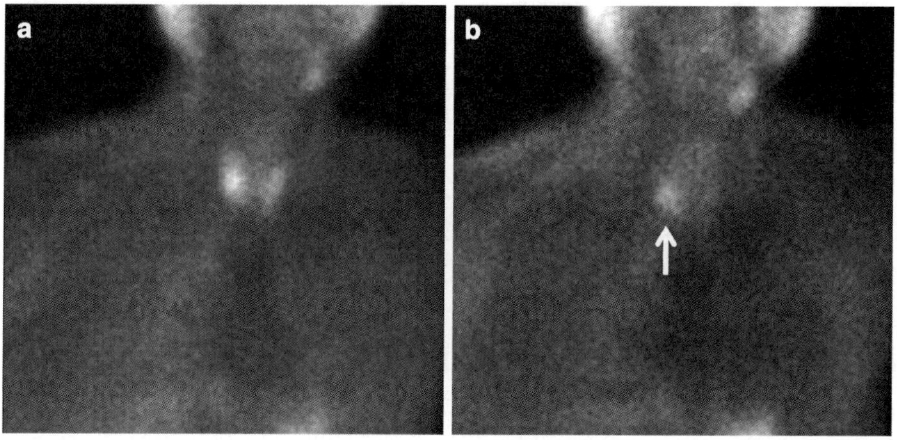

Fig. 6.1 ^{99m}Tc-sestamibi scan localizing a right lower parathyroid adenoma. (**a**) Early image illustrates uptake of radiotracer by thyroid and parathyroid tissue. (**b**) Late image shows delayed clearance of radiotracer from the right lower parathyroid gland (*arrow*)

that obtained by ^{99m}Tc-sestamibi. Ultrasound can be performed in the operating room immediately prior to incision and can optimize the location and size of the incision and minimize the amount of dissection of neck tissues. Additionally, ultrasound can readily distinguish between thyroid nodules and abnormal parathyroids, a distinction that is sometimes impossible to make with nuclear imaging studies. Lastly, ultrasound can identify intrathyroidal parathyroid glands and is particularly useful in the reoperative setting. Like ^{99m}Tc-sestamibi, ultrasound has been shown to be up to 88% specific for the detection of solitary parathyroid adenomas [9] (Fig. 6.2).

Intraoperative Adjuncts

Radioguided Surgery

Like ^{99m}Tc-sestamibi scanning, radioguided surgery exploits the differential uptake of radiotracer by abnormal parathyroid tissue. Patients receive an intravenous dose of ^{99m}Tc-sestamibi 1–4 h prior to surgery. In the operating room, a background level of radioactivity is measured by placing the gamma probe over the thyroid isthmus. The probe can then be used transcutaneously to optimize the location of the incision and intraoperatively to direct the actual dissection. After removal of the abnormal parathyroid, the gland itself is placed on the gamma probe. Counts >20% of background are diagnostic for parathyroid tissue [12]. This technology is particularly useful for distinction between parathyroid tissue and thyroid nodules, a distinction that can be difficult to make on ^{99m}Tc-sestamibi scans, as well as for intraoperative

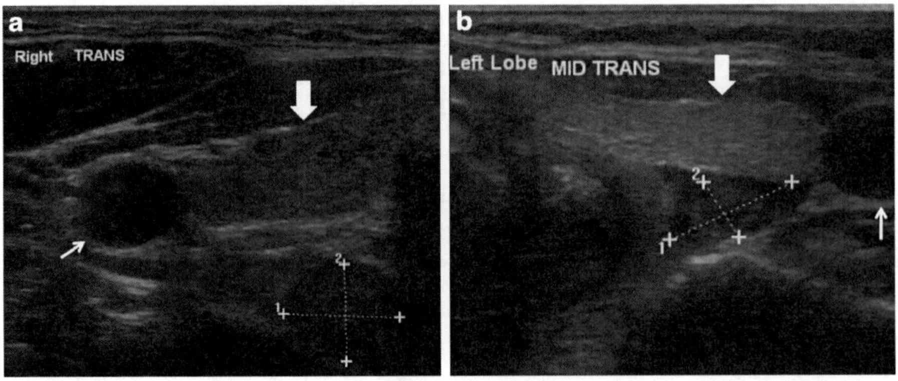

Fig. 6.2 Ultrasound images demonstrating right-sided (**a**) and left-sided (**b**) parathyroid adenomas. (**a**) demonstrates a round, adenoma (*dashed lines*) situated posterior to the right thyroid lobe (*large arrow*) and posteromedial to the right carotid artery (*small arrow*). Exposure of this deeply posterior adenoma would require opening the plane between the right carotid artery and the right lobe of the thyroid, and retracting the right lobe medially. (**b**) shows an adenoma situated slightly more laterally behind the left thyroid lobe (*large arrow*), just medial to the left carotid artery (*small arrow*). This particular adenoma could be easily approached by opening the plane between the left carotid artery and the left lobe of the thyroid

localization of ectopic parathyroid tissue. Another benefit of radioguided surgery is that it can successfully localize parathyroid adenomas and gland hyperplasia [13]. Lastly, this technology can be used to locate hyperplastic parathyroid tissue that has been previously autotransplanted in the forearm [14].

Intraoperative PTH Monitoring

PTH levels can be monitored intraoperatively to predict the success of parathyroidectomy. Because the half life of PTH is only 2–4 min, levels drop significantly as early as 5 min after resection of a hyperfunctioning gland. Peripheral blood samples are typically drawn at 5, 10, and 15 min after the removal of a suspicious gland. With the rapid intraoperative PTH (ioPTH) assay, results are available within 12–15 min. A drop in PTH level of 50% from baseline is considered indicative of a curative parathyroidectomy. Lew and colleagues demonstrated that in PHPT patients with discordant sestamibi scan and ultrasound results, ioPTH findings changed management in 30% of cases and resulted in an operative success rate of 93% [15]. They concluded that the addition of ioPTH is of minimal benefit in PHPT patients with concordant imaging studies, but is essential for successful resection in patients with discordant imaging studies. Chen et al. evaluated the relative accuracy of sestamibi scanning, radioguided surgery, and ioPTH and found that ioPTH to be the most sensitive and accurate test with a PPV of 99.5% [10].

Bilateral Internal Jugular Venous Sampling

Bilateral Internal Jugular PTH sampling (BIJ PTH) is an additional method which can localize the side of a parathyroid adenoma. This procedure can be performed in the operating room immediately prior to surgery. Differences in PTH levels of 5–10% between the right and left internal jugular vein blood samples are considered positive for lateralization. Ito and colleagues demonstrated a sensitivity of 80% and PPV of 71% for localization of parathyroid adenomas in patients with PHPT [16]. They found that BIJ PTH resulted in successful localization in nearly 60% of patients with negative ^{99m}Tc-sestamibi studies but with parathyroid adenomas. BIJ PTH has been shown to be particularly useful for localization of hypersecreting glands in multiglandular disease cases where intraoperative peripheral PTH levels did not fall by 50% after removal of one abnormal gland. For these reasons, BIJ PTH can be a useful adjunct to ^{99m}Tc-sestamibi and ioPTH monitoring.

Principles of Management

Surgery is the only curative therapy available for PHPT. Focused parathyroidectomy of a single hyperfunctioning gland or subtotal parathyroidectomy for multiglandular disease results in normalization of PTH secretion and of serum calcium levels. Surgery is clearly indicated for all PHPT patients with any of the above-mentioned associated morbidities. Surgery for patients with "asymptomatic" or mild PHPT, however, is more controversial. Some feel that these patients should not be exposed to the risks of surgery for a clinically insignificant disease. The counter argument, however, is that asymptomatic PHPT will develop into symptomatic or complicated disease in 23–62% of patients by 10 years [17–19]. In addition, studies have shown that patients with so-called "asymptomatic" PHPT do report numerous symptoms (i.e. depression, insomnia, weakness/easy fatigue, memory loss, etc.) related to their hyperparathyroidism and approximately 80% of these symptoms resolve or diminish after successful parathyroidectomy [20–22].

In 1990, the NIH and National Institute of Diabetes and Digestive and Kidney Diseases set forth consensus guidelines for recommending parathyroidectomy in asymptomatic PHPT patients and these were revised at workshops in 2002 and more recently in 2008. Parathyroidectomy is currently recommended in asymptomatic patients meeting any of the following criteria: (1) <50 years of age, (2) serum calcium level >1.0 mg/dL above normal, (3) the presence of kidney stones, (4) estimated GFR < 60 mL/min/1.73 m^2, (5) osteoporosis (T-score -2.5 or less at any site and/or fragility fracture in patients ≥50, or Z-score of -2.5 or less in premenopausal women or men <50), [17], or (6) inability to participate in adequate follow up [23] (Table 6.2).

Many groups have recommended broadening these guidelines. They argue that medical follow up for PHPT patients not treated with surgery is expensive and time-consuming. It has been shown that parathyroidectomy is cost-effective relative to

Table 6.2 A comparison of guidelines for parathyroidectomy in patients with asymptomatic PHPT

Clinical factors	1990 NIH criteria	2002 workshop guidelines	2008 workshop guidelines
Age	<50 years	<50 years	<50 years
Serum calcium	>1.6 mg/dL above normal	>1 mg/dL above normal	>1 mg/dL above normal
Urinary calcium	>400 mg/24 h	>400 mg/24 h or nephrocalcinosis	not indicated
Renal function	Creatinine clearance decreased by ≥30%	Creatinine clearance decreased by ≥30%	Estimated GFR <60 mL/min/1.73 m^2
BMD	Z-score <−2 at forearm	T-score <−2.5 at hip, Lumbar spine, or distal 1/3 radius	T-score ≤−2.5 at any site in pts ≥50, premenopausal women or men <50, and/or previous fragility fracture

observation for management of both asymptomatic and symptomatic PHPT patients with life expectancy >6.5 years [24–26].

Additionally, the majority of PHPT patients are at risk for the development of complications. There are currently no known laboratory values or markers that predict which asymptomatic PHPT patients will progress to having symptomatic and/or complicated disease [17]. Lastly, it is important to remember that although these patients are referred to as having "asymptomatic" disease, the vast majority of them are, in fact, symptomatic. They experience the vague complaints mentioned previously including weakness, fatigue, insomnia, memory loss, constipation, depression, etc. They are still classified as "asymptomatic" because these symptoms are not tangible and they do not meet biochemical criteria nor do they have associated morbid conditions requiring immediate treatment. It has been shown that up to 65% of "asymptomatic" PHPT patients have left ventricular hypertrophy that is thought to be a direct effect of elevated serum PTH [27]. At present, however, echocardiography is not a standard part of the work up for PHPT and most patients are therefore not assessed for left ventricular hypertrophy. Because both medical and surgical management are currently appropriate treatment options for PHPT, we will discuss both here.

Medical Management

Medical management is generally chosen for PHPT patients who refuse surgery, those considered high-risk for surgery, and those with asymptomatic or mild disease not meeting consensus guidelines for parathyroidectomy. Medical management entails an initial evaluation with a base-line evaluation with serum calcium, PTH, and creatinine levels, and a bone scan at three sites. Follow up then consists of yearly assessment of serum calcium and creatinine levels and assessment of bone mineral density (BMD) at three sites (lumbar spine, hip, and forearm) every 1–2 years [23, 28]. It is important to check BMD at cortical bone as several studies have demonstrated that cancellous bone is somewhat protected from the catabolic effects of PTH relative to cortical bone [29].

These patients should be instructed to stay well-hydrated and to avoid prolonged immobilization. They should avoid medications that can increase serum calcium levels such as thiazide diuretics and lithium. Estrogen replacement therapy and raloxifene have been shown to have modest effects at decreasing bone resorption in postmenopausal women with PHPT [30–32].

Bisphosphonates can reduce serum calcium levels in patients with PHPT by inhibition of osteoclasts and bone resportion, but refractory cases unresponsive to bisphosphonate therapy have been reported [33]. Additionally, bisphosphonates must be administered cautiously as serious adverse effects may result from their use. Cases of severe muscle and joint pain, acute systemic inflammatory response syndrome (SIRS), nephrotic syndrome, renal failure, and osteonecrosis of the jaw have been reported with bisphosphonate therapy [34, 35].

Calcimimetics are agents that stimulate the CaSR on cells within the parathyroid glands and thereby inhibit the secretion of PTH. Cinacalcet is a calcimimetic agent that is FDA-approved for treatment of secondary hyperparathyroidism and parathyroid carcinoma. It has recently been shown to normalize serum calcium and decrease PTH levels in patients with PHPT and to do so over a sustained period of time [36]. Cinacalcet, however, has not been shown to improve BMD or prevent complications of PHPT in medically managed patients.

In summary, it has been shown that most patients with PHPT not meeting criteria for parathyroidectomy will have stable disease over a period of 10 years [18]. A worsening of laboratory values and/or worsening cortical bone loss, however, may occur in up to 37% of patients over 15 years and there is no way to predict which patients will progress [29]. Furthermore, the use of antiresorptive agents does not affect the progressive cortical bone loss observed in PHPT patients treated without surgery. All patients with PHPT not undergoing surgery, therefore, must be followed indefinitely to monitor for the development of complications.

Surgical Management

The first successful parathyroidectomy was performed by Felix Mandl in 1925. For decades since that time, the conventional surgical treatment of choice for PHPT has been a bilateral neck exploration with identification and inspection of all 4 glands. The parathyroids are inspected for size, color, and consistency. Normal glands are flat or ovoid in shape and are dark yellow/tan in color. They weigh approximately 30–40 mg. Abnormal glands are more globular and are generally larger, often weighing >150 mg. In addition, abnormal glands tend to be more red in color. Bilateral neck exploration and 4 gland inspection has a success rate of >95% when performed by experienced surgeons [37–40]. Bilateral neck exploration can be performed alone or in combination with the previously described preoperative imaging modalities for localization of abnormal parathyroid tissue. Upon inspection of all 4 glands, the decision is made whether to proceed with removal of a single or double adenoma, or for the finding of 4-gland disease, subtotal parathyroidectomy, or total parathyroidectomy with autotransplantation.

The development of preoperative parathyroid localization studies and intraoperative localization techniques has led to the development of a new operative approach to PHPT by focused, or minimally invasive, parathyroidectomy. With this technique abnormal glands (whether isolated or multiple) are resected while normal glands are left completely undisturbed. Benefits of this technique include that it requires a smaller neck incision, it involves less dissection of the neck, and therefore theoretically decreases the risk of complications like bilateral recurrent laryngeal nerve injury or devascularization of all 4 glands that may occur with bilateral exploration. Additional benefits of this technique include decreased operating room time and cost. Patients can often go home the same day after focused parathyroidectomy whereas they are frequently observed overnight with calcium levels checked on postoperative day 1 after 4 gland exploration. It is also feasible to perform focused parathyroidectomy with local anesthesia if desired. Fang and colleagues performed a prospective study of 33 PHPT patients with poor anesthesia risk. One group received medical treatment with bisphosphonates while the other underwent focused parathyroidectomy under local anesthesia. They found that the medically managed group had significantly higher incidence of hypercalcemia episodes, deterioration of renal function, bone fractures, increased medical costs, and decreased overall survival compared to the group treated surgically [33]. Recently, McGill and colleagues have shown that conventional 4 gland exploration identifies multiglandular disease more frequently than focused parathyroidectomy (16.5% incidence vs. 11.1%, respectively), but that operative success (defined by normocalcemia 6 months postoperatively) were equivalent at >95% for both approaches [40].

Following parathyroidectomy, patients must be monitored for signs and symptoms of hypocalcemia. Hypocalcemia can occur because of devascularization of parathyroid glands (after a bilateral exploration) secondary to operative manipulation, suppression of remaining normal parathyroid glands or because of bone hunger. Bone hunger is a phenomenon of severe hypocalcemia that can occur because of the immediate uptake of calcium by the bone after successful parathyroidectomy. Symptoms of hypocalcemia include numbness and tingling of the hands, feet, and perioral skin. Untreated severe hypocalcemia can lead to EKG changes, most often a prolongation of the Q-T interval. Physical examination including testing for positive Chvostek sign can be performed to evaluate for hypocalcemia. The Trousseau sign is no longer recommended in the physical examination because it is very unpleasant for patients. Postoperative hypocalcemia should be treated with oral calcium supplementation. In patients with significant hypocalcemia or hypoparathyroidism, an activated form of vitamin D (calcitriol) can be administered, which increases the absorption of calcium from the GI tract. Vitamin D deficiency can also be a cause of postoperative hypocaclemia. Postoperative vitamin D supplementation is important for vitamin D deficient patients after parathyroidectomy as it decreases the incidence of postoperative eucalcemic PTH elevation [41]. Recently, it has been shown that preoperative vitamin D supplementation in patients with PHPT is also safe and does not significantly increase serum calcium levels [42].

Patients should be evaluated in the clinic 1–4 weeks postoperatively for serum calcium levels. Monitoring of postoperative PTH levels is somewhat controversial. Elevated PTH (ePTH) levels with normocalcemia following parathyroidectomy are found in up to 40% of patients and in most cases do not signify operative failure. Yen and colleagues found that postoperative PTH measurements may be misleading and are not indicated in normocalcemic patients [43]. More recently, however, we have shown that recurrent disease is significantly more common in patients with postoperative ePTH and that it was always associated with a serum calcium level ≥9.7 mg/dL [44]. We therefore advocate monitoring serum calcium and PTH levels 4 weeks postoperatively to identify this subgroup of patients at risk for the development of recurrent disease for appropriate surveillance. Operative cure of PHPT is defined as normocalcemia 6 months after surgery. After successful parathyroidectomy, patients are typically followed up with annual calcium levels for the rest of their lives.

Risks and Benefits of Parathyroidectomy

Benefits

The currently reported cure rate of parathyroidectomy is 96–98% for both 4-gland exploration and focused parathyroidectomy approaches. After successful parathyroidectomy, PHPT patients experience significant improvement in symptoms and quality of life, improved BMD and decreased fracture risk, cardiovascular benefits, and decreased overall mortality [45]. Multiple studies have shown dramatic improvement in symptomatology and quality of life in PHPT patients after parathyroidectomy [46, 47]. Of note, Eigelberger et al. looked at symptomatic improvement with parathyroidectomy in PHPT patients with mild disease not meeting NIH criteria for surgery and in those with classic PHPT meeting these criteria. They reported equal and dramatic improvement in nonspecific somatic and neuropsychiatric symptoms and quality of life in these two groups [48]. Adler and colleagues demonstrated that patients undergoing focused parathyroidectomy experienced an even greater improvement in quality of life after surgery than those undergoing bilateral neck exploration [49].

BMD has been shown to improve gradually over time in PHPT patients after successful parathyroidectomy. Silverberg and colleagues reported a significant improvement in BMD at the lumbar spine and femoral neck at 1 and 10 years after curative parathyroidectomy [18]. In more extended follow up of this same cohort of patients, Rubin et al. demonstrated sustained postoperative increases in BMD at both cancellous and cortical sites 15 years after surgery despite the expectation of age-related bone loss [29]. Vestergaard et al. confirmed that this improvement in BMD does translate into a decreased fracture risk. They found that PHPT patients have an increased fracture risk relative to age-matched controls without hyperparathyroidism as early as 10 years prior to surgery and this increased risk was not associated with the degree of hypercalcemia. After successful parathyroidectomy, however, fracture risk returned to normal [50].

Another common problem among PHPT patients is the development of kidney stones. In following PHPT patients with a history of kidney stones treated either with or without surgery, Silverberg et al. found no recurrence of kidney stones after parathyroidectomy versus recurrence in 75% of patients managed without surgery [18].

Parathyroidectomy also results in cardiac benefits for PHPT patients. Left ventricular hypertrophy in PHPT resolves by 6 months after curative parathyroidectomy. Similarly, the increased risk of myocardial infarction in PHPT patients decreases to normal after surgery [51].

Lastly, the increased risk of death associated with PHPT decreases after parathyroidectomy. Palmer and colleagues followed a cohort of 441 PHPT patients who underwent parathyroidectomy for a period of 22 years. They found that the increased risk of death associated with PHPT does decrease gradually, by 5–8 years after surgery [6].

Risks

The major risks associated with parathyroidectomy include injury to the recurrent laryngeal nerve, hypoparathyroidism/hypocalcemia, hemorrhage, wound complications, and failure to cure hyperparathyroidism. The risk of recurrent laryngeal nerve injury is on the order of 1%. Transient postoperative hypocalcemia does occur in a significant number of patients after parathyroidectomy and this is due to devosulavization, suppression of the remaining glands, or bone hunger as described previously. Permanent hypocalcemia secondary to hypoparathyroidism occurs rarely, (<1%). Cryopreservation of parathyroid tissue is often performed for patients undergoing surgery for recurrent or persistent hyperparathyroidism or for those undergoing subtotal or total parathyroidectomy. Cryopreserved tissue can be used for delayed autotransplantation if persistent postoperative hypocalcemia develops, and can result in normocalcemia in approximately 45% of patients [52]. Graft success in the setting of delayed autotransplantation is indirectly proportional to the duration of cryopreservation. Cohen and colleagues have found no functional autografts after 22 months of cryopreservation [52].

To date, no study has demonstrated a significant difference in overall complication rate between standard bilateral neck exploration and focused parathyroidectomy. Bergenfelz and colleagues, however, demonstrated a higher incidence of biochemical and severe symptomatic postoperative hypocalcemia in patients undergoing bilateral neck exploration [53].

Management of Persistent/Recurrent PHPT

Approximately 5% of patients undergoing parathyroidectomy for PHPT will require further intervention for either persistent or recurrent disease. Hypercalcemia within 6 months of resection is considered persistent disease because of failure to identify and remove all hyperfunctioning glands. Recurrent disease is characterized by the development of hypercalcemia more than 6 months postoperatively. Recurrent PHPT is most commonly because of re-growth of abnormal parathyroid tissue after a subtotal resection. This can occur after resection of what appear to be single or double adenomas that are, in fact, dominant glands in 4-gland hyperplasia. Similarly, re-growth can occur after a 3.5-gland resection or after total parathyroidectomy with autotransplantation of abnormal parathyroid tissues. Less often, recurrent disease can be a manifestation of parathyromatosis or development of metastases from parathyroid carcinoma.

Once a biochemical diagnosis of persistent or recurrent pHPT is made, the radiology, pathology, and operative reports from the initial surgery should be reviewed thoroughly. Noninvasive imaging studies should then be employed to localize the abnormal parathyroid tissue and provide a directed approach for the reoperation. Ultrasound, sestamibi, and MRI are all potentially useful in this regard. A diagnosis of persistent/recurrent disease should be confirmed by at least two concordant studies. When noninvasive imaging studies are discordant or equivocal, invasive tests such as selective venous sampling for PTH levels are necessary [54]. ioPTH assays and intraoperative localization techniques are also important adjuncts for reoperative parathyroid surgery. These studies can aid in localization of ectopic tissue or abnormal tissue left behind in the neck or autotransplanted in a previous procedure. Sippel and colleagues reported successful use of radioguided surgery for localization of hyperplastic parathyroid tissue after autotransplantation to the forearm. In this case, no clips or other identifiers were placed at the original operation to aid with localization of the autotransplanted tissue. With ^{99m}Tc injection and use of a hand-held gamma probe, however, two foci of re-grown hyperplastic parathyroid tissue were readily identified [14].

The risk/benefit profile of reoperative surgery for persistent or recurrent PHPT is not as favorable as that of initial neck exploration. Recurrent laryngeal nerve injury causing vocal cord paralysis occurs in up to 10% of reoperative cases [55, 56]. Permanent hypoparathyroidism also occurs more frequently at reoperation, with reported incidence ranging from 10 to 35% [57]. Cure rate for reoperation for PHPT is 90–95% which means that 5–10% of patients will have failed operations [55, 58]. These factors should be discussed with patients.

Summary

PHPT is a disease that has the potential to cause serious morbidity and yet remains relatively innocuous in some patients. Parathyroidectomy, whether via bilateral neck exploration or a focused approach, offers cure and unequivocal long-term benefits in symptomatic improvement and decreased risk of developing associated comorbid conditions. There is a current trend toward broadening the indications for parathyroidectomy in PHPT patients because medical follow up for this disease is time-consuming, expensive, and does not protect patients from developing associated comorbid conditions. The 2005 AACE/AAES position statement states that "Operative management should be considered and recommended for all asymptomatic patients with PHPT who have a reasonable life expectancy and suitable operative risk factors. Consultation with an experienced endocrinologist and surgeon can help clarify the patient's risk/benefit ratio" [17]. With the availability of multiple technologies for localization of abnormal parathyroid tissue, focused parathyroidectomy can be performed successfully in experienced hands with very little operative risk to patients. We therefore feel that every patient with a diagnosis of PHPT should be considered for parathyroidectomy.

References

1. Surgery of the Thyroid and Parathyroid Glands: Springer; 2007.
2. Carneiro-Pla DM, Irvin GL III, Chen H (2007) Consequences of parathyroidectomy in patients with "mild" sporadic primary hyperparathyroidism. Surgery 142(6):795–799; discussion 9 e1–e2
3. Ogard CG, Engholm G, Almdal TP, Vestergaard H (2004) Increased mortality in patients hospitalized with primary hyperparathyroidism during the period 1977–1993 in Denmark. World J Surg 28(1):108–111
4. Hedback G, Oden A (1998) Increased risk of death from primary hyperparathyroidism – an update. Eur J Clin Invest 28(4):271–276
5. Sambrook PN, Chen JS, March LM et al (2004) Serum parathyroid hormone is associated with increased mortality independent of 25-hydroxy vitamin d status, bone mass, and renal function in the frail and very old: a cohort study. J Clin Endocrinol Metab 89(11):5477–5481
6. Palmér M, Adami HO, Bergstrom R, Akerstrom G, Ljunghall S (1987) Mortality after surgery for primary hyperparathyroidism: a follow-up of 441 patients operated on from 1956 to 1979. Surgery 102(1):1–7
7. Wermers RA, Khosla S, Atkinson EJ et al (1998) Survival after the diagnosis of hyperparathyroidism: a population-based study. Am J Med 104(2):115–122
8. Palazzo FF, Delbridge LW (2004) Minimal-access/minimally invasive parathyroidectomy for primary hyperparathyroidism. Surg Clin North Am 84(3):717–734
9. Siperstein A, Berber E, Barbosa GF et al (2008) Predicting the success of limited exploration for primary hyperparathyroidism using ultrasound, sestamibi, and intraoperative parathyroid hormone: analysis of 1158 cases. Ann Surg 248(3):420–428
10. Chen H, Mack E, Starling JR (2005) A comprehensive evaluation of perioperative adjuncts during minimally invasive parathyroidectomy: which is most reliable? Ann Surg 242(3):375–380; discussion 80–83
11. Moure D, Larranaga E, Dominguez-Gadea L et al (2008) 99MTc-sestamibi as sole technique in selection of primary hyperparathyroidism patients for unilateral neck exploration. Surgery 144(3):454–459
12. Chen H (2004) Radioguided parathyroid surgery. Adv Surg 38:377–392
13. Chen H, Mack E, Starling JR (2003) Radioguided parathyroidectomy is equally effective for both adenomatous and hyperplastic glands. Ann Surg 238(3):332–337; discussion 7–8

14. Sippel RS, Bianco J, Chen H (2003) Radioguided parathyroidectomy for recurrent hyperparathyroidism caused by forearm graft hyperplasia. J Bone Miner Res 18(5):939–942
15. Lew JI, Solorzano CC, Montano RE, Carneiro-Pla DM, Irvin GL III (2008) Role of intraoperative parathormone monitoring during parathyroidectomy in patients with discordant localization studies. Surgery 144(2):299–306
16. Ito F, Sippel R, Lederman J, Chen H (2007) The utility of intraoperative bilateral internal jugular venous sampling with rapid parathyroid hormone testing. Ann Surg 245(6):959–963
17. The American Association of Clinical Endocrinologists and the American Association of Endocrine Surgeons (2005) Position statement on the diagnosis and management of primary hyperparathyroidism. Endocr Pract 11(1):49–54
18. Silverberg SJ, Shane E, Jacobs TP, Siris E, Bilezikian JP (1999) A 10-year prospective study of primary hyperparathyroidism with or without parathyroid surgery. N Engl J Med 341(17):1249–1255
19. Silverberg SJ, Brown I, Bilezikian JP (2002) Age as a criterion for surgery in primary hyperparathyroidism. Am J Med 113(8):681–684
20. Clark OH, Wilkes W, Siperstein AE, Duh QY (1991) Diagnosis and management of asymptomatic hyperparathyroidism: safety, efficacy, and deficiencies in our knowledge. J Bone Miner Res 6 Suppl 2:S135–S142; discussion 51–52
21. Talpos GB, Bone HG III, Kleerekoper M, et al (2000) Randomized trial of parathyroidectomy in mild asymptomatic primary hyperparathyroidism: patient description and effects on the SF-36 health survey. Surgery 128(6):1013–1020;discussion 20–21
22. Rao DS (2001) Parathyroidectomy for asymptomatic primary hyperparathyroidism (PHPT): is it worth the risk? J Endocrinol Invest 24(2):131–134
23. Bilezikian JP, Khan AA, Potts JT Jr (2009) Guidelines for the management of asymptomatic primary hyperparathyroidism: summary statement from the third international workshop. J Clin Endocrinol Metab 94(2):335–339
24. Udelsman R, Pasieka JL, Sturgeon C, Young JE, Clark OH (2009) Surgery for asymptomatic primary hyperparathyroidism: proceedings of the third international workshop. J Clin Endocrinol Metab 94(2):366–372
25. Zanocco K, Angelos P, Sturgeon C (2006) Cost-effectiveness analysis of parathyroidectomy for asymptomatic primary hyperparathyroidism. Surgery 140(6):874–881; discussion 81–82
26. Zanocco K, Sturgeon C (2008) How should age at diagnosis impact treatment strategy in asymptomatic primary hyperparathyroidism? A cost-effectiveness analysis. Surgery 144(2):290–298
27. Piovesan A, Molineri N, Casasso F, et al (1999) Left ventricular hypertrophy in primary hyperparathyroidism. Effects of successful parathyroidectomy. Clin Endocrinol (Oxf) 50(3):321–328
28. Bilezikian JP, Potts JT Jr, Fuleihan Gel H et al (2002) Summary statement from a workshop on asymptomatic primary hyperparathyroidism: a perspective for the 21st century. J Clin Endocrinol Metab 87(12):5353–5361
29. Rubin MR, Bilezikian JP, McMahon DJ et al (2008) The natural history of primary hyperparathyroidism with or without parathyroid surgery after 15 years. J Clin Endocrinol Metab 93(9):3462–3470
30. Boucher A, D'Amour P, Hamel L et al (1989) Estrogen replacement decreases the set point of parathyroid hormone stimulation by calcium in normal postmenopausal women. J Clin Endocrinol Metab 68(4):831–836
31. Selby PL, Peacock M (1986) Ethinyl estradiol and norethindrone in the treatment of primary hyperparathyroidism in postmenopausal women. N Engl J Med 314(23):1481–1485
32. Rubin MR, Lee KH, McMahon DJ, Silverberg SJ (2003) Raloxifene lowers serum calcium and markers of bone turnover in postmenopausal women with primary hyperparathyroidism. J Clin Endocrinol Metab 88(3):1174–1178
33. Fang WL, Tseng LM, Chen JY, et al (2008) The management of high-risk patients with primary hyperparathyroidism – minimally invasive parathyroidectomy vs. medical treatment. Clin Endocrinol (Oxf) 68(4):520–528

34. Tanvetyanon T, Stiff PJ (2006) Management of the adverse effects associated with intravenous bisphosphonates. Ann Oncol 17(6):897–907
35. Wong P, Carmeci C, Jeffrey RB, Weigel RJ (2001) Parathyroid crisis in a 20 year old – an unusual cause of hypercalcaemic crisis. Postgrad Med J 77(909):468–470
36. Peacock M, Bilezikian JP, Klassen PS, Guo MD, Turner SA, Shoback D (2005) Cinacalcet hydrochloride maintains long-term normocalcemia in patients with primary hyperparathyroidism. J Clin Endocrinol Metab 90(1):135–141
37. Kaplan EL, Yashiro T, Salti G (1992) Primary hyperparathyroidism in the 1990s. Choice of surgical procedures for this disease. Ann Surg 215(4):300–317
38. Sosa JA, Powe NR, Levine MA, Udelsman R, Zeiger MA (1998) Profile of a clinical practice: thresholds for surgery and surgical outcomes for patients with primary hyperparathyroidism: a national survey of endocrine surgeons. J Clin Endocrinol Metab 83(8):2658–2665
39. Eigelberger MS, Clark OH (2000) Surgical approaches to primary hyperparathyroidism. Endocrinol Metab Clin North Am 29(3):479–502
40. McGill J, Sturgeon C, Kaplan SP, Chiu B, Kaplan EL, Angelos P (2008) How does the operative strategy for primary hyperparathyroidism impact the findings and cure rate? A comparison of 800 parathyroidectomies. J Am Coll Surg 207(2):246–249
41. Beyer TD, Solorzano CC, Prinz RA, Babu A, Nilubol N, Patel S (2007) Oral vitamin D supplementation reduces the incidence of eucalcemic PTH elevation after surgery for primary hyperparathyroidism. Surgery 141(6):777–783
42. Grubbs EG, Rafeeq S, Jimenez C, et al (2008) Preoperative vitamin D replacement therapy in primary hyperparathyroidism: safe and beneficial? Surgery 144(6):852–858; discussion 8–9
43. Yen TW, Wilson SD, Krzywda EA, Sugg SL (2006) The role of parathyroid hormone measurements after surgery for primary hyperparathyroidism. Surgery 140(4):665–672; discussion 72–74
44. Ning L SR, Schaefer S, and Chen H (2009) What is the clinical significance of an elevated parathyroid hormone level after curative surgery for primary hyperparathyroidism? Ann Surg 249(3):469–472
45. Egan KR, Adler JT, Olson JE, Chen H (2007) Parathyroidectomy for primary hyperparathyroidism in octogenarians and nonagenarians: a risk-benefit analysis. J Surg Res 140(2):194–198
46. Burney RE, Jones KR, Peterson M, Christy B, Thompson NW (1998) Surgical correction of primary hyperparathyroidism improves quality of life. Surgery 124(6):987–991; discussion 91–92
47. Roman S, Sosa JA (2007) Psychiatric and cognitive aspects of primary hyperparathyroidism. Curr Opin Oncol 19(1):1–5
48. Eigelberger MS, Cheah WK, Ituarte PH, Streja L, Duh QY, Clark OH (2004) The NIH criteria for parathyroidectomy in asymptomatic primary hyperparathyroidism: are they too limited? Ann Surg 239(4):528–535
49. Adler JT, Sippel RS, Chen H (2008) The influence of surgical approach on quality of life after parathyroid surgery. Ann Surg Oncol 15(6):1559–1565
50. Vestergaard P, Mollerup CL, Frokjaer VG, Christiansen P, Blichert-Toft M, Mosekilde L (2000) Cohort study of risk of fracture before and after surgery for primary hyperparathyroidism. BMJ 321(7261):598–602
51. Vestergaard P, Mollerup CL, Frokjaer VG, Christiansen P, Blichert-Toft M, Mosekilde L (2003) Cardiovascular events before and after surgery for primary hyperparathyroidism. World J Surg 27(2):216–222
52. Cohen MS, Dilley WG, Wells SA Jr, et al (2005) Long-term functionality of cryopreserved parathyroid autografts: a 13-year prospective analysis. Surgery 138(6):1033–1040; discussion 40–41
53. Bergenfelz A, Lindblom P, Tibblin S, Westerdahl J (2002) Unilateral versus bilateral neck exploration for primary hyperparathyroidism: a prospective randomized controlled trial. Ann Surg 236(5):543–551

54. Caron NR, Sturgeon C, Clark OH (2004) Persistent and recurrent hyperparathyroidism. Curr Treat Options in Oncol 5(4):335–345
55. Shen W, Duren M, Morita E, et al (1996) Reoperation for persistent or recurrent primary hyperparathyroidism. Arch Surg 131(8):861–867; discussion 7–9
56. Mariette C, Pellissier L, Combemale F, Quievreux JL, Carnaille B, Proye C (1998) Reoperation for persistent or recurrent primary hyperparathyroidism. Langenbecks Arch Surg 383(2):174–179
57. Lo CY, Kung AW, Lam KS (1997) Surgical treatment for primary hyperparathyroidism. Chin Med J (Engl) 110(8):612–616
58. Jaskowiak N, Norton JA, Alexander HR, et al (1996) A prospective trial evaluating a standard approach to reoperation for missed parathyroid adenoma. Ann Surg 224(3):308–320; discussion 20–21

Chapter 7
Parathyromatosis and Parathyroid Cancer

Wen T. Shen

Introduction

Parathyroid carcinoma is a rare entity, accounting for less than 1% of all cases of primary hyperparathyroidism [1–5]. This chapter provides an overview of the clinical presentation, pathophysiology, and medical and surgical management of parathyroid carcinoma and highlights some of the ongoing controversies and areas of current research interest involving this uncommon disease, including: difficulties in distinguishing benign from malignant disease both macroscopically and histologically; recent developments in the understanding of the genetic basis for this disease; the use of calcimimetics and other medical therapies for nonoperative management; and the utility of multiple reoperations in patients with recurrent disease. This chapter also summarizes the current state of knowledge regarding parathyromatosis, defined as an overgrowth of multiple hyperfunctioning nodules of the parathyroid tissue, a condition which may develop after capsular fracture and intraoperative seeding during parathyroid tumor resection.

Demographics

Parathyroid carcinoma accounts for 0.005% of all cancers and in most published series is found in less than 1% of all cases of primary hyperparathyroidism [1–5]. Some centers in Japan and Italy have reported parathyroid cancer incidence rates of up to 5% of all patients with primary hyperparathyroidism [6–9]. This variability in incidence rates may reflect demographic and geographic differences but may also be due to differences in histopathologic criteria for defining parathyroid cancer as well

W.T. Shen (✉)
Department of Surgery, Section of Endocrine Surgery, Mt. Zion Medical Center,
University Of California San Francisco, Hellman Bldg. Room C-349,
Campus Box 1674, San Francisco, CA, 94115, USA
e-mail: wen.shen@ucsfmedctr.org

C. Sturgeon (ed.), *Endocrine Neoplasia*, Cancer Treatment and Research, vol 153,
DOI 10.1007/978-1-4419-0857-5_7, © Springer Science+Business Media, LLC 2010

as selection bias, since the reporting authors work at high-volume referral centers. Despite its rarity, parathyroid carcinoma does appear to be increasing in incidence, perhaps mirroring the overall increase in the diagnosis of primary hyperparathyroidism that has been witnessed in the decades after the introduction of improved immunoassays for detection of PTH. Prior to 1992, fewer than 300 cases of parathyroid carcinoma had been described in the literature [3]; more than 100 cases have been reported in the subsequent decade and a half [3]. A review of the multicenter national cancer databases confirms this trend: a 1999 report from the National Cancer Database reported 286 cases of parathyroid cancer diagnosed between 1985 and 1995 [10], and a 2007 examination of the SEER database revealed an overall 60% increase in parathyroid cancer incidence between 1988 and 2003 [2].

The gender distribution for parathyroid carcinoma is different from that of benign primary hyperparathyroidism; men and women are equally affected by parathyroid carcinoma, whereas women are disproportionately affected by benign primary hyperparathyroidism by a 4:1 ratio [2, 4, 6]. The peak age of incidence for both parathyroid carcinoma and benign primary hyperparathyroidism is similar, with both diseases most commonly affecting patients in the fifth decade of life [2, 3, 10]. There have been no reported differences in parathyroid carcinoma incidence or severity of disease in African-American, white, or other ethnicities.

Clinical Presentation

The presenting signs and symptoms of parathyroid carcinoma are typically those of hypercalcemia, and are not usually symptoms of local invasion or compression; the patient presentation can be virtually indistinguishable from the "classic" signs and symptoms of hypercalcemia caused by benign primary hyperparathyroidism. The most frequently reported symptoms are fatigue, weakness, polyuria, polydipsia, depression, and nausea [3]. Patients with more severe hypercalcemia may have kidney stones and pathologic fractures. It is important to note that very few patients with parathyroid carcinoma will be asymptomatic, while most patients with primary hyperparathyroidism are now diagnosed quite early and will not have the "classic" symptoms of advanced hypercalcemia. Patients with parathyroid carcinoma will almost always present themselves with a higher serum calcium level than patients with benign primary hyperparathyroidism; it is not uncommon for patients with parathyroid carcinoma to have serum calcium 2–4 mg/dL higher than the upper limit of the normal [11]. Similarly, PTH levels are generally much higher in patients with parathyroid carcinoma when compared to patients with benign primary hyperparathyroidism. Therefore, suspicion for parathyroid carcinoma should be raised in patients with severe symptoms and markedly elevated serum calcium and PTH levels. Nonfunctioning parathyroid cancers are relatively rare, accounting for approximately 5% of parathyroid cancers [12]. These patients will not manifest the biochemical features of primary hyperparathyroidism but will instead present themselves with neck mass and symptoms of local compression or invasion.

Physical examination findings are usually not reliable in distinguishing parathyroid carcinoma from benign primary hyperparathyroidism. Palpable cervical mass is found in only 5% of cases [1], and symptoms of local compression or invasion are seen only in the advanced disease.

If there is strong preoperative suspicion for parathyroid carcinoma based on clinical or biochemical findings, further workup with localization studies for preoperative planning should be undertaken (see following section). Fine-needle aspiration biopsy of the neck mass should not be performed unless it would alter clinical management (i.e., tissue diagnosis is needed in a patient with obvious distant metastases); there is a risk of needle-tract seeding with subsequent parathyromatosis, which makes operative intervention much more difficult [13].

Preoperative Localization Studies

The algorithm for preoperative workup of primary hyperparathyroidism has changed in the past two decades with the introduction of improved imaging studies and the widespread adoption of minimally invasive parathyroidectomy in lieu of bilateral four-gland neck exploration [14]. Almost all patients with primary hyperparathyroidism will undergo some form of preoperative imaging, usually neck ultrasound and Sestamibi scan, with the aim of identifying abnormal parathyroid glands and planning for either focused or bilateral exploration [15]. Since the diagnosis of parathyroid carcinoma is not usually made preoperatively, patients with this entity will usually undergo the same preoperative imaging studies as patients with benign primary hyperparathyroidism. An ultrasound of the neck can provide useful information regarding the number of enlarged parathyroid glands, the location of the parathyroid tumor in relation to adjacent structures, and the coexistence of thyroid nodules or other abnormalities, and is helpful in guiding the operative approach. Sestamibi scanning provides evidence of hyperfunctioning parathyroid tissue and is especially useful for parathyroid tumors located in ectopic positions.

While imaging studies are useful in directing first-time operations for patients with benign or malignant primary hyperparathyroidism, they are essential for operative planning in patients with persistent or recurrent disease [16, 17]. Patients with parathyroid carcinoma will usually recur locally, and neck ultrasound provides invaluable information regarding the precise location of the tumor recurrence and the involvement of adjacent structures [17]. Sestamibi scanning confirms the location of functioning parathyroid tumor and can also detect distant metastases (Fig. 7.1) [17–19]. In patients with negative or equivocal localization with ultrasound and Sestamibi scan, CT or MRI can be useful for identifying recurrent tumor in the neck or mediastinum [17, 19]. If multiple clips were used in the prior operation or operations, clip artifact may reduce the accuracy of CT scan to detect tumor recurrence. Selective venous catheterization is an invasive study that is utilized only if noninvasive imaging is inconclusive for identifying recurrent parathyroid carcinoma [17].

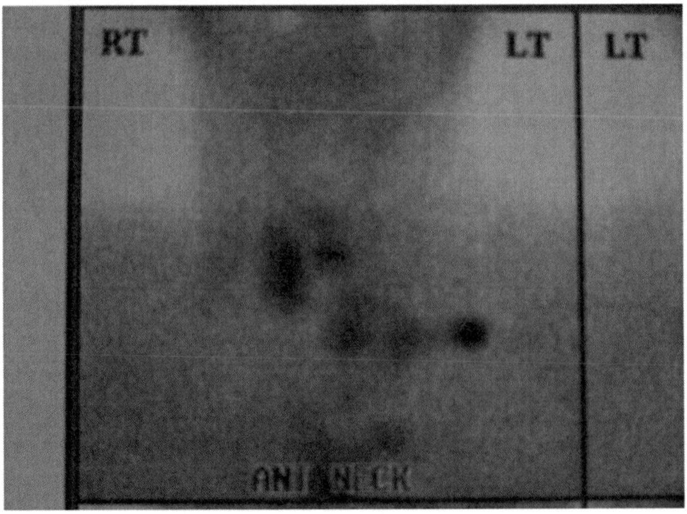

Fig. 7.1 Sestamibi scan demonstrating parathyroid carcinoma with primary disease in the neck and metastatic disease in the mediastinum

Pathology

Clinical suspicion for parathyroid carcinoma may be raised by findings on physical examination or diagnostic evaluation such as palpable cervical mass, markedly elevated calcium or PTH, or symptoms of local invasion, but these features are not reliably present, and the diagnosis may not be confirmed until operation is undertaken. Certain intraoperative features can help to distinguish parathyroid carcinomas from benign parathyroid tumors. Parathyroid cancers differ from benign parathyroid adenomas or hyperplasia both in visual appearance and in consistency on palpation. While benign parathyroid tumors are typically soft, beefy red-brown in color, well-encapsulated and minimally adherent to surrounding structures, parathyroid cancers are frequently hard, whitish-gray, poorly encapsulated, and stuck to or invading into adjacent structures [1, 4, 20–24]. Some authors have suggested that large tumor size is a distinguishing feature for parathyroid cancer; the median gland weight in one series was greater than 4 g [25]. However, just as tumor size has not been shown to correlate with preoperative serum calcium or PTH level, tumor size alone is not reliably predictive of malignancy.

The diagnosis of parathyroid cancer is difficult to make definitively based on clinical or macroscopic features; unfortunately, the histopathologic diagnosis of parathyroid cancer is also difficult. Controversy exists regarding the criteria for classification of parathyroid tissue as benign or malignant [22, 24, 26, 27]. Among the histopathologic features that are attributed to parathyroid carcinoma, include dense fibrous sheets with trabeculae; cellular atypia (Fig. 7.2); infiltrative growth pattern; capsular or vascular invasion (Figs. 7.3 and 7.4); and mitotic figures [26]. However, apart from capsular and vascular invasion, all of these features have been

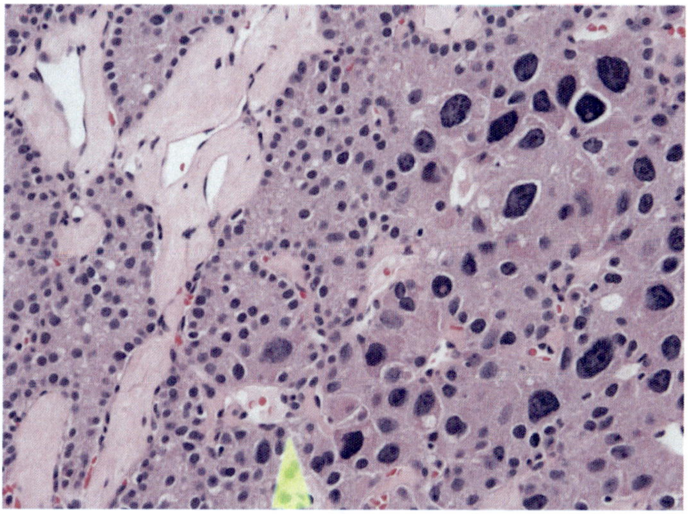

Fig. 7.2 Histopathologic section of parathyroid carcinoma showing cellular atypia

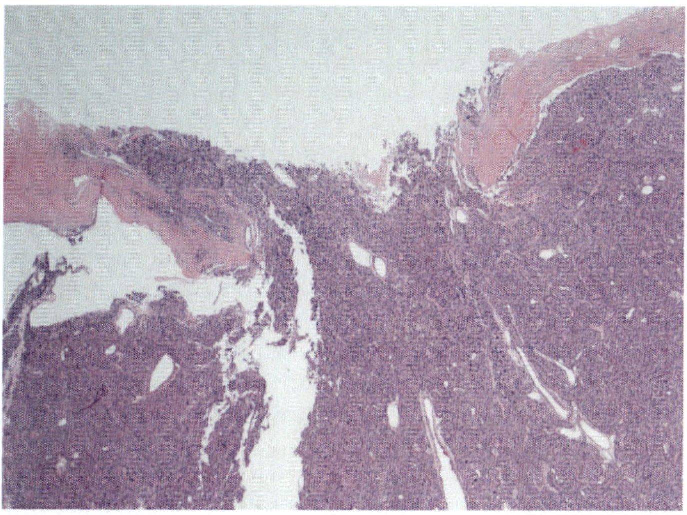

Fig. 7.3 Histopathologic section of parathyroid carcinoma showing capsular invasion

documented in benign parathyroid tumors as well [22]. Because of the lack of reliable microscopic features differentiating benign and malignant parathyroid tumors, frozen section analysis has been found to be minimally useful for distinguishing between the two entities [22].

Because of the inaccuracy of standard histopathologic criteria for malignancy, investigators have proposed multiple molecular and genetic tests for distinguishing benign from malignant parathyroid tumors. Mean nuclear DNA content on flow

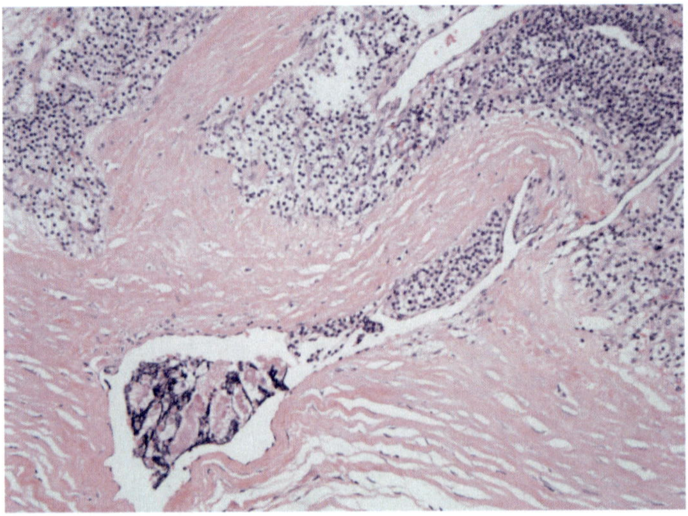

Fig. 7.4 Histopathologic section of parathyroid carcinoma showing vascular invasion

cytometry analysis is elevated in malignant parathyroid tissue as compared to benign [25]. DNA aneuploidy is characteristic of malignant parathyroid tissue [25]. Immunohistochemistry performed on malignant parathyroid tissue reveals absence of retinoblastoma (Rb) protein, whereas Rb protein is usually present in benign parathyroid tissue [28]. The coding region for Rb is located on chromosome 13, and loss of this region has been identified in several patients with parathyroid carcinoma. Ki-67, a cell-cycle antigen that serves as a marker of cellular proliferative activity, demonstrates more intense immunohistochemical staining in malignant than benign parathyroid tumors [29]. The PRAD1 oncogene, which codes for cyclin D1 and is active in cell cycle regulation, has been demonstrated to be overexpressed in patients with parathyroid carcinoma [30]. Most recently, mutations in the tumor suppressor gene HRPT2 have been identified in certain patients with sporadic parathyroid carcinoma [31]. HRPT2 is known to be associated with the familial hyperparathyroidism-jaw tumor syndrome. Mutations of HRPT2 may be early events in parathyroid oncogenesis and may serve as a useful predictor of malignancy in patients with atypical parathyroid tumors. In addition, small-molecule targeted therapies may be designed and utilized for patients with HRPT2 mutations and parathyroid carcinoma.

Management: Operative

The only effective long-term therapy for parathyroid carcinoma is operative resection with complete extirpation of all malignant tissue. When parathyroid carcinoma is suspected from preoperative clinical or biochemical features or intraoperative findings, the recommended operation is en bloc resection of the parathyroid tumor with complete ipsilateral thyroid lobectomy and isthmusectomy; in addition, a complete ipsilateral central neck dissection from the upper mediastinum to the larynx should be performed, with the goal of removing all potential tumor-bearing tissues on the tracheo-esophageal groove [4, 6, 20, 32]. Any structures to which the parathyroid cancer is adherent should be removed in continuity with the primary tumor; capsular disruption should be avoided if at all possible so that tumor recurrence from seeding and parathyromatosis can be prevented. If the recurrent laryngeal nerve is definitively invaded by tumor then it should be sacrificed; however, if the parathyroid cancer is merely abutting the nerve then it can be shaved off of the nerve so that vocal cord function is preserved.

In some cases the diagnosis of parathyroid cancer is made postoperatively on pathologic examination after parathyroidectomy is performed for presumed benign primary hyperparathyroidism. If the patient still has elevated serum calcium or parathyroid hormone, or if the pathology specimen harbors gross capsular or vascular invasion, then the patient should be re-explored, with ipsilateral thyroid lobectomy, central neck lymph node dissection and removal of all potential tumor-bearing tissue of the tracheo-esophageal groove [17, 33]. If the patient is normocalcemic and the pathology reveals only microscopic evidence of parathyroid cancer, then the patient may be followed closely with serial laboratory evaluation of calcium and PTH, supplemented by neck ultrasound to look for recurrence.

Patients who develop local recurrence will benefit from reoperation unless their metabolic state or overall health precludes operation. While definitive cure is rarely achieved in patients with parathyroid cancer, reoperation is intended to provide biochemical and symptomatic palliation. Unfortunately, several authors have noted that the best biochemical results occur after the first one or two reoperations, and that subsequent operations are less effective in lowering calcium and PTH levels [4, 6, 17, 20, 33–35]. Nevertheless, some patients will undergo ten or more total operations over the course of several years before succumbing to the disease. The decision whether to pursue further operation in cases of recurrent parathyroid cancer should be made after in-depth discussion of the goals and expectations of care with the patient and patient's family, as well as the endocrinologist or primary care physician.

Management: Calcium-Lowering Medications/Chemotherapy/ Radiation

While the only definitive treatment for parathyroid carcinoma remains operative resection of hyperfunctioning malignant parathyroid tissue, medical therapy remains a cornerstone of management for patients with severe hypercalcemia prior to operation as well as for patients who have unresectable disease. The treatment of acute hypercalcemia is aimed towards correcting biochemical abnormalities and preventing cardiovascular, renal, and neuromuscular dysfunction. Aggressive volume replacement with saline and repletion of other electrolytes is initiated; once the volume status is normalized then loop diuretics can be administered.

There are several types of medications that function to lower serum calcium. Calcitonin promotes urinary calcium excretion and inhibits osteoclast activity, but is quite short-acting [36]; plicamycin is another osteoclast inhibitor but has multiple gastrointestinal side effects [37]. Bisphosphonates are more potent osteoclast inhibitors and are longer-acting and better tolerated than either calcitonin or plicamycin. Bisphosphonates have been shown to effectively lower serum calcium in patients with parathyroid cancer [38].

The latest calcium-lowering medication to be introduced was cinacalcet (Sensipar), which was approved by the United States FDA in 2004 for the treatment of secondary hyperparathyroidism in chronic kidney disease and hypercalcemia associated with parathyroid cancer. Cinacalcet therapy has transformed the treatment of patients with hypercalcemia from secondary hyperparathyroidism [39]. Several authors have now reported on its use in patients with parathyroid carcinoma [40, 41]. Cinacalcet is a calcimimetic which binds directly to the calcium-sensing receptors of the parathyroid gland and lowers the secretion of parathyroid hormone, with consequent reduction in the serum calcium level. The case reports in the literature of cinacalcet use in parathyroid carcinoma have reported remission periods of up to 3 years with continued treatment [40, 41]. Larger series and more long-term data are pending, but for the present, cinacalcet therapy appears to be the most effective mode of medical therapy for patients with hypercalcemia and unresectable or metastatic parathyroid carcinoma.

Multiple chemotherapy agents have been studied for the treatment of patients with advanced parathyroid carcinoma who are not candidates for operation. These include regimens consisting of dacarbazine alone; dacarbazine, 5-FU, and cyclophosphamide; adriamycin alone; vincristine, cyclophosphamide and actinomycin D [3, 36, 42]. Because of the small number of overall cases of parathyroid carcinoma, virtually all of the experience with chemotherapy treatment of parathyroid carcinoma comes from small series or case reports. Most chemotherapy regimens have had limited effect on controlling either tumor growth or biochemical secretion. The best results obtained come from a case report of an 18-month remission after treatment with methotrexate, doxorubicin, cyclophosphamide, and lomustine [43]. Large-scale trials of chemotherapy for patients with parathyroid carcinoma are probably not feasible given the low incidence of the disease. Recent insights into the genetic basis of parathyroid carcinoma may yield targeted small-molecule therapies for the treatment of this disease.

As parathyroid carcinoma is usually a slow-growing, indolent tumor, radiation therapy is minimally effective in controlling tumor growth or biochemical function in existing recurrent tumor. Small case series have reported some success in controlling future recurrence of the disease after operative resection and adjuvant radiotherapy [4, 20, 32, 44]. This approach may be useful for preventing future recurrence and merits further study; one potential concern with this approach is the increased risk and difficulty of operating in a radiated field in patients who develop recurrence after operation and radiotherapy.

Prognosis/Outcomes

Perhaps because of the lack of agreement on strict pathologic definitions of parathyroid carcinoma, published series from different institutions worldwide vary in terms of patient outcomes and prognosis. Five-year survival rates vary widely, from 46% to 90%, with some authors even questioning whether parathyroid cancer should be considered a lethal disease [45]. Recent data obtained from the SEER database revealed an all-cause 5-year mortality rate of 16% and a 10-year mortality rate of 33% [2]. The National Cancer Database mortality rates were less favorable, with a 10-year overall survival rate of 49% [10]. Swedish Cancer Registry mortality rates were 70% for 10 years [25]. Reports from smaller patient cohorts describe a variety of possible clinical courses for patients diagnosed with parathyroid carcinoma: some patients enjoy lengthy disease-free periods lasting decades (prompting some authors to report "curative" one-stage operations for this disease [32]), while others will recur within weeks to months and undergo multiple reoperations in attempt to control the disease. In patients requiring multiple reoperations to control the disease, the interval of time between recurrences will typically decrease as the disease progresses. The cause of death from parathyroid carcinoma is typically metabolic in nature, with uncontrolled malignant hypercalcemia and its attendant effects on the renal, cardiovascular, and neurologic systems. Recurrence is usually local, with tumor invasion of central neck structures, including the trachea, esophagus, recurrent laryngeal nerve, and the strap muscles. Metastases may occur in the late stages of the disease in the cervical lymph nodes, lungs, liver, and bones (Fig. 7.5).

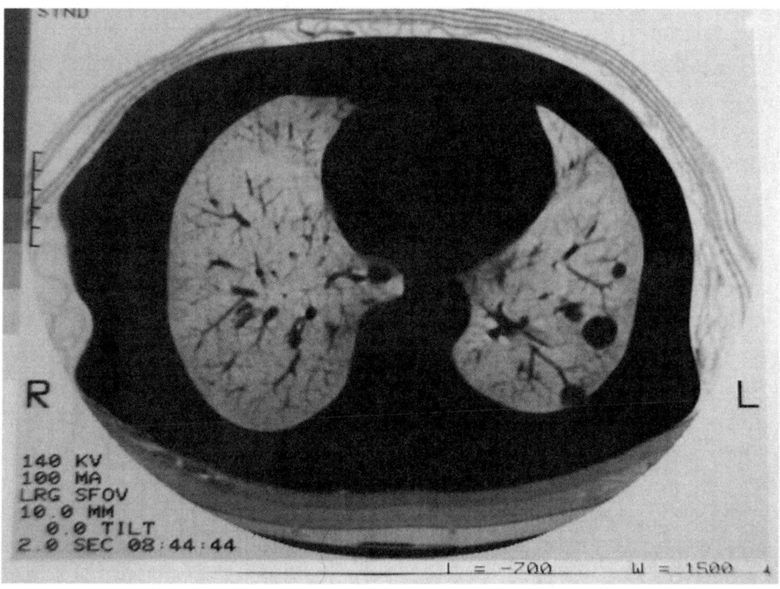

Fig. 7.5 CT scan demonstrating pulmonary metastases of parathyroid carcinoma

Parathyromatosis

Parathyromatosis is defined as the overgrowth of multiple small hyperfunctioning nodules of parathyroid tissue. It is a rare entity that can be difficult to manage. Parathyromatosis may occur as a primary phenomenon, with overgrowth of multiple small embryologically derived parathyroid rests, but this is exceedingly uncommon [46]. Parathyromatosis usually develops after capsular fracture and intraoperative seeding during parathyroid tumor resection. This condition is most frequently reported in patients with secondary hyperparathyroidism who have undergone subtotal or total parathyroidectomy [47]; however, parathyromatosis may occur after capsular fracture of either benign parathyroid adenoma or parathyroid carcinoma in patients with primary hyperparathyroidism [22, 48, 49]. Controversy exists regarding the precise defining features of parathyromatosis and whether this condition represents overgrowth of seeded benign parathyroid tissue or disseminated parathyroid cancer. Recent research efforts have focused on identifying clinical characteristics, histopathologic features, and molecular markers that may distinguish parathyromatosis from parathyroid cancer or atypical benign parathyroid adenoma [22].

The diagnosis of parathyromatosis is made based on the biochemical evidence of parathyroid hyperfunction and either preoperative imaging demonstrating multiple foci of abnormal parathyroid tissue or intraoperative findings of multiple nodules of the parathyroid tissue. Ultrasound is the most accurate preoperative imaging study for identifying parathyromatosis; sonographic findings include multiple hypoechoic or hypervascular nodules that appear atypical for benign lymph nodes or normal parathyroid glands [49]. However, the nodules of parathyromatosis may be too small or too well-incorporated into the surrounding tissues to be detected by ultrasound. Sestamibi scanning will demonstrate abnormal uptake in hyperfunctioning parathyroid tissue, but as with ultrasound, the small size of the nodules seen in parathyromatosis may render them undetectable by Sestamibi scan. However, when positive, preoperative imaging studies can help to guide operative planning, for surgical treatment of this condition.

Parathyromatosis is more frequently diagnosed on neck exploration than on preoperative imaging. The abnormal tissue of parathyromatosis will appear similar to that of solitary parathyroid adenoma, with a beefy red appearance and firm texture; however, the tumor foci typically measure less than 5 mm and will thus be smaller than the usual parathyroid adenoma. In addition, the tumor foci may be incorporated into adjacent tissues such as the strap muscles, and may be difficult to distinguish from the scar tissues from prior operation. The aim of surgical therapy is to remove all hyperfunctioning parathyroid tissue; this may be especially difficult in the reoperative setting when the tumor nodules can be incorporated into scar tissue or surrounding structures and en bloc resection is required. Careful dissection, avoidance of capsular fracture, and preservation of structures such as the recurrent laryngeal nerve are the keys to successful operation. Intraoperative parathyroid hormone measurement can assist in determining whether resection of hyperfunctioning tissue is complete, but is not likely to predict long-term cure since this condition will frequently recur.

References

1. Sandelin K (2005) Parathyroid carcinoma. In: Clark OH (ed) Textbook of endocrine surgery, 2nd edn. Elsevier Saunders, Philadelphia, pp 549–554
2. Lee PK, Jarosek SL, Virnig BA, Evasovich M, Tuttle TM (2007) Trends in the incidence and treatment of parathyroid cancer in the United States. Cancer 109:1736–1741
3. Shane E (2001) Clinical review 122: parathyroid carcinoma. J Clin Endocrinol Metab 86:485–493
4. Busaidy NL, Jimenez C, Habra MA et al (2004) Parathyroid carcinoma: a 22-year experience. Head Neck 26:716–726
5. Kebebew E (2001) Parathyroid carcinoma. Curr Treat Options Oncol 2:347–354
6. Iihara M, Okamoto T, Suzuki R et al (2007) Functional parathyroid carcinoma: long-term treatment outcome and risk factor analysis. Surgery 142:936–943; discussion 43 e1
7. Obara T, Okamoto T, Kanbe M, Iihara M (1997) Functioning parathyroid carcinoma: clinicopathologic features and rational treatment. Semin Surg Oncol 13:134–141
8. Favia G, Lumachi F, Polistina F, D'Amico DF (1998) Parathyroid carcinoma: sixteen new cases and suggestions for correct management. World J Surg 22:1225–1230
9. Iacobone M, Lumachi F, Favia G (2004) Up-to-date on parathyroid carcinoma: analysis of an experience of 19 cases. J Surg Oncol 88:223–228
10. Hundahl SA, Fleming ID, Fremgen AM, Menck HR (1999) Two hundred eighty-six cases of parathyroid carcinoma treated in the U.S. between 1985-1995: a National Cancer Data Base Report. The American College of Surgeons Commission on Cancer and the American Cancer Society. Cancer 86:538–544
11. Kebebew E (2008) Parathyroid carcinoma, a rare but important disorder for endocrinologists, primary care physicians, and endocrine surgeons. Thyroid 18:385–386
12. Fernandez-Ranvier GG, Jensen K, Khanafshar E et al (2007) Nonfunctioning parathyroid carcinoma: case report and review of literature. Endocr Pract 13:750–757
13. Agarwal G, Dhingra S, Mishra SK, Krishnani N (2006) Implantation of parathyroid carcinoma along fine needle aspiration track. Langenbecks Arch Surg 391:623–626
14. Lee JA, Inabnet WB 3rd (2005) The surgeon's armamentarium to the surgical treatment of primary hyperparathyroidism. J Surg Oncol 89:130–135
15. Arici C, Cheah WK, Ituarte PH et al (2001) Can localization studies be used to direct focused parathyroid operations? Surgery 129:720–729
16. Yen TW, Wang TS, Doffek KM, Krzywda EA, Wilson SD (2008) Reoperative parathyroidectomy: an algorithm for imaging and monitoring of intraoperative parathyroid hormone levels that results in a successful focused approach. Surgery 144:611–619; discussion 9–21
17. Kebebew E, Arici C, Duh QY, Clark OH (2001) Localization and reoperation results for persistent and recurrent parathyroid carcinoma. Arch Surg 136:878–885
18. Placzkowski K, Christian R, Chen H (2007) Radioguided parathyroidectomy for recurrent parathyroid cancer. Clin Nucl Med 32:358–360
19. Clark P, Wooldridge T, Kleinpeter K, Perrier N, Lovato J, Morton K (2004) Providing optimal preoperative localization for recurrent parathyroid carcinoma: a combined parathyroid scintigraphy and computed tomography approach. Clin Nucl Med 29:681–684
20. Clayman GL, Gonzalez HE, El-Naggar A, Vassilopoulou-Sellin R (2004) Parathyroid carcinoma: evaluation and interdisciplinary management. Cancer 100:900–905
21. Wiseman SM, Rigual NR, Hicks WL Jr et al (2004) Parathyroid carcinoma: a multicenter review of clinicopathologic features and treatment outcomes. Ear Nose Throat J 83:491–494
22. Fernandez-Ranvier GG, Khanafshar E, Jensen K et al (2007) Parathyroid carcinoma, atypical parathyroid adenoma, or parathyromatosis? Cancer 110:255–264
23. Lumachi F, Basso SM, Basso U (2006) Parathyroid cancer: etiology, clinical presentation and treatment. Anticancer Res 26:4803–4807
24. Chang YJ, Mittal V, Remine S et al (2006) Correlation between clinical and histological findings in parathyroid tumors suspicious for carcinoma. Am Surg 72:419–426
25. Sandelin K, Auer G, Bondeson L, Grimelius L, Farnebo LO (1992) Prognostic factors in parathyroid cancer: a review of 95 cases. World J Surg 16:724–731

26. Kameyama K, Takami H (2005) Proposal for the histological classification of parathyroid carcinoma. Endocr Pathol 16:49–52
27. Stojadinovic A, Hoos A, Nissan A et al (2003) Parathyroid neoplasms: clinical, histopathological, and tissue microarray-based molecular analysis. Hum Pathol 34:54–64
28. Cryns VL, Thor A, Xu HJ et al (1994) Loss of the retinoblastoma tumor-suppressor gene in parathyroid carcinoma. N Engl J Med 330:757–761
29. Farnebo F, Auer G, Farnebo LO et al (1999) Evaluation of retinoblastoma and Ki-67 immunostaining as diagnostic markers of benign and malignant parathyroid disease. World J Surg 23:68–74
30. Tahara H, Smith AP, Gaz RD, Arnold A (1996) Loss of chromosome arm 9p DNA and analysis of the p16 and p15 cyclin-dependent kinase inhibitor genes in human parathyroid adenomas. J Clin Endocrinol Metab 81:3663–3667
31. Shattuck TM, Valimaki S, Obara T et al (2003) Somatic and germ-line mutations of the HRPT2 gene in sporadic parathyroid carcinoma. N Engl J Med 349:1722–1729
32. Kirkby-Bott J, Lewis P, Harmer CL, Smellie WJ (2005) One stage treatment of parathyroid cancer. Eur J Surg Oncol 31:78–83
33. Iacobone M, Ruffolo C, Lumachi F, Favia G (2005) Results of iterative surgery for persistent and recurrent parathyroid carcinoma. Langenbecks Arch Surg 390:385–390
34. Dotzenrath C, Goretzki PE, Sarbia M, Cupisti K, Feldkamp J, Roher HD (2001) Parathyroid carcinoma: problems in diagnosis and the need for radical surgery even in recurrent disease. Eur J Surg Oncol 27:383–389
35. Sheehan JJ, Hill AD, Walsh MF, Crotty TB, McDermott EW, O'Higgins NJ (2001) Parathyroid carcinoma: diagnosis and management. Eur J Surg Oncol 27:321–324
36. Bukowski RM, Sheeler L, Cunningham J, Esselstyn C (1984) Successful combination chemotherapy for metastatic parathyroid carcinoma. Arch Intern Med 144:399–400
37. Bilezikian JP (1992) Management of acute hypercalcemia. N Engl J Med 326:1196–1203
38. Phitayakorn R, McHenry CR (2008) Hyperparathyroid crisis: use of bisphosphonates as a bridge to parathyroidectomy. J Am Coll Surg 206:1106–1115
39. Block GA, Martin KJ, de Francisco AL et al (2004) Cinacalcet for secondary hyperparathyroidism in patients receiving hemodialysis. N Engl J Med 350:1516–1525
40. Szmuilowicz ED, Utiger RD (2006) A case of parathyroid carcinoma with hypercalcemia responsive to cinacalcet therapy. Nat Clin Pract Endocrinol Metab 2:291–296; quiz 7
41. Silverberg SJ, Rubin MR, Faiman C et al (2007) Cinacalcet hydrochloride reduces the serum calcium concentration in inoperable parathyroid carcinoma. J Clin Endocrinol Metab 92:3803–3808
42. Calandra DB, Chejfec G, Foy BK, Lawrence AM, Paloyan E (1984) Parathyroid carcinoma: biochemical and pathologic response to DTIC. Surgery 96:1132–1137
43. Chahinian AP, Holland JF, Nieburgs HE, Marinescu A, Geller SA, Kirschner PA (1981) Metastatic nonfunctioning parathyroid carcinoma: ultrastructural evidence of secretory granules and response to chemotherapy. Am J Med Sci 282:80–84
44. Munson ND, Foote RL, Northcutt RC et al (2003) Parathyroid carcinoma: is there a role for adjuvant radiation therapy? Cancer 98:2378–2384
45. Kleinpeter KP, Lovato JF, Clark PB et al (2005) Is parathyroid carcinoma indeed a lethal disease? Ann Surg Oncol 12:260–266
46. Fitko R, Roth SI, Hines JR, Roxe DM, Cahill E (1990) Parathyromatosis in hyperparathyroidism. Hum Pathol 21:234–237
47. Matsuoka S, Tominaga Y, Sato T et al (2007) Recurrent renal hyperparathyroidism caused by parathyromatosis. World J Surg 31:299–305
48. Kollmorgen CF, Aust MR, Ferreiro JA, McCarthy JT, van Heerden JA (1994) Parathyromatosis: a rare yet important cause of persistent or recurrent hyperparathyroidism. Surgery 116:111–115
49. Tublin ME, Yim JH, Carty SE (2007) Recurrent hyperparathyroidism secondary to parathyromatosis: clinical and imaging findings. J Ultrasound Med 26:847–851

Part III
Adrenal

Chapter 8
Incidentaloma

Jacob Moalem, Insoo Suh, and Quan-Yang Duh

Introduction

Incidentalomas, unsuspected tumors of the adrenal gland that are found during radiographic testing that is done for unrelated causes, are among the most common solid organ tumors. Incidentaloma has a very broad differential diagnosis that spans the spectrum of aggressiveness (Table 8.1). Most incidentalomas are benign and require no intervention, but adrenocortical carcinoma is among the most aggressive cancers in man. Beyond the risk of malignancy, some incidentalomas autonomously oversecrete hormones of the adrenal cortex or medulla, and failure to diagnose and treat these could lead to morbidity and possible mortality for patients.

With the increasing utilization of cross-sectional, sonographic, and other imaging technologies, incidentalomas are likely to be diagnosed even more frequently in the future. Once identified, these tumors must be characterized as hypersecretory or nonhypersecretory, and as benign or malignant (and if malignant, as primary vs. metastatic). Because the majority of incidentalomas are ultimately managed non-surgically, the follow up of incidentalomas is likely to become an even more difficult diagnostic, logistic, and financial challenge for physicians and patients, and for our healthcare system. This chapter will discuss the prevalence, differential diagnosis, and diagnostic and therapeutic strategies for adrenal incidentalomas.

Embryology of the Adrenal Glands

The anatomic and functional division of the adrenal gland into the cortex and medulla recapitulates fetal development of the organ. Aberrant migration results in ectopic adrenal tissue called adrenal rests, which are usually located in the retroperitoneum, broad ligament, ovaries, testes, or inguinal regions [1].

Q.-Y. Duh (✉)
Department of Surgery, Veterans Affairs Medical Center,
University of California, San Francisco, CA, USA
e-mail: quan-yang.duh@va.gov

C. Sturgeon (ed.), *Endocrine Neoplasia*, Cancer Treatment and Research, vol 153,
DOI 10.1007/978-1-4419-0857-5_8, © Springer Science+Business Media, LLC 2010

Table 8.1 The most common incidentally found adrenal tumors and their relative frequency in the literature

Adrenal cortex	
Adenoma	36–94%
Nodular hyperplasia	7–68%
Carcinoma	0–25%
Adrenal medulla	
Pheochromocytoma	0–11%
Ganglioneuroma	0–6%
Metastases	
patients without prior cancer diagnosis	0–21%
patients with known cancer diagnosis	32–73%
Other adrenal masses:	
Cysts	0–22%
Hematoma	0–4%
Lipoma	0–11%
Myelolipoma	7–15%
Pseudoadrenal masses	0–10%

The fetal adrenal cortex matures during the fifth to eighth week of gestation [2]. Cells of the coelomic mesoderm of the urogenital ridge proliferate and form the primitive adrenal cortex. A second layer of mesothelial cells that surround the primitive cortex proliferates 1 week later to form the definitive adult cortex. The cortical tissue separates from the rest of the mesoderm in the eighth week. Differentiation of the cortex into its three distinct zones – the zona glomerulosa, fasciculata, and reticularis – does not occur until the third year of life, and structural maturation is not fully achieved until puberty.

Unlike the mesothelial origins of the cortex, the medulla is derived from ectodermal cells of the neural crest [3]. These cells, termed chromaffin cells because of their yellow-brown staining with chrome salts, are located in the sympathetic ganglion at the level of the celiac plexus. The chromaffin cells migrate toward the adrenal cortex at the seventh week of gestation, and then invade into it along the central vein until the medulla is eventually situated in the inner medial adrenal gland. By late fetal development, the definitive medulla is encapsulated and completely surrounded by the cortex.

Partial fragmentation of the developing adrenal gland can form ectopic adrenal tissue or adrenal rests. Fragmentation appears to be relatively common, as evidenced by a 50% incidence of adrenal rests in newborns; however, they are found in only 1% of adults, implying atrophy and regression of ectopic adrenal tissue during life [4]. All adrenal rests contain cortical tissue from the urogenital ridge, and are usually found along the course of gonadal descent. Rest tissue contains medulla only if the fragmentation event occurred after medullary migration towards the cortex; therefore, rests with medullary tissue are necessarily close to the original position of the main adrenal gland.

Prevalence

First described in the early 1980s [5], the term "incidentaloma" refers to clinically unapparent adrenal tumors that are incidentally discovered by imaging studies that are done for other indications. Large, symptomatic adrenal tumors and tumors that are discovered during the initial or follow up assessment of patients with nonadrenal malignancies are excluded from this definition. The prevalence of incidentaloma ranges from 0.35 to 5% [6], depending on the sensitivity of the radiologic examination and inclusion criteria; thin-cut helical CT scanning and high-resolution MRI regularly identify subcentimeter adrenal lesions that were previously undetectable. Moreover, studies that include a large number of older patients or patients with symptoms that can retrospectively be attributed to their adrenal tumors will report a higher prevalence of incidentalomas, and also have a higher prevalence of metastatic and primary cancer of the adrenal gland.

The large variation in the prevalence of adrenal incidentaloma that is reported by radiologic tests is also reported in autopsy series. Depending on inclusion criteria, the reported prevalence of adrenal tumors is between 1.05% [7] and 32% [8]. Autopsies of hypertensive patients reveal an even higher prevalence of adrenal tumors, as high as 68% in one series [9]. A recent report of pooled autopsy data suggested that the overall prevalence of adrenal tumors is 5.9%. This prevalence increases with age. Adrenal tumors were found in only 0.2% of those younger than 30, but in 6.9% of those older than 70 [10].

Biochemical Evaluation

Independent of their malignant risk, all adrenal tumors must be evaluated for hormonal hypersecretion. Biopsy or manipulation of an unsuspected pheochromocytoma during an operation can cause hemodynamic instability and death (mortality rate as high as 80% in one series [9, 11]). Resection of a cortisol secreting adrenal tumor that was not recognized as such and therefore not treated with perioperative glucocorticoids may lead to postoperative Addisonian crisis, which can be fatal.

Small, radiographically benign-appearing lesions with biochemical hypersecretion should be resected laparoscopically. Suspicion of malignancy or plans for open resection do not obviate the need for biochemical testing. A recent review of seven studies with a total of more than 600 patients with ACC found 65% to have hormonal hypersecretion [12]. Because most adrenocortical cancers (ACCs) are hormonally active and cortisol is frequently elaborated, the patients are at risk for postoperative Addisonian crisis [12].

Pheochromocytoma

While the prevalence of pheochromocytomas in the general population is only 2–8 per million [13], they account for up to 11–23% of incidentalomas [6, 9, 14, 15]. The classic symptoms attributable to pheochromocytoma are the triad of sweating, headaches, and palpitation, but this symptom complex is present in only approximately 40% of patients with an established diagnosis [16, 17]. Partly because pheochromocytomas may be clinically silent [16, 17], up to three-fourths are not diagnosed until after the patients' death [11]. The stimulation of an undiagnosed pheochromocytoma by the induction of anesthesia [18], percutaneous biopsy, or surgery is associated with mortality rates up to 80% [9, 11]. For 10% of all pheochromocytomas, the first manifestation will be pheochromocytoma crisis, because of spontaneous hemorrhage or rupture [16].

Because the consequences of failure to recognize a pheochromocytoma are so dire, this diagnosis must be definitively established or excluded in any patient who has an adrenal mass, irrespective of symptoms or radiographic characteristics. Thus, there has been considerable research to determine which of the multiple biochemical and radiographic tests is best for making the diagnosis.

A recent multicenter cohort study compared all available biochemical (urine and plasma) tests for the diagnosis of pheochromocytoma [19]. The authors concluded that plasma free metanephrines, with sensitivity of 99% and specificity of 89%, was the single best test for the confirmation or exclusion of pheochromocytoma. In their series, the addition of a second diagnostic test did little to improve the diagnostic accuracy in patients with negative plasma metanephrines. They therefore recommended against the utilization of confirmatory tests for most cases. This study formed the basis for the recent recommendations made at the NIH consensus conference that plasma metanephrines alone be used to diagnose pheochromocytoma [20].

Others [13] disagreed. They pointed out the impact of pretest probability (prevalence) in the predictive value of a diagnostic test, and suggested that for the general population, routinely using plasma metanephrines, with its relatively poor specificity, would result in too many false positive tests. They therefore recommended that the plasma metanephrine test be reserved only for situations with high pretest probability of pheochromocytoma (patients with a genetic syndrome, family history, or radiologic features of pheochromocytoma). For the more typical scenario of patients with a clinical suspicion (based upon difficult to control hypertension, palpitations, or a low – attenuation incidentaloma) they suggested that 24-h urinary metanephrines and catecholamines, with significantly higher specificity and minimally lower sensitivity than plasma free metanephrines be used.

On the basis of these studies, our practice is to use plasma metanephrines as a screening test only. When negative, pheochromocytoma is excluded. We confirm positive plasma catecholamine levels using 24 h urine metanephrine measurements. Recently, we studied a group of 10 patients who had an adrenal incidentaloma and borderline-elevated (not more than twice the upper-limit of normal) urine or plasma metanephrine levels [21]. Among this group of completely asymptomatic patients, three (30%) had a pheochromocytoma, highlighting the need for preoperative α-blockade in all patients who have any elevation in metanephrines.

Cushing's

Although ACTH-independent adrenal Cushing's syndrome is rare in the general population [22], studies in specific high-risk subpopulations revealed an unexpectedly high prevalence: In newly diagnosed diabetic patients, poorly controlled diabetic patients, and in obese patients with hypertension, diabetes, or polycystic ovary syndrome, the frequency of Cushing's syndrome was 2–3.3, 1, and 5.8%, respectively [23–25]. Even among patients whose only comorbidity was hypertension, screening studies have found a 0.5–1% prevalence of unsuspected Cushing's syndrome [26, 27].

Biochemical Evaluation

There are a variety of biochemical tests available for the evaluation of patients with suspected Cushing's syndrome, and they are all designed to detect abnormalities in the normal hypothalamic–pituitary–adrenal (HPA) axis. In normal individuals with typical sleep-wake cycles, serum ACTH and cortisol levels begin to rise in the early morning, peak between 7 and 9 AM, and fall to a nadir for the remainder of the day as long as the patient is unstressed or asleep. In these patients, the delivery of large supraphysiologic doses of glucocorticoids will suppress ACTH and cortisol release. On the other hand, patients with Cushing's syndrome have no diurnal variation in ACTH and cortisol release, and their serum cortisol level remains persistently elevated throughout the day [28, 29]. Moreover, cortisol release in these patients is autonomous (either because of a primary adrenal tumor or because of an ACTH-secreting mass), and is not suppressible by low-dose glucocorticoid administration [30].

Serum Cortisol Levels

Because the measurement of serum cortisol is directly affected by albumin and cortisol binding globulin (CBG) levels, this test is prone to false positive and false negative results under a variety of conditions. Birth control pills that contain estrogen increase CBG levels, causing 50% of women taking these medicines to have a falsely elevated cortisol [31]. They should therefore be advised to undergo testing after a 6 week withdrawal, whenever possible [32]. On the other hand, hypoalbuminemic patients (because of malnutrition, critical illness, or the nephrotic syndrome) will have falsely decreased serum cortisol levels [33, 34]. Furthermore, because the degree of hypercortisolism varies in these patients, duplicated testing is recommended to increase the accuracy of the test [22].

Dexamethasone Suppression Test

The dexamethasone suppression test (DST) is the most commonly used test to evaluate patients with suspected Cushing's syndrome. While there are a number of published protocols for the performance and interpretation of the DST [35–38], most clinicians use the overnight (1 mg) test. This is the simplest version of the DST, and involves the oral administration of 1 mg of dexamethasone between 11 PM and midnight, and measuring serum cortisol between 8 and 9 o'clock on the following morning. Because patients with Cushing's syndrome characteristically manifest variable degrees of suppression in response to dexamethasone administration, some researchers have recommended that a low threshold (postsuppression cortisol level <1.8 μg/dl) be used to enhance the sensitivity of the test [22, 38].

Some endocrinologists prefer the 48 h, 2 mg/d (low dose) DST because of its improved specificity over the 1 mg test [22]. This exam can be administered in the outpatient setting; the patient takes 0.5 mg of dexamethasone every 6 h for 2 days, and the final serum cortisol level is measured 6 h after the last dose. As in the 1 mg test, a postsuppression cortisol level <1.8 μg/dl is considered a normal response and excludes Cushing's syndrome.

Urinary Free Cortisol Levels

Unlike serum cortisol measurements, urinary free cortisol (UFC) measurements are unaffected by patients' CBG or albumin levels. Measured over a 24 h period, UFC provides an integrated measurement of the patient's daily cortisol secretion. Falsely low measurements of UFC occur in patients whose creatinine clearance is less than 60 ml/min [39], and elevated UFC measurements are seen in patients with excessive (more than 5 l/day) fluid intake [40], or in patients with other conditions that are known to increase cortisol levels such as pregnancy, depression, alcoholism, morbid obesity, or poorly controlled diabetes [22].

To optimize this test's reliability, patients should be carefully instructed to avoid all glucocorticoid-containing medications during the collection period, and to avoid excessive fluid intake. In addition, the collection should begin with an empty bladder, excluding the first morning's void, and include all subsequent voids for the next 24 h including the first morning void of the second day. During the test period, the specimen should be refrigerated. The test should be duplicated to increase its accuracy, particularly in children [22].

Late Night Salivary Cortisol Level

This test is usually performed at midnight on two consecutive nights, and relies on the fact that in Cushing's syndrome there is an absence of the normal late night cortisol nadir. Free serum cortisol rapidly (within a few minutes) equilibrates with salivary cortisol [41]. Saliva is collected either actively while the patient chews on a salivette, or passively. The finding of elevated midnight salivary cortisol is consistent with the loss of diurnal variation in cortisol levels that is seen in Cushing's syndrome. There are many assays for the measurement of salivary cortisol, the ELISA- and mass spectrometry (LC-MS/MS)-based tests are best validated, and are the most commonly used [22]. With a sensitivity and specificity between 92 and 100% for the detection of Cushing's syndrome, late night salivary cortisol has similar accuracy to UFC [42] and is commonly used in children. This test's accuracy may be decreased in critically ill patients, patients in whom the circadian rhythm is blunted, and in elderly men, smokers, or heavy drinkers [22].

Aldosteronoma

Primary hyperaldosteronism is the most frequent cause of secondary hypertension, and when due to a unilateral aldosterone producing adenoma is curable or improved by adrenalectomy. Among all hypertensive patients, the prevalence of aldosteronoma was estimated to be approximately 1% [43]. More recent reports suggest that the true prevalence of aldosteronoma is far higher than initially thought, even among normokalemic patients [44]. Among patients with incidentaloma, however, aldosteronoma is a relatively infrequent diagnosis: aldosteronoma accounted for only 1.4% of tumors in a recent series of more than 1,000 incidentalomas [45]. This low frequency is likely due to patient selection, as most aldosteronomas are discovered as part of a workup for hypertension, and even very small and barely detectable aldosteronomas can cause significant hypertension and hypokalemia.

While the hallmark of primary hyperaldosteronism (Conn's disease) is hypertension and hypokalemia, hypokalemia is not necessary for the diagnosis: Dr. Conn himself described a large number of patients with normokalemia in the setting of an aldosteronoma [46, 47], and there are even reports of normotensive patients with primary hyperaldosteronism [48]. Nevertheless, the absence of hypertension essentially rules out the presence of an aldosterone secreting tumor, and most endocrinologists do not recommend biochemical workup to exclude aldosteronoma if the patient is normotensive [9, 14].

The biochemical test with the highest sensitivity and specificity for identifying patients with primary hyperaldosteronism is the measurement of the urinary or plasma aldosterone excretion rate during salt loading, where a rate greater than 14 μg/24 h is diagnostic [49]. A simpler test that is more commonly used is the plasma aldosterone concentration (PAC)/plasma renin activity (PRA) ratio which, if greater than 30, is highly suggestive of aldosteronoma [50]. Drugs such as beta blockers and antisympathetic medications can lower renin, and thereby falsely elevate the PAC/PRA ratio, and may lead to false-positive results [51]. Some authors [6, 14, 51] advocate liberal use of a confirmatory test (such as the saline suppression test), to verify the diagnosis. In patients with aldosteronoma, serum aldosterone level should not decrease in response to the infusion of 2 l of normal saline.

Aldosteronomas are typically solitary and small (most are smaller than 2 cm), but larger tumors are occasionally seen. Malignant mineralocorticoid-secreting tumors of the adrenal have been reported [52], but pure mineralocorticoid-secreting tumors are exceedingly rare, as most adrenal cancers also hypersecrete glucocorticoid, and these tumors are typically large and locally invasive.

Some controversy exists as to the necessity of routine adrenal vein sampling (AVS) to confirm unilateral hypersecretion (adenoma instead of hyperplasia) in patients with a unilateral solitary adrenal mass. AVS is only used in patients with an established biochemical diagnosis of primary hyperaldosteronism and is specifically for discriminating bilateral adrenal hyperplasia from unilateral aldosterone producing adenoma. AVS is not used to confirm the diagnosis of primary hyperaldosteronism. Some authors view AVS as the gold standard localization test and advocate liberal use of this test prior to adrenalectomy [53, 54]. Others [55] report excellent surgical outcomes when a single unilateral adrenal lesion (larger than 1 cm) is resected in patients with biochemically proven primary hyperaldosteronism. Those who advocate selective use of AVS reserve AVS for patients with primary hyperaldosteronism who have questionable findings on CT, such as bilateral adrenal nodules, no adrenal abnormality identified, or the adrenal tumor smaller than 1.0 cm. Using these criteria, about 30% of patients will require AVS and, as a group, 95% of patients with hyperaldosteronism will improve after adrenalectomy.

Radiographic Evaluation

Because of its widespread use, CT scanning is the most common radiographic test that leads to the discovery of an incidentaloma [56]. Irrespective of the imaging modality used, the most common tumor characteristic that has been used to differentiate ACC from other benign or malignant tumors of the adrenal gland is size. A recent review from the SEER database [57] demonstrated that the mean size of malignant adrenal tumors was significantly larger than the mean size of benign adrenal tumors (11.2 ± 5.4 vs. 4.2 ± 1.9 cm). Overall, ACC accounts for 5% of all incidentalomas found [58]. When stratified by size, ACC accounts for less than 2% of all adrenal tumors that are smaller than 4 cm, 6% of those 4.1–6 cm, and 25% of those larger than 6 cm. Conversely, benign cortical adenomas account for 65% of all incidentalomas smaller than 4 cm, and only 18% of incidentalomas larger than 6 cm [20].

Because there is significant overlap in the size distribution of benign and malignant adrenal tumors, no sharp diagnostic size cutoff exists: ACC's smaller than 2 cm have been described [57], but lowering the cutoff for resection of adrenal tumors to 4 cm to maximize sensitivity would lower specificity to 52%. Conversely, choosing a higher size cutoff (≥8 cm) would improve specificity to 95%, but would markedly diminish sensitivity to 79% [57].

Other radiologic features that are highly suggestive of malignancy include the presence of local invasion, regional lymphadenopathy, or tumor metastases. When present, these findings should prompt expeditious open resection.

CT Scan

Beyond morphologic features that may suggest the presence of ACC, there has been much interest as to whether CT scanning could accurately provide the exact diagnosis of an incidentally discovered adrenal tumor. Much of this research relies upon differences in cellular water and lipid content among the various tumors of the adrenal gland.

Benign adrenal adenomas, in contrast to cancers, commonly have high intracellular lipid content, and therefore lower attenuation by unenhanced CT [59], and a less - bright appearance on T2-weighted MRI images [60]. In a recent metaanalysis, Boland [56] reviewed 10 studies that evaluated the ability of unenhanced CT scan to differentiate between 272 benign adenomas and 223 malignant lesions. When a threshold of 10 Hounsfield Units (HU) was applied, unenhanced CT had sensitivity and specificity of 71% and 98% for the diagnosis of cancer. In a later series [59], the attenuation values averaged 8 HU for adenomas and 68.6 HU for other lesions. Thus, most authorities agree that an enhancement value of 10 HU or less (on a noncontrast CT) is diagnostic of a benign adrenal adenoma, and that no further radiologic diagnostic workup is necessary [61–63]. Nevertheless, annual screening for subclinical Cushing's is still recommended.

Unfortunately, the ability of unenhanced CT to differentiate the nonadenomatous adrenal lesions by attenuation value alone is poor, as mean enhancement values of ACC, pheochromocytoma, and metastasis from nonadrenal cancer are 39, 44, and 34 HU, respectively, and have significant overlap. Moreover, because up to 40% of benign adrenal adenomas are lipid-poor [64], these cannot be differentiated from nonadenomas by noncontrast CT. In addition, some (relatively rare) fatty tumors can metastasize to or originate from the adrenal glands; these might be confused with benign adenomas.

Interestingly, adding IV contrast does little to improve the ability of CT to segregate adrenal neoplasms [59], because both adenomas and nonadenomas demonstrate rapid enhancement. A recent study demonstrated that 60 s post injection, mean enhancement values for adenomas, ACCs, pheochromocytomas, and metastatic lesions were 60, 83, 94, and 81 HU. Fifteen minutes later, the enhancement values were 32, 72, 83, and 66. These findings confirmed those from an earlier report [63], which demonstrated that while both adenomas and nonadenomas had rapid enhancement following contrast administration, nonadenomas have a longer washout phase than adenomas. As a result, adenomas have a faster washout (percent loss of enhancement compared to initial enhancement) [59]. As all nonadenomas have similar retention of IV contrast, the loss of enhancement ratio alone cannot discriminate these tumors [59].

A more recent study was conducted to assess whether the combination of unenhanced CT and enhancement ratios obtained from contrast-enhanced CT could improve the diagnostic accuracy of adrenal lesions [62]. Using a dedicated adrenal CT scanning protocol that combined unenhanced and enhanced CT scans, the authors were able to correctly diagnose 124 of 127 cortical adenomas and 36 of 39 nonadenomas. In this study, adenomas were diagnosed if they had attenuation values of 10 HU or less on noncontrast CT, or if they had greater than 60% enhancement washout at 15 min postinjection.

A proposed algorithm [64] is to begin the evaluation with a noncontrast CT scan, and if the attenuation value of the adrenal mass is less than 10 HU, the diagnosis of adenoma is made. In all other cases, IV contrast is administered and the scan is repeated at 1 and 15 min intervals. Enhancement washout calculations are then performed; if the absolute enhancement ratio is greater than 60%, the lesion is characterized as an adenoma. If the enhancement ratio is less than 60%, additional testing is recommended.

Adrenal masses that contain grossly visible fatty components (attenuation values of −30 HU) can be definitively diagnosed as myelolipomas [62]. Unless symptomatic, these lesions may be safely observed and require no specific treatment.

MRI

MRI also utilizes differences in intracellular lipid and water content to differentiate adrenal tumors. Pheochromocytomas, ACC's, and metastases have higher water content than adenomas, so they appear brighter on T2-weighted images. By standardizing the signal intensity of the adrenal tumor to the intensity of the liver, Reining et al. [60] demonstrated that three subsets of adrenal tumors exist. Pheochromocytomas had the highest adrenal/liver signal intensity ratios, other tumors, especially cancers (ACC and metastases), had intermediate intensity ratios, and adenomas had the lowest intensity ratios.

Unfortunately, while pheochromocytomas could be definitively diagnosed by MRI (all had intensity ratios greater than 3.4, and no other tumor had a ratio greater than 2.7), the differentiation between adenoma and cancer was less conclusive. All adrenal masses with intensity ratios between 1.4 and 2.6 were malignant (metastases), and all adrenal masses with intensity ratios less than 1.2 were adenomas. However, 21% of the nonpheochromocytoma adrenal masses had an adrenal/liver intensity ratio in the indeterminate range between 1.2 and 1.4, and could not be definitively diagnosed by these criteria [65]. In these cases, if the patient had a known extra-adrenal primary cancer, its appearance on the T2 image was compared with that of the adrenal tumor. An adrenal tumor that appeared less bright than the known extraadrenal cancer was considered more likely to be an adenoma.

PET Scan

Unlike CT and MRI, which attempt to differentiate adrenal lesions on the basis of histology (water and fat content), positron emission tomography (PET) scanning differentiates lesions on the basis of their glucose metabolism. Malignant lesions and pheochromocytomas are characterized by their high metabolic rates, which cause increased fluorodeoxyglucose (FDG) uptake and bright appearance on PET scan (high standardized uptake value; SUV). Pheochromocytomas, in turn, are readily diagnosed by biochemical testing.

Many studies have evaluated the ability of FDG-PET to differentiate between benign and malignant adrenal lesions in patients with a history of cancer. These have reported a sensitivity close to 100% and specificity ranging between 80 and 100% [66]. A recent prospective study broadened the scope, and looked at the ability of PET scanning to differentiate benign from malignant tumors in patients without biochemical hypersecretion or a recent (5 year) history of malignancy: [67] In 41 adrenal incidentalomas, PET scan had a 100% sensitivity and negative predictive value, and was 86% specific.

Operative Approach

Since the introduction of laparoscopic adrenalectomy [68], there have been more than 30 studies (totaling more than 1,600 patients) comparing open vs. laparoscopic adrenalectomy [51]. Although most of these studies were retrospective and some were marred by large variations in methodology and patient selection, it is apparent that laparoscopic surgery is associated with a shortened operative time and postoperative hospital stay, and less blood loss. Excellent results have been reported for laparoscopic surgery in the setting of incidentaloma, aldosteronoma [69], Cushing's [70], pheochromocytoma [16], and metastatic lesions to the adrenal gland [71]. Moreover, some authors have reported excellent results for laparoscopic adrenalectomy in the setting of bilateral disease [70], or large (larger than 6 cm) adrenal tumors [17, 72]. Because the results of laparoscopic surgery are excellent, a prospective comparison study is unlikely to ever be conducted. Studies of less commonly utilized approaches to adrenalectomy (such as posterior open and laparoscopic, robotic, and needlescopic) are also published, but are beyond the scope of this chapter.

Because of early reports of loco-regional and port-site metastasis of ACC following laparoscopic resection, and the soft, friable nature of ACC, laparoscopic adrenalectomy is contraindicated in this setting. Therefore, if preoperative imaging is obvious for ACC (large, locally invasive lesion; retroperitoneal lymphadenopathy), open adrenalectomy should be performed.

Natural History and Long-Term Follow Up

While the workup and management of incidentalomas is fairly well standardized, the extent of follow up for apparently benign, nonhypersecretory adrenal tumors remains controversial. Recommendations vary regarding the interval of biochemical evaluations and radiographic examinations. Some authors suggest that hormonal behavior and size of benign adenomas are unlikely to change [73], while others recommend serial biochemical testing and imaging [74, 75]. Moreover, there is no consensus regarding the duration of follow up.

The Mayo Clinic recently reported a series of 224 patients with incidentaloma who were followed for an average of 7 years [73]. The average tumor size in their cohort was 2 cm, and only 9 of the patients had tumors larger than 4 cm on initial imaging. Ninety one of the patients had a follow-up CT scan (at an average of 49 months), and only four tumors had grown. Although repeat biochemical testing was not routinely done, no patient who was originally euadrenal developed symptoms of adrenal hypersecretion. Moreover, none of the patients developed ACC.

Another recent study, however, reported on 75 patients with incidentaloma who were followed for a mean of 4.6 years with serial imaging and biochemical evaluations. The authors reported that 17 (29%) of the tumors either grew ($n=11$), became hormonally active ($n=3$), or both ($n=3$) [76]. In this cohort, the cumulative risk for mass enlargement or for adrenal hyperfunction was 22.8% and 9.5% at 10 years. The majority of this risk was in the first 3 years after diagnosis, and did not continue to increase substantially after the first 5 years from the diagnosis. Initial tumor larger than 3 cm was predictive of future hyperfunction.

The NIH consensus statement reflects the paucity of data on this subject [20]. Currently, the recommendation is for a single, short interval (6–12 months) CT scan. There are no data to support further radiographic surveillance for lesions that do not change in size. Because the risk for development of adrenal hyperfunction is greatest in lesions larger than 3 cm, and cortisol hypersecretion is the most likely disorder to be diagnosed, our recommendation is to perform an annual 1 mg DST and reserve biochemical testing for pheochromocytoma and aldosteronoma for the rare patients who develop suggestive symptoms.

Patients with a History of Cancer

Patients with a history of cancer who are found to have an adrenal lesion on follow-up imaging are a particularly challenging group. Although these are technically not considered to be incidentalomas, the workup should be conducted in a similar fashion. Even in this selected population, many of the adrenal lesions are benign and nonsecreting [67], but a comprehensive functional evaluation is still necessary. A recent study of a group of 33 patients who had a history of cancer and who underwent adrenalectomy for isolated adrenal masses [77] found 8 (24%) to be pheochromocytomas.

While some authors [9, 10, 20, 51] have suggested fine needle aspiration (FNA) to differentiate benign from malignant adrenal lesions, we believe it is rarely helpful. FNA biopsy of the adrenal gland is associated with an up to 50% nondiagnostic rate, and excluding these, its sensitivity rate is only about 80% [51]. FNA of a pheochromocytoma is dangerous; FNA of a cortical tumor cannot reliably distinguish adenoma from carcinoma, and FNA of ACC risks tumor seeding. Moreover,

FNA is associated with a variety of complications, including pneumothorax or hemothorax, fever and bacteremia, adrenal, renal, and hepatic hematomas, hypotension, and pain. PET scanning is more accurate in differentiating benign from malignant lesions without the associated risks in patients with a history of nonadrenal cancer.

References

1. Barwick TD, Malhotra A, Webb JA, Savage MO, Reznek RH (2005) Embryology of the adrenal glands and its relevance to diagnostic imaging. Clin Radiol 60(9):953–959
2. Langman J, Sadler TW (1995) Langman's medical embryology, 7th edn. Williams & Wilkins, Baltimore
3. Avisse C, Marcus C, Patey M, Ladam-Marcus V, Delattre JF, Flament JB (2000) Surgical anatomy and embryology of the adrenal glands. Surg Clin North Am 80(1):403–415
4. Souverijns G, Peene P, Keuleers H, Vanbockrijck M (2000) Ectopic localisation of adrenal cortex. Eur Radiol 10(7):1165–1168
5. Geelhoed GW, Druy EM (1982) Management of the adrenal "incidentaloma". Surgery 92(5):866–874
6. Mantero F, Arnaldi G (2000) Management approaches to adrenal incidentalomas. A view from Ancona, Italy. Endocrinol Metab Clin North Am 29(1):107–125, ix
7. Kokko JP, Brown TC, Berman MM (1967) Adrenal adenoma and hypertension. Lancet 1(7488):468–470
8. Dobbie JW (1969) Adrenocortical nodular hyperplasia: the ageing adrenal. J Pathol 99(1):1–18
9. Kloos RT, Gross MD, Francis IR, Korobkin M, Shapiro B (1995) Incidentally discovered adrenal masses. Endocr Rev 16(4):460–484
10. Thompson GB, Young WF Jr (2003) Adrenal incidentaloma. Curr Opin Oncol 15(1):84–90
11. Sutton MG, Sheps SG, Lie JT (1981) Prevalence of clinically unsuspected pheochromocytoma. Review of a 50-year autopsy series. Mayo Clin Proc 56(6):354–360
12. Ng L, Libertino JM (2003) Adrenocortical carcinoma: diagnosis, evaluation and treatment. J Urol 169(1):5–11
13. Kudva YC, Sawka AM, Young WF Jr (2003) Clinical review 164: The laboratory diagnosis of adrenal pheochromocytoma: the Mayo Clinic experience. J Clin Endocrinol Metab 88(10):4533–4539
14. Brunt LM, Moley JF (2001) Adrenal incidentaloma. World J Surg 25(7):905–913
15. Aso Y, Homma Y (1992) A survey on incidental adrenal tumors in Japan. J Urol 147(6):1478–1481
16. Cheah WK, Clark OH, Horn JK, Siperstein AE, Duh QY (2002) Laparoscopic adrenalectomy for pheochromocytoma. World J Surg 26(8):1048–1051
17. Kebebew E, Siperstein AE, Clark OH, Duh QY (2002) Results of laparoscopic adrenalectomy for suspected and unsuspected malignant adrenal neoplasms. Arch Surg 137(8):948–951; discussion 952–943
18. Hartley L, Perry-Keene D (1985) Phaeochromocytoma in Queensland – 1970–83. Aust NZ J Surg 55(5):471–475
19. Lenders JW, Pacak K, Walther MM et al (2002) Biochemical diagnosis of pheochromocytoma: which test is best? JAMA 287(11):1427–1434
20. Grumbach MM, Biller BM, Braunstein GD et al (2003) Management of the clinically inapparent adrenal mass ("incidentaloma"). Ann Intern Med 138(5):424–429
21. Lee JA, Zarnegar R, Shen WT, Kebebew E, Clark OH, Duh QY (2007) Adrenal incidentaloma, borderline elevations of urine or plasma metanephrine levels, and the "subclinical" pheochromocytoma. Arch Surg 142(9):870–873; discussion 873–874

22. Nieman LK, Biller BM, Findling JW et al (2008) The diagnosis of Cushing's syndrome: an endocrine society clinical practice guideline. J Clin Endocrinol Metab 93(5):1526–1540
23. Catargi B, Rigalleau V, Poussin A et al (2003) Occult Cushing's syndrome in type-2 diabetes. J Clin Endocrinol Metab 88(12):5808–5813
24. Reimondo G, Pia A, Allasino B et al (2007) Screening of Cushing's syndrome in adult patients with newly diagnosed diabetes mellitus. Clin Endocrinol (Oxf) 67(2):225–229
25. Ness-Abramof R, Nabriski D, Apovian CM et al (2002) Overnight dexamethasone suppression test: a reliable screen for Cushing's syndrome in the obese. Obes Res 10(12):1217–1221
26. Anderson GH Jr, Blakeman N, Streeten DH (1994) The effect of age on prevalence of secondary forms of hypertension in 4429 consecutively referred patients. J Hypertens 12(5):609–615
27. Omura M, Saito J, Yamaguchi K, Kakuta Y, Nishikawa T (2004) Prospective study on the prevalence of secondary hypertension among hypertensive patients visiting a general outpatient clinic in Japan. Hypertens Res 27(3):193–202
28. Glass AR, Zavadil AP III, Halberg F, Cornelissen G, Schaaf M (1984) Circadian rhythm of serum cortisol in Cushing's disease. J Clin Endocrinol Metab 59(1):161–165
29. Refetoff S, Van Cauter E, Fang VS, Laderman C, Graybeal ML, Landau RL (1985) The effect of dexamethasone on the 24-hour profiles of adrenocorticotropin and cortisol in Cushing's syndrome. J Clin Endocrinol Metab 60(3):527–535
30. Orth DN (1995) Cushing's syndrome. N Engl J Med 332(12):791–803
31. Nickelsen T, Lissner W, Schoffling K (1989) The dexamethasone suppression test and long-term contraceptive treatment: measurement of ACTH or salivary cortisol does not improve the reliability of the test. Exp Clin Endocrinol 94(3):275–280
32. Qureshi AC, Bahri A, Breen LA et al (2007) The influence of the route of oestrogen administration on serum levels of cortisol-binding globulin and total cortisol. Clin Endocrinol (Oxf) 66(5):632–635
33. Klose M, Lange M, Rasmussen AK et al (2007) Factors influencing the adrenocorticotropin test: role of contemporary cortisol assays, body composition, and oral contraceptive agents. J Clin Endocrinol Metab 92(4):1326–1333
34. Hamrahian AH, Oseni TS, Arafah BM (2004) Measurements of serum free cortisol in critically ill patients. N Engl J Med 350(16):1629–1638
35. Liddle GW (1960) Tests of pituitary–adrenal suppressibility in the diagnosis of Cushing's syndrome. J Clin Endocrinol Metab 20:1539–1560
36. Pecori Giraldi F, Pivonello R, Ambrogio AG et al (2007) The dexamethasone-suppressed corticotropin-releasing hormone stimulation test and the desmopressin test to distinguish Cushing's syndrome from pseudo-Cushing's states. Clin Endocrinol (Oxf) 66(2):251–257
37. Invitti C, Pecori Giraldi F, de Martin M, Cavagnini F (1999) Diagnosis and management of Cushing's syndrome: results of an Italian multicentre study. Study Group of the Italian Society of Endocrinology on the Pathophysiology of the Hypothalamic–Pituitary–Adrenal Axis. J Clin Endocrinol Metab 84(2):440–448
38. Wood PJ, Barth JH, Freedman DB, Perry L, Sheridan B (1997) Evidence for the low dose dexamethasone suppression test to screen for Cushing's syndrome – recommendations for a protocol for biochemistry laboratories. Ann Clin Biochem 34(Pt 3):222–229
39. Chan KC, Lit LC, Law EL et al (2004) Diminished urinary free cortisol excretion in patients with moderate and severe renal impairment. Clin Chem 50(4):757–759
40. Mericq MV, Cutler GB Jr (1998) High fluid intake increases urine free cortisol excretion in normal subjects. J Clin Endocrinol Metab 83(2):682–684
41. Read GF, Walker RF, Wilson DW, Griffiths K (1990) Steroid analysis in saliva for the assessment of endocrine function. Ann N Y Acad Sci 595:260–274
42. Elamin MB, Murad MH, Mullan R et al (2008) Accuracy of diagnostic tests for Cushing's syndrome: a systematic review and metaanalyses. J Clin Endocrinol Metab 93(5):1553–1562
43. Melby JC (1985) Diagnosis and treatment of primary aldosteronism and isolated hypoaldosteronism. Clin Endocrinol Metab 14(4):977–995

44. Gordon RD, Stowasser M, Tunny TJ, Klemm SA, Rutherford JC (1994) High incidence of primary aldosteronism in 199 patients referred with hypertension. Clin Exp Pharmacol Physiol 21(4):315–318
45. Mantero F, Terzolo M, Arnaldi G et al (2000) A survey on adrenal incidentaloma in Italy. Study Group on Adrenal Tumors of the Italian Society of Endocrinology. J Clin Endocrinol Metab 85(2):637–644
46. Conn JW (1967) Diagnosis of Normokalemic primary aldosteronism, a new form of curable hypertension. Science 158(3800):525–526
47. Conn JW, Cohen EL, Rovner DR, Nesbit RM (1965) Normokalemic primary aldosteronism. A detectable cause of curable "essential" hypertension. JAMA 193:200–206
48. Vantyghem MC, Ronci N, Provost F et al (1999) Aldosterone-producing adenoma without hypertension: a report of two cases. Eur J Endocrinol 141(3):279–285
49. Bravo EL (1994) Primary aldosteronism. Issues in diagnosis and management. Endocrinol Metab Clin North Am 23(2):271–283
50. Young WF Jr, Hogan MJ, Klee GG, Grant CS, van Heerden JA (1990) Primary aldosteronism: diagnosis and treatment. Mayo Clin Proc 65(1):96–110
51. Mansmann G, Lau J, Balk E, Rothberg M, Miyachi Y, Bornstein SR (2004) The clinically inapparent adrenal mass: update in diagnosis and management. Endocr Rev 25(2):309–340
52. Weingartner K, Gerharz EW, Bittinger A, Rosai J, Leppek R, Riedmiller H (1995) Isolated clinical syndrome of primary aldosteronism in a patient with adrenocortical carcinoma. Case report and review of the literature. Urol Int 55(4):232–235
53. Doppman JL, Gill JR Jr (1996) Hyperaldosteronism: sampling the adrenal veins. Radiology 198(2):309–312
54. Young WF, Stanson AW, Thompson GB, Grant CS, Farley DR, van Heerden JA (2004) Role for adrenal venous sampling in primary aldosteronism. Surgery 136(6):1227–1235
55. Zarnegar R, Bloom AI, Lee J et al (2008) Is adrenal venous sampling necessary in all patients with hyperaldosteronism before adrenalectomy? J Vasc Interv Radiol 19(1):66–71
56. Boland GW, Lee MJ, Gazelle GS, Halpern EF, McNicholas MM, Mueller PR (1998) Characterization of adrenal masses using unenhanced CT: an analysis of the CT literature. AJR Am J Roentgenol 171(1):201–204
57. Sturgeon C, Shen WT, Clark OH, Duh QY, Kebebew E (2006) Risk assessment in 457 adrenal cortical carcinomas: how much does tumor size predict the likelihood of malignancy? J Am Coll Surg 202(3):423–430
58. Terzolo M, Ali A, Osella G, Mazza E (1997) Prevalence of adrenal carcinoma among incidentally discovered adrenal masses. A retrospective study from 1989 to 1994. Gruppo Piemontese Incidentalomi Surrenalici. Arch Surg 132(8):914–919
59. Szolar DH, Korobkin M, Reittner P et al (2005) Adrenocortical carcinomas and adrenal pheochromocytomas: mass and enhancement loss evaluation at delayed contrast-enhanced CT. Radiology 234(2):479–485
60. Reinig JW, Doppman JL, Dwyer AJ, Frank J (1986) MRI of indeterminate adrenal masses. AJR Am J Roentgenol 147(3):493–496
61. Caoili EM, Korobkin M, Francis IR, Cohan RH, Dunnick NR (2000) Delayed enhanced CT of lipid-poor adrenal adenomas. AJR Am J Roentgenol 175(5):1411–1415
62. Caoili EM, Korobkin M, Francis IR et al (2002) Adrenal masses: characterization with combined unenhanced and delayed enhanced CT. Radiology 222(3):629–633
63. Korobkin M, Brodeur FJ, Francis IR, Quint LE, Dunnick NR, Londy F (1998) CT time-attenuation washout curves of adrenal adenomas and nonadenomas. AJR Am J Roentgenol 170(3):747–752
64. Al-Hawary MM, Francis IR, Korobkin M (2005) Non-invasive evaluation of the incidentally detected indeterminate adrenal mass. Best Pract Res Clin Endocrinol Metab 19(2):277–292
65. Reinig JW, Doppman JL, Dwyer AJ, Johnson AR, Knop RH (1986) Adrenal masses differentiated by MR. Radiology 158(1):81–84
66. Yun M, Kim W, Alnafisi N, Lacorte L, Jang S, Alavi A (2001) 18F-FDG PET in characterizing adrenal lesions detected on CT or MRI. J Nucl Med 42(12):1795–1799

67. Tessonnier L, Sebag F, Palazzo FF et al (2008) Does (18)F-FDG PET/CT add diagnostic accuracy in incidentally identified non-secreting adrenal tumours? Eur J Nucl Med Mol Imaging (11):2018–2025
68. Gagner M, Lacroix A, Prinz RA et al (1993) Early experience with laparoscopic approach for adrenalectomy. Surgery 114(6):1120–1124; discussion 1124–1125
69. Shen WT, Lim RC, Siperstein AE et al (1999) Laparoscopic vs open adrenalectomy for the treatment of primary hyperaldosteronism. Arch Surg 134(6):628–631; discussion 631–622
70. Fernandez-Cruz L, Saenz A, Benarroch G, Astudillo E, Taura P, Sabater L (1996) Laparoscopic unilateral and bilateral adrenalectomy for Cushing's syndrome. Transperitoneal and retroperitoneal approaches. Ann Surg 224(6):727–734; discussion 734–726
71. Duh QY (2007) Laparoscopic adrenalectomy for isolated adrenal metastasis: the right thing to do and the right way to do it. Ann Surg Oncol 14(12):3288–3289
72. Henry JF, Sebag F, Iacobone M, Mirallie E (2002) Results of laparoscopic adrenalectomy for large and potentially malignant tumors. World J Surg 26(8):1043–1047
73. Barry MK, van Heerden JA, Farley DR, Grant CS, Thompson GB, Ilstrup DM (1998) Can adrenal incidentalomas be safely observed? World J Surg 22(6):599–603; discussion 603–594
74. Jockenhovel F, Kuck W, Hauffa B et al (1992) Conservative and surgical management of incidentally discovered adrenal tumors (incidentalomas). J Endocrinol Invest 15(5):331–337
75. Staren ED, Prinz RA (1995) Selection of patients with adrenal incidentalomas for operation. Surg Clin North Am 75(3):499–509
76. Barzon L, Scaroni C, Sonino N, Fallo F, Paoletta A, Boscaro M (1999) Risk factors and long-term follow-up of adrenal incidentalomas. J Clin Endocrinol Metab 84(2):520–526
77. Adler JT, Mack E, Chen H (2007) Isolated adrenal mass in patients with a history of cancer: remember pheochromocytoma. Ann Surg Oncol 14(8):2358–2362

Chapter 9
Pheochromocytoma and Paraganglioma

Goswin Y. Meyer-Rochow and Stan B. Sidhu

Introduction

Pheochromocytomas and extra-adrenal sympathetic paragangliomas are catecholamine-secreting neuroendocrine tumors derived from the chromaffin cells of the embryonic neural crest. Parasympathetic paragangliomas are related tumors which most often arise within the head and neck, and are anatomically associated with the parasympathetic nervous system. Patients with pheochromocytomas and extra-adrenal sympathetic paragangliomas generally present with symptoms resulting from excessive production and secretion of catecholamines whereas parasympathetic paragangliomas usually present as a solitary and progressively enlarging mass without catecholamine secretion.

The greatest recent development with regard to the management of pheochromocytoma and paraganglioma is undoubtedly the discovery of the hereditable germline mutations responsible for the familial syndromes associated with these tumors. A number of pheochromocytoma/paraganglioma susceptibility genes have now been identified, providing further insights into molecular pathways involved in pheochromocytoma/paraganglioma oncogenesis.

Because of the unique nature and specific management required for the treatment of catecholamine-producing tumors, aspects of clinical management in this chapter will focus on pheochromocytoma and extra-adrenal sympathetic paraganglioma.

Nomenclature

Pheochromocytomas and paragangliomas are tumors that occur within the neural crest-derived clusters of neuroendocrine cells known as paraganglia. These tumors can be further classified by anatomical location, autonomic system derivation, and

S.B. Sidhu (✉)
Department of Endocrine and Oncology Surgery, Royal North Shore Hospital,
St Leonards, NSW, 2065, Australia
e-mail: stansidhu@nebsc.com.au

C. Sturgeon (ed.), *Endocrine Neoplasia*, Cancer Treatment and Research, vol 153,
DOI 10.1007/978-1-4419-0857-5_9, © Springer Science+Business Media, LLC 2010

Adrenal medullary tumours
Malignant pheochromocytoma
Benign pheochromocytoma
Composite pheochromocytoma/paraganglioma

Extra-adrenal paraganglioma
Extra-adrenal sympathetic paraganglioma
Extra-adrenal parasympathetic paraganglioma
- Carotid body
- Jugulotympanic
- Vagal
- Laryngeal
- Aortico-pulmonary
- Gangliocytic
- Cauda equina
- Orbital
- Nasopharangeal
- Superior and inferior para-aortic paraganglioma

Fig. 9.1 WHO histological classification of adrenal medullary tumors and extra-adrenal paragangliomas

endocrine function with respect to catecholamine production. Historically, the term pheochromocytoma is derived from the color change that occurs when tumor tissue is treated with a chromate salt solution, which is seen with both intra- and extra-adrenal sympathetic paragangliomas (i.e., chromaffin tumors), whereas tumors derived from parasympathetic ganglia are negative for the chromaffin reaction (i.e., nonchromaffin tumors).

The World Health Organization (WHO) Classification of Tumours, updated in 2004, has proposed a classification to define these tumors according to their anatomical location (intra- or extra-adrenal paragangliomas), and whether they are sympathetic- or parasympathetic-derived (Fig. 9.1). Extra-adrenal parasympathetic paragangliomas are further defined by anatomical site of origin and it is suggested that the term pheochromocytoma be reserved only for sympathetic intra-adrenal paragangliomas [1]. The nomenclature in the literature, however, remains inconsistent and many clinicians still prefer to refer to functional intra- and extra-adrenal sympathetic paragangliomas collectively as pheochromocytomas as the presentation and clinical management of the catecholamine-secreting tumors are very similar.

In this chapter, the WHO classification will generally be adhered to, however unless specified, the term pheochromocytomas will be used to collectively describe intra- and extra-adrenal sympathetic paragangliomas.

Epidemiology

Population-based studies suggest that the annual incidence of pheochromocytoma is between 2 and 9 per million [2–4], however, this appears to be an underestimation as the prevalence of pheochromocytoma in autopsy studies is 0.05% [5, 6], suggesting that many tumors are either clinically silent or are not being diagnosed premortem. In patients with secondary hypertension, the prevalence of pheochromocytoma is between 0.2 and 0.6% [7, 8], making this an important group to consider screening for the presence of a pheochromocytoma. Median age of presentation is 44.5 years [9], however, pheochromocytoma can occur at both extremes of age and has even been documented to occur in a neonate [10].

Embryology

The embryological origins and development of the adrenal medulla and paraganglia offer insights into the etiology and relationship of pheochromocytomas to parasympathetic paragangliomas, particularly with regard to the patterns of disease seen with germline mutations, and is paramount for an understanding of the anatomical sites at which extra-adrenal paragangliomas can occur.

The adrenal medulla and paraganglia have a common embryological origin from the neural crest. The neural crest can be divided into four main, but overlapping, functional categories. The cranial neural crest cells give rise to the craniofacial mesenchyme and the sensory ganglia of the fifth, seventh, ninth, and tenth cranial nerves. Vagal and sacral neural crest cells generate parasympathetic enteric ganglia which supply the gut and other abdominal organs. The cardiac neural crest overlaps the vagal neural crest and provides connective tissue elements to the great vessels of the heart and also gives rise to pre-aortic (mesenteric) ganglia, melanocytes, neurons, and connective tissue elements to the third, fourth, and sixth pharyngeal arches. The trunk neural crest lies between the vagal and sacral crest. Cells from this region that migrate along the ventral pathway give rise to the dorsal root ganglia and sympathoadrenal progenitor cells (which form the adrenal medulla and sympathetic ganglia), whereas trunk neural crest cells migrate along the dorsolateral pathway and give rise to melanocytes and Merkel cells. Bone morphogenetic proteins derived from the dorsal aorta appear to play a central role in the differentiation of sympathoadrenal cells. Other transcription factors, which also appear to be involved in sympathoadrenal cell development, include MASH-1/CASH-1, Phox2a/b, Hand2, and GATA2/3 [11].

Anatomy

The migration of sympathoadrenal progenitor cells during embryological development explains the anatomic location at which catecholamine-producing sympathetic paragangliomas occur. Approximately 90% of sympathetic paragangliomas arise within the adrenal medulla. The remaining extra-adrenal sympathetic paragangliomas occur most commonly within the paravertebral ganglia of the sympathetic chain in the abdomen and thorax, however, they may also occasionally arise from collateral sympathetic ganglia within the neck, chest, abdomen, and pelvis. Parasympathetic paragangliomas occur most often in the head and neck, and are associated with vascular structures and branches of the glossopharyngeal and vagus nerves, however, they may also arise from parasympathetic-associated tissue of the heart, great vessels, and sacral region, albeit rarely.

Pathology

Pheochromocytomas are variable in size, however, at the time of diagnosis they typically measure between 3 and 5 cm [12]. Macroscopically, pheochromocytomas are usually well circumscribed and appear encapsulated due to the presence of a pseudocapsule. On sectioning, the cut surface usually appears gray to tan in color. Areas of hemorrhage, central degenerative or cystic change, fibrosis, and calcification may be present (Fig. 9.2a). Microscopic examination demonstrates an organoid pattern wherein nests ("zellballen" = cannonball) of tumor cells (Fig. 9.2b) are surrounded by bland spindled cells known as sustentacular cells (Fig. 9.2c). Tumor cells are usually polygonal with prominent granular cytoplasm [13] and invariably show positive immunohistochemical staining for the neuroendocrine marker chromogranin A (Fig. 9.2d). The electron microscopic demonstration of ectoplasmatic processes containing dense neurosecretory granules is a characteristic feature of catecholamine-producing cells of the sympathoadrenal lineage and may occasionally be useful when there is uncertainty over the definitive diagnosis of pheochromocytoma. Although not invariably present, the sustentacular cells are negative for chromogranin but positive for S-100 by immunohistochemistry (Fig. 9.2c, d). The combination of an organoid growth pattern and positive chromogranin staining of nests of tumor cells surrounded by sustentacular cells positive for S-100 is pathognomonic of pheochromocytoma.

Parasympathetic paragangliomas are essentially histologically identical to adrenal and extra-adrenal pheochromocytomas. However, these tumors do not stain with chromate salt solutions and are, therefore, also commonly referred to as nonchromaffin tumors [14].

Catecholamine Synthesis and Metabolism

Pheochromocytomas and paragangliomas are members of the amine precursor uptake and decarboxylation (APUD) family. These cells have the common ability to synthesize biogenic amines and polypeptide hormones. Catecholamines are derived from the amino acid tyrosine by a process of hydroxylation and decarboxylation (Fig. 9.3). The rate-limiting step in catecholamine synthesis is the conversion of tyrosine to L-dihydroxyphenylalanine (L-DOPA) by the enzyme tyrosine hydroxylase. Dopamine is the first catecholamine to be synthesized from

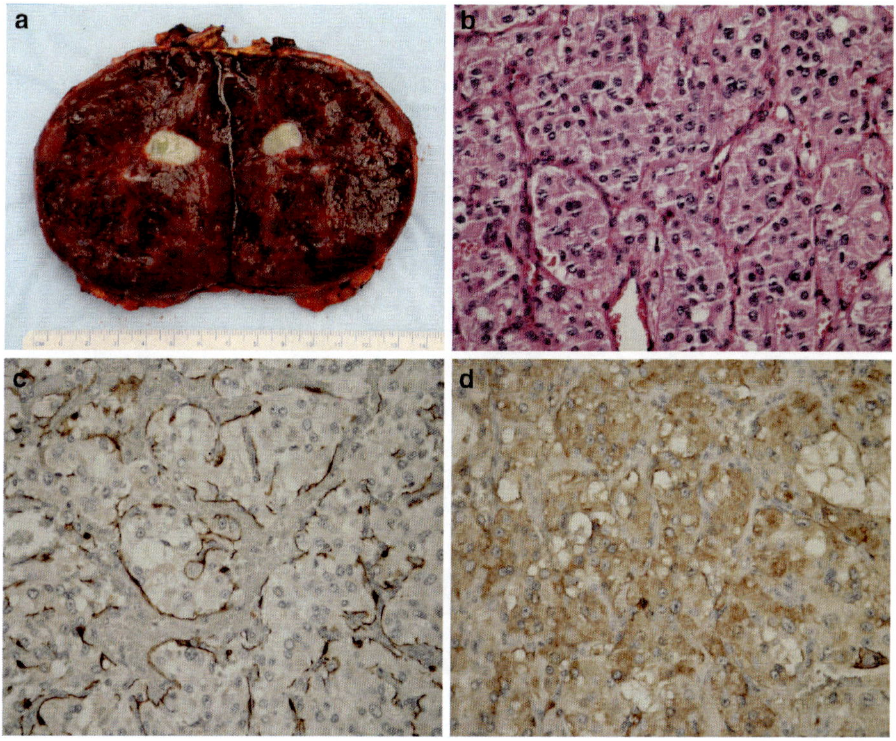

Fig. 9.2 (**a**) Pheochromocytoma with regions of hemorrhage, cystic degeneration, and central fibrosis. Residual normal adrenal remnant present above the tumor. (**b**) Zellballen architecture seen with medium power hematoxylin and eosin tissue staining. Photo courtesy of Dr. Anthony Gill. (**c**) S-100 immunohistochemistry demonstrating sustentacular cells. Photo courtesy of Dr. Anthony Gill. (**d**) Chromogranin immunohistochemistry with staining of the tumor cells. Photo courtesy of Dr. Anthony Gill

tyrosine. Norepinephrine and epinephrine are synthesized in a stepwise fashion by further modifications of dopamine and the enzyme phenylethanolamine-*N*-methyltransferase (PNMT) is required for the conversion of norepinephrine to epinephrine [15]. Whilst adrenal pheochromocytoma usually express PNMT and secrete both epinephrine and norepinephrine, extra-adrenal sympathetic paragangliomas, malignant tumors, and *VHL*-associated tumors generally lack PNMT expression and, therefore, predominantly secrete norepinephrine rather than epinephrine [16].

Epinephrine and norepinephrine are metabolized to metanephrine and normetanephrine by the enzyme catechol-*O*-methyl transferase (COMT). These metabolites are more stable than the catecholamines and are produced continuously by the tumor cells. Fractionated metanephrine measurements, therefore, have a higher sensitivity and specificity for the diagnosis of pheochromocytoma compared to catecholamines which are secreted in a variable and episodic manner [17, 18].

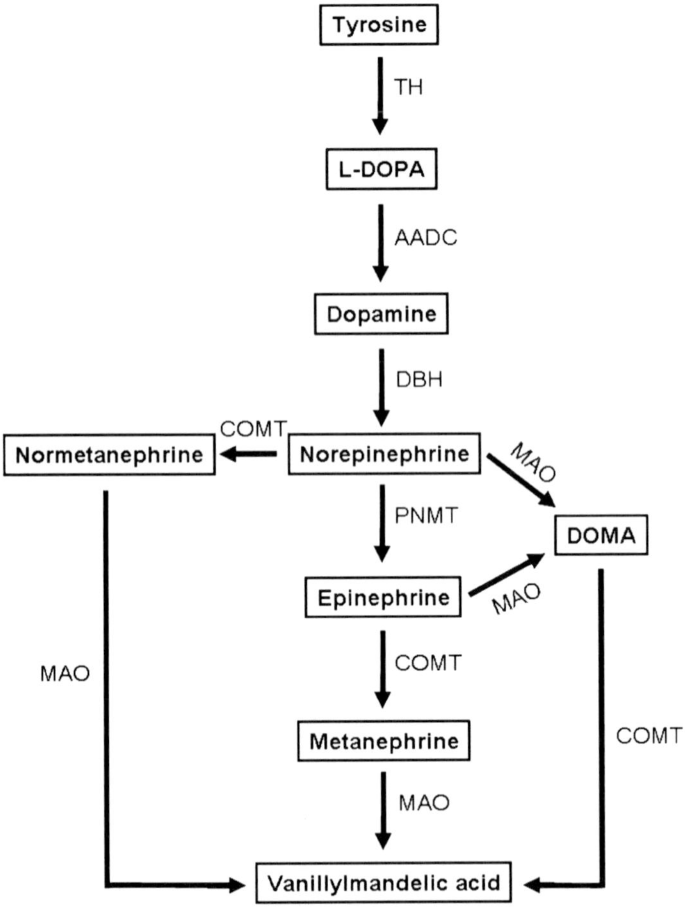

Fig. 9.3 Biosynthetic pathway and metabolism of catecholamines. Tyrosine is converted to 3,4-dihydroxyphenylalanine (L-DOPA) by tyrosine hydroxylase (TH). Aromatic L-amino acid decarboxylase (AADC) converts L-DOPA to dopamine which is hydroxylated to norepinephrine by dopamine β-hydroxylase (DBH). Norepinephrine is converted to epinephrine by phenylethanolamine-*N*-methyltransferase (PNMT). Metabolism of catecholamines can occur by two pathways: (1) meta-*O*-methylation of epinephrine and norepinephrine to metanephrine and normetanephrine by catechol-*O*-methyltransferase (COMT) and further oxidized by monoamine oxidase (MAO) to vanillylmandelic acid (VMA) or (2) MAO may oxidize epinephrine and norepinephrine to dihydroxymandelic acid (DOMA) which is then converted to VMA by COMT

Clinical Presentation

Classic

The signs and symptoms of pheochromocytomas result from the hypersecretion of the catecholamines norepinephrine, epinephrine, and dopamine. Catecholamine secretion by the tumors is episodic, resulting in paroxysmal symptoms in approximately half of all patients [19]. The classic symptom triad in patients with pheochromocytoma consists of episodic headaches, sweating, and palpitations. Other associated symptoms may include visual blurring, severe anxiety, heat intolerance, constipation, polyuria, polydipsia, weight loss, chest or abdominal pain, and postural symptoms. Hypertension and tachycardia are the most common clinical signs, however, orthostatic hypotension, tremor, pallor, pyrexia, leukocytosis, hyperglycemia, and transitory electrocardiographic changes may also be present [20].

Hypertension caused by pheochromocytoma may be sustained or paroxysmal and is frequently resistant to standard antihypertensive drugs. Malignant hypertension with retinopathy, proteinuria, and encephalopathy may occur. Approximately 13% of patients will remain normotensive and tumors which predominantly secrete epinephrine may result in sustained hypotension rather than hypertension [19, 21].

Whilst the actual incidence of truly asymptomatic pheochromocytoma is unclear, autopsy studies have demonstrated a prevalence of occult pheochromocytoma at 0.05% [5, 6]. With the increasing use and improving resolution of imaging technology, an increasing number of patients are being diagnosed with pheochromocytoma incidentally whilst being investigated for an unrelated cause. Approximately 6–30% of adrenal tumors incidentally discovered by imaging will subsequently be diagnosed as adrenal pheochromocytomas after further investigations [22, 23].

Pheochromocytoma (Adrenergic) Crisis

Severe and acute presentations of pheochromocytoma can also occur. Features of a pheochromocytoma crisis may include malignant hypertension, cardiac arrhythmia, cardiac arrest, cardiomyopathy, and multiorgan failure [24, 25]. Potential precipitants include hemorrhage into the tumor, direct or indirect tumor manipulation, anesthetic induction, endotracheal intubation, surgical/dental procedures, exercise, labor, intravenous or intra-arterial radiographic contrast, and a number of drugs (sympathomimetics, monoamine oxidase inhibitors, β-blockers, tricyclic antidepressants, volatile anesthetic agents, histamine releasing drugs, suxamethonium, metoclopramide, steroids, nicotine, naloxone, phenothiazines, and glucagon) [26, 27]. Mechanical pressure on the tumor can induce catecholamine release and is the likely cause for paroxysmal symptoms during micturition or coitus seen with bladder pheochromocytomas [19].

Pediatric

Pheochromocytomas and parasympathetic paragangliomas in children are rare, however, among hypertensive children the incidence of pheochromocytoma has been reported to be 0.5–2.0% [28]. The average age at presentation is 11 years with a male-to-female ratio of 2:1. In children with pheochromocytoma, approximately

40% will be associated with a known germline mutation [29]. Multifocal tumors occur in 43%, 25% have bilateral adrenal disease at presentation and extra-adrenal lesions are present in 25–40%. In children, extra-adrenal sympathetic paragangliomas often arise within the bladder (10%). Unlike adults, the incidence of malignant disease is low and only 3% of children will have a malignant pheochromocytoma [10, 30–32].

Familial

It is now recognized that an occult germline mutation will be present in approximately 24% of patients presenting with an apparently sporadic pheochromocytoma [33]. Four inherited disorders have thus far been identified: multiple endocrine neoplasia type 2 (MEN2), von Hippel–Lindau disease, neurofibromatosis type 1, and familial pheochromocytoma/paraganglioma syndrome. These syndromes are caused by mutations in the RET, VHL, NF1, and SDH (SDHD, SDHB, and SDHC) genes, respectively, and will be discussed in detail below. Patients with familial pheochromocytoma usually present at a younger age than sporadic pheochromocytomas, however, classic symptoms are only present in about half of patients with familial disease [34, 35]. The possibility of familial disease should be strongly suspected in any patient with a family history of pheochromocytoma or paraganglioma, presentation <35 years of age, extra-adrenal lesions, multifocal tumors, bilateral adrenal pheochromocytomas, the presence of syndrome-related tumors, and recurrent or malignant disease [36].

Malignant Disease

Definition

The WHO tumor definition for malignant pheochromocytoma is the presence of metastases. In order to avoid any confusion with multifocal primary tumors, a metastasis is defined as the presence of chromaffin tissue in a region where it would not be expected to be found [1]. Metastases may appear as long as 20 years after initial presentation and the most frequent site of metastasis are bone, liver, and lungs [37, 38]. Currently, there are no prognostic investigations that can reliably predict or detect which patients are at risk of developing metastatic disease; however, certain clinical, biochemical, histological features, and cytological markers are associated with a higher risk of malignant disease.

Locally invasive tumors are considered benign by WHO criteria. Local invasion is a poor predictor for metastases [39], however, further subclassification of benign pheochromocytoma may be helpful to describe the different biological behavior of invasive and noninvasive tumors.

Clinical Features

Functioning malignant tumors have a similar presentation to benign pheochromocytomas; however, with nonfunctioning tumors symptoms may not be present or may result from local mass effect or metastasis [37, 40]. Unlike adrenocortical lesions, the size of a pheochromocytoma does not appear to be a predictive factor for malignancy [41]. Malignant tumors may be associated with dopamine or neuropeptide Y secretion and generally secrete norepinephrine rather than epinephrine [42, 43]. The overall risk of malignant disease is approximately 10%; however, adrenal pheochromocytomas appear to have a lower risk of malignancy than extra-adrenal tumors (5% vs. 20%) [44]. Malignant disease is uncommon with the familial pheochromocytoma syndromes, with the exception of *SDHB* germline mutations in which retrospective studies suggest that the risk of malignancy may be as high as 70% [45–48].

Pathology

Several different scoring systems have suggested that the combinations of various cytological and architectural features are associated with an increased risk of aggressive behavior [49]. However, the predictive value of these systems is inconsistent and there is currently no accepted way of distinguishing benign from malignant pheochromocytomas or paragangliomas based on histopathological features. The diagnosis of malignant disease is, therefore, often only made in retrospect once distant metastases become clinically evident. Tumor histological features which are suggestive of a more aggressive tumor with potential for malignant behavior include vascular or capsular invasion, periadrenal adipose tissue invasion, diffuse growth or large nests of tumor cells, focal or confluent necrosis, high cellularity, cell spindling, tumor monotony, increased or atypical mitotic figures, profound nuclear pleomorphism, and hyperchromasia [49].

Cancer-associated markers such as p53, p21, Bcl-2, mdm-2, cyclin D1, MIB-1, Ki-67, HSP90, telomerase, and neuroendocrine- and catecholamine-related markers such as chromogranin A and 3,4-dihydroxyphenylalanine have not shown to be reliable prognostic markers [50, 51].

Prognosis

Once an individual has developed metastatic disease, overall survival is 50% at 5 years although progression of disease is highly variable and some patients with metastatic disease have been documented to survive up to 20 years. Morbidity and mortality is generally related to tumor burden resulting in high circulating catecholamines and mass effect from metastases [47, 52]. Malignant pheochromocytomas are generally resistant to chemotherapy and radiotherapy [47, 53], therefore, treatment is aimed at palliative control of symptoms.

Approach to Diagnosis

Any patient with suggestive symptoms or signs should be evaluated for a pheochromocytoma. A thorough medical and family history should be taken to determine any features that may imply familial disease. The diagnosis is generally confirmed by biochemical analysis, followed by radiological imaging and localization prior to deciding definitive treatment.

Biochemical Evaluation

The initial biochemical evaluation for pheochromocytoma should include measurements of catecholamines (epinephrine, norepinephrine, and dopamine) and metanephrines (metanephrine and normetanephrine). Plasma and urinary measurements of metanephrines have now been well established to have greater sensitivity and specificity than catecholamines for the detection of pheochromocytoma. The increased sensitivity of metanephrines compared with catecholamines is due to the production of *O*-methylated metabolites by the tumors which is independent of the variable and episodic release of catecholamines [17]. Plasma-free metanephrines provide an overall diagnostic sensitivity of 98% and specificity of 92% and urinary-fractionated metanephrines have a sensitivity of 97% and specificity of 69% [54, 55]. As well as being highly accurate, the collection of a blood sample for plasma metanephrines also removes potential patient compliance issues related to 24 h urine collection.

Plasma or urinary levels of chromogranin A, neuropeptide Y, and vanillylmandelic acid (VMA) have comparatively low sensitivity and specificity, and are no longer used for the diagnosis of pheochromocytoma as they have been superseded by metanephrine measurements. Provocative testing with glucagon, histamine, metoclopramide, or tyramine are no longer required as they have a comparatively low sensitivity and have the risk of inducing a potentially lethal adrenergic crisis [56, 57]. Clonidine and phentolamine suppression tests may still have a role when false positive increases in metanephrines and catecholamines are suspected. Clonidine and phentolamine are centrally acting alpha2-adrenergic receptor agonists that normally suppress the release of catecholamines from neurons but are unable to suppress the secretion of catecholamines in pheochromocytomas. The clonidine suppression test is reported to have a diagnostic accuracy of 92% for the diagnosis of pheochromocytomas [58, 59].

Pharmacologic agents which may interfere with biochemical testing include caffeine, β-blockers, sympathomimetics, tricyclic antidepressants, monoamine oxidase inhibitors, methyldopa, and levodopa. In order to avoid false positive results, these agents should be ceased at least 2 weeks prior to biochemical testing [55].

Tumor Localization

Once pheochromocytoma has been diagnosed, localization of the tumor by radiological imaging should be initiated to determine the site and size of the lesion, and the presence of synchronous lesions or metastatic disease. Localization modalities include computed tomography (CT), magnetic resonance imaging (MRI), metaiodobenzylguanidine (MIBG) or octreotide scintigraphy, and positron emission imaging (PET).

CT and MRI have a sensitivity of 98–100% for the detection of pheochromocytoma; however, due to the frequency of adrenal incidentalomas, both have a lower specificity of between 70 and 80% [55, 60, 61]. Since the majority of extra-adrenal pheochromocytomas occur within the abdomen, imaging of the entire abdomen and pelvis should be performed [60]. CT imaging has the advantage of being a rapid, widely available and relatively inexpensive imaging tool; however, T2-weighted MRI is preferred for the localization of extra-adrenal tumors and in patients with allergies to intravenous contrast. Because there is no radiation exposure with MRI, it is also the preferred imaging modality for pheochromocytoma in pregnancy and for children [32, 62].

MIBG is a norepinephrine analog preferentially taken up and concentrated by hyperfunctioning chromaffin tissue. The isotopes most commonly used for scintigraphy are ^{123}I-MIBG or ^{131}I-MIBG. ^{123}I-MIBG is superior to ^{131}I-MIBG for the evaluation of metastases, but is a less stable compound and is less widely available [63]. Both have a specificity of near 100%, however, the sensitivity of ^{123}I-MIBG is greater (90% vs. 77%) [64]. MIBG scintigraphy may be used as a confirmatory test for the diagnosis of pheochromocytoma, however, it is probably unnecessary when a solitary lesion is identified in the presence of an unequivocal biochemical diagnosis of pheochromocytoma [18]. As MIBG scintigraphy is usually done as a full body image, MIBG is a more useful tool for the detection of multifocal or metastatic disease compared to CT or MRI [65]. Prior to MIBG imaging, oral iodine must be administered to block uptake of radioactive iodine by the thyroid gland.

Neuroendocrine tissue has a high density of somatostatin receptors. Indium-111 OctreoScan is a radiolabeled somatostatin analog and can, therefore, be used as an alternative agent for scintigraphy in patients with pheochromocytoma, particularly for the scintigraphic imaging of pheochromocytoma that do not take up MIBG [18].

PET imaging with ^{18}F-fluorodopamine, ^{18}F-fluorodopa, ^{18}F-dihydroxyphenylalanine, ^{11}C-hydroxyephedrine, and ^{11}C-epinephrine are other functional imaging methods that can be used as an alternative or additional imaging procedure when scintigraphy is negative. Unlike ^{18}F-fluorodeoxyglucose (^{18}F-FDG), these agents are highly specific for pheochromocytoma because they depend on the uptake into the tumor cells by norepinephrine transporters unique to chromaffin tissues. While studies have shown remarkably high sensitivity and specificity, the series have been small and many of the agents are not yet in widespread clinical use [18, 55, 64, 66].

Treatment of Pheochromocytoma

Medical Preparation for Surgery

Adequate medical preparation is crucial prior to embarking on therapeutic intervention for pheochromocytoma, and has been a significant contributing factor in the reduction of perioperative mortality of pheochromocytoma from 18% to less than 2% [67, 68]. The role of pharmacological management is to limit the cardiovascular instability, particularly at the time of surgery, as anesthetic induction and surgical manipulation of the tumor can result in massive surges of catecholamines, risking a potentially lethal adrenergic crisis [69]. Due to the lack of randomized prospective controlled trials, there is no clear consensus regarding the drug of choice, however alpha-adrenoceptor antagonists, dihydropyridine calcium channel receptor blockers, the tyrosine hydroxylase inhibitor α-methyltyrosine, and the competitive α- and ß-receptor blocking drug labetalol have all been successfully used in an oral form for the preoperative treatment of pheochromocytoma [21, 70–72].

The traditional and most widely used preoperative pharmaceutical agent is the nonselective, noncompetitive α-adrenergic antagonist phenoxybenzamine. Treatment is usually started at the time of diagnosis and commenced at least 10–14 days preoperatively to allow blood pressure normalization and volume expansion to occur. Common side effects with phenoxybenzamine include nasal stuffiness, central sedation, dizziness, and orthostatic hypotension. Dosage is usually commenced at 20–40 mg daily and titrated until normal blood pressure with mild orthostatic hypotension is achieved. Due to the reflex tachycardia that may result from nonselective α-adrenergic blockade, the subsequent addition of a ß-adrenergic blocker is often required [55]. Doxazosin is a more recently developed selective α_1-adrenergic antagonist which does not result in a reflex tachycardia, however, as a competitive antagonist can be displaced by high levels of endogenous catecholamines [73]. Both of these agents have a plasma half-life of approximately 24 h which may contribute to postoperative hypotension often present in the early postoperative period.

Dihydropyridine calcium channel receptor blockers are useful alternatives for patients unable to tolerate α-adrenergic blocking agents or as an adjunct for patients in whom ß-adrenergic blocking agents are contraindicated. They are particularly useful for patients with catecholamine-associated coronary artery spasm or myocarditis as they do not cause tachycardia and may also reduce the catecholamine-associated coronary artery spasm [74–76].

Unopposed α-adrenergic receptor stimulation can induce a catastrophic hypertensive crisis, therefore, β-adrenergic blockers should never be used alone and only commenced after adequate pretreatment with α-adrenergic blockade [75–77]. Labetalol is a mixed α- and ß-receptor antagonist and has been successfully used as a single pharmaceutical agent in the preoperative management of pheochromocytoma. Labetalol can also be administered intravenously and titrated for a desired effect, and is therefore a useful agent for the control of blood pressure intraoperatively or in the intensive care setting [78]. Other intravenous pharmacologic agents that may be used to control blood pressure intraoperatively include phentolamine, sodium nitroprusside, nitroglycerine, magnesium sulfate, or urapidil.

Alpha-methyltyrosine is a competitive inhibitor of tyrosine hydroxylase, the enzyme which catalyzes the rate-limiting step of catecholamine synthesis. Treatment with α-methyltyrosine will, therefore, reduce the synthesis and secretion of catecholamines from a pheochromocytoma. Because it is centrally acting, it has significant side effects including diarrhea, sedation, psychic disturbance, and extrapyramidal side effects that may be exacerbated by the concurrent use of a dopamine antagonist. It can be used for the preoperative preparation of pheochromocytoma patients as well as for patients with widespread metastatic disease. Its use, however, is limited by the side effects that occur with α-methyltyrosine at high doses [75–77].

Operative Approach

The optimal outcome for the surgical management of a pheochromocytoma requires a team approach, with an endocrinologist, an experienced surgeon, and an anesthetist. Despite aggressive preoperative pharmacological management, blood pressure may be labile and the anesthetist must be prepared to respond rapidly to any major fluctuations of blood pressure. Cardiovascular lability can be minimized by adequate preoperative pharmacological preparation, patient volume expansion, and minimal tumor manipulation during surgical resection.

Laparoscopic resection has become the accepted standard surgical approach for adrenal pheochromocytomas and for accessible extra-adrenal pheochromocytomas. The laparoscopic approach is associated with superior surgical access to the adrenal gland and vessels, a shorter hospital stay, less postoperative pain, quicker recovery, superior cosmesis, and fewer postoperative complications compared to an open approach [79]. The size of an adrenal pheochromocytoma correlates poorly with the risk of malignancy and should, therefore, not be the deciding factor when considering a laparoscopic approach. Tumors of 10 cm or greater can be removed safely via a laparoscopic approach by experienced hands [41, 80, 81].

Laparoscopic adrenalectomy can be performed either by a transperitoneal or retroperitoneal approach depending on the surgeon's preference and experience. The advantages of a transperitoneal approach include easier positioning of the patient in a lateral decubitus position, larger operating space, and greater familiarity of the anatomic landmarks to the operating surgeon as most other open and laparoscopic abdominal operations are also performed by this approach. This is the preferred approach for large adrenal lesions. A retroperitoneal approach is generally performed with the patient in a supine position. The advantages of a retroperitoneal approach include a more direct access to the adrenal gland and vessels, avoiding adhesions from previous intra-abdominal surgery and the ability to use greater gas pressures, thus impeding venous bleeding and improving visibility of the operative field. The retroperitoneal approach is preferred for lesions <6 cm and for bilateral adrenal lesions as the contra-lateral adrenal gland can be easily accessed without repositioning the patient [41, 75, 80, 81]. An open procedure can be performed via an anterior or posterior approach, and conversion from a laparoscopic to an open approach should be considered when a difficult dissection, uncontrolled bleeding, or suspicion of a malignant lesion is encountered.

The standard operation for an adrenal lesion is a complete adrenalectomy, however, cortical sparing adrenalectomy should be considered for any patient with bilateral adrenal pheochromocytomas. Preservation of at least one-third of a gland with an adequate blood supply will allow 65% of patients to remain corticosteroid-independent; however, this is at the cost of a 10–20% long-term rate of recurrent pheochromocytoma from the adrenal remnant [82, 83].

Postoperative Management

In the early postoperative period, monitoring in a high dependency or intensive care setting may be required for the first 12–24 h. Hypotension may result from the withdrawal of chronic high levels of circulating catecholamines and from the lingering effect of long-acting antihypertensives used in the perioperative period. Volume expansion and support of blood pressure with vasopressors may be required for significant postoperative hypotension. Any hypotensive patient must be carefully evaluated for the possibility of postoperative hemorrhage.

Biochemical testing is usually repeated at least 2 weeks postoperatively to confirm successful resection and biochemical cure of a pheochromocytoma, although normal biochemical tests will not exclude the presence of small synchronous lesions or microscopic disease [38]. Patients should be followed up indefinitely with annual biochemical screening, as recurrence rates of up to 17% have been reported and approximately 10% will be found to have malignant disease [75, 84].

Treatment Options for Malignant Disease

Currently, there are no therapeutic options that will cure malignant pheochromocytoma; therefore, treatment is aimed at palliative control of symptoms. Surgical resection should be considered if technically feasible, as this will reduce the tumor burden and circulating catecholamine levels, and may improve the response rate of any residual disease to subsequent radio- or chemotherapy. Long-term pharmacologic treatment is necessary to control the effects of high levels of circulating catecholamines.

Combination chemotherapy with cyclophosphamide, vincristine, and dacarbazine (CVD) is able to achieve partial and complete tumor response rates of 44% and 11%, and partial and complete biochemical response rates of 55% and 17% [85]. Targeted radiotherapy with high dose ^{131}I-MIBG will provide similar partial and complete tumor response rates of 50% and 13%, and partial and complete biochemical response rates of 32% and 13%, respectively [86, 87]. Although both treatments provide improved quality of life for patients with metastatic disease and reduce the need for antihypertensive treatment, neither treatment modality appears to improve the overall survival. External beam radiotherapy is useful for relieving pain and inhibiting growth of bony metastases, but will abolish the tumor avidity to MIBG and should, therefore, not be used if ^{131}I-MIBG treatment is planned [88, 89].

The radiolabeled somatostatin analog, DOTATOC, has recently been shown to be another treatment option for somatostatin receptor positive pheochromocytoma. Although less effective, DOTATOC may be particularly useful for tumors that do not show sufficient MIBG uptake to qualify for treatment with ^{131}I-MIBG [90].

Pheochromocytoma/Paraganglioma Syndromes

It is now recognized that up to 24% of patients with apparently sporadic pheochromocytomas will have a germline mutation which suggests that the overall rate of hereditary pheochromocytomas may be as high as 34% [33, 36, 84]. Although additional pheochromocytoma susceptibility genes may be identified, currently germline mutations in six genes are associated with familial pheochromocytoma: *von Hippel–Lindau* (*VHL*) which causes von Hippel–Lindau syndrome, *RET* leading to MEN2, *neurofibromatosis type* 1 (*NF1*) associated with von Recklinghausen's disease, and the genes encoding subunits B, D, and C of mitochondrial succinate dehydrogenase (SDH) (*SDHB, SDHD,* and *SDHC*) which are associated with Familial Paraganglioma/Pheochromocytoma syndromes (Table 9.1) [91–94]. More recently *KIF1Bbeta*, a member of the kinesin superfamily proteins, has been identified as a tumor suppressor implic7ated in the pathogenesis of pheochromocytoma [95].

The Carney triad is a rare non-hereditary syndrome for which a mutation has not yet been identified, however, the paraganglioma–gastrointestinal stromal tumor (GIST) dyad also known as the Carney–Stratakis syndrome, which was previously thought to be a familial variant of the Carney triad, has now been demonstrated to be associated with germline mutations of the SDH genes [96, 97].

Von Hippel–Lindau Syndrome

Von Hippel–Lindau disease is an autosomal dominant inherited tumor syndrome with an estimated prevalence of 2–3 per 100,000. This syndrome is characterized by the development of a spectrum of highly vascularized tumors in different organs including

Table 9.1 Features of familial syndromes associated with pheochromocytoma (Reprinted from Adler et al. (2008), with permission from AlphaMed Press)

Syndrome	Gene	Inheritance	Syndrome clinical features	Age of presentation (years)	Frequency of mutation (%)	Penetrance of disease	Frequency of malignant disease	Catecholamines	Common site of disease
VHL	*VHL* (3p25-26)	Autosomal dominant	Renal cell cysts and carcinomas Retinal and CNS hemangioblastomas Endolymphatic sac tumors Epididymal cystadenomas Pancreatic neoplasms and cysts Pheochromocytomas	30 (5–54)	2–9	7–18%	<10%	Norepinephrine-producing tumors only	Adrenal (predominates) and extra-adrenal abdominal and thoracic. Often multifocal or bilateral adrenal disease
MEN type 2	*RET* (10q11.2)	Autosomal dominant	Type 2A Medullary thyroid carcinoma Pheochromocytoma Hyperparathyroidism Cutaneous lichen amyloidosis Type 2B Medullary thyroid carcinoma Pheochromocytoma Multiple neuromas Marfanoid habitus	39.5 (14–68) 32.4 (15–41)	3–5	50%	<5%	Epinephrine producing tumors predominate	Adrenal. Bilateral disease common. Extra-adrenal disease rare
NF1	*NF1* (17q11.2)	Autosomal dominant	Multiple neurofibromas Café au lait skin spots Pheochromocytomas	40 (25–69)	2–4	0.1–5.5%	<10%	Epinephrine and Norepinephrine-producing tumors	Adrenal. Bilateral disease common. Extra-adrenal disease rare

PGL4	*SDHB* (1p36.13)	Autosomal dominant	No clinical phenotypic features Pheochromocytoma/ paraganglioma	34 (10–58)	2–7	50% by 35 years 77% by 50 years	34–70%	Norepinephrine-producing tumors predominate	Extra-adrenal (generally solitary) abdominal and thoracic pheochromocytoma predominates. If adrenal then commonly bilateral disease
PGL1	*SDHD* (11q23)	Maternal imprinting	No clinical phenotypic features Paraganglioma/ pheochromocytoma	31.2 (17–59)	3–5	50% by 31 years80% by 50 years	<5%	Norepinephrine-producing tumors predominate	Head and neck paragangliomas predominate (glomus tumors). If adrenal, then commonly bilateral disease. Often multifocal disease
PGL3	*SDHC* (1q21)	Autosomal dominant	No clinical phenotypic features Head and neck paraganglioma	46 (13–73)	<0.1	Unknown	Uncertain (<5%)	Non-functioning	Head and neck paragangliomas

retinal and central nervous system (CNS) haemangioblastomas, clear cell renal cell carcinoma, pheochromocytoma, pancreatic and renal cysts, endolymphatic sac tumors, and papillary cystadenomas of the epididymis or broad ligament [98, 99].

VHL disease is classified into four subtypes. Type 1 VHL patients do not develop pheochromocytoma, whereas 7–18% of type 2A, B, and C will develop pheochromocytoma at a mean age of 30 years (range 5–54). Patients with type 2A have a low risk of renal cell carcinoma (RCC) while type 2B patients have a high risk of RCC. Type 2C VHL patients have an increased risk of pheochromocytomas without other manifestations of the disease [33, 35, 100]. A *VHL* germline mutation will be identified in 3–11% of patients presenting with an apparently sporadic pheochromocytoma. *VHL*-associated pheochromocytomas predominantly secrete norepinephrine rather than epinephrine and frequently present with bilateral adrenal or multiple extra-adrenal lesions [16, 35]. Long-term morbidity and mortality are usually related to complications from retinal and CNS haemangioblastomas and metastatic renal cell carcinoma [99, 101].

Multiple Endocrine Neoplasia Type 2

Activating germline mutations of the *RET* proto-oncogene result in MEN2A, MEN2B, or familial medullary thyroid cancer (FMTC) syndromes and have an estimated prevalence of 2 per 100,000. MEN2A is characterized by the development of medullary thyroid cancer (MTC), hyperparathyroidism, and pheochromocytoma. MEN2B is characterized by MTC and pheochromocytoma but has a distinctive clinical phenotype with mucosal ganglioneuromas and a marfanoid habitus. Patients with FMTC develop MTC but without any other manifestations of MEN2. Inheritance occurs in an autosomal dominant fashion and 50% of germline mutation carriers develop pheochromocytoma by a mean age of 36 years (range 14–68) [102]. MTC is usually the first manifestation of MEN2 as it has a high penetrance, however, in 9–27% of patients pheochromocytoma is the first manifestation of the syndrome [102, 103]. MEN2-associated pheochromocytoma are usually adrenal in location and predominantly secrete epinephrine in contrast to VHL-associated tumors. Malignant pheochromocytomas are rare [104]. Bilateral adrenal pheochromocytomas occur in approximately 50% of patients [16, 102].

Neurofibromatosis Type 1

NF1 results from inactivating mutations of the tumor suppressor gene, neurofibromin. The overall frequency of pheochromocytoma with NF1 is relatively low with an estimated lifetime incidence of 0.1–5.7%; however, in hypertensive patients with NF1 the frequency of pheochromocytoma rises to 20–50% [105]. Diagnosis is usually made on clinical grounds by the finding of two or more of the following features: greater than six café-au-lait spots, more than two neurofibromas, axillary or inguinal freckling, two or more iris hamartomas (Lisch nodules), a least one optic nerve glioma, dysplasia of sphenoid bone or pseudoarthrosis, and a first degree relative with NF1 [106]. Pheochromocytomas in NF1 are usually benign, adrenal in location, and bilateral in approximately 10% of cases. Extra-adrenal lesions are rare [105, 106].

Familial Pheochromocytoma/Paraganglioma Syndromes

Inactivating germline mutations of *SDHB, SDHD, SDHC*, encoding three subunits of the SDH enzyme, were recently identified as a cause of familial pheochromocytoma or familial paraganglioma.

SDHD was the first of these genes to be identified, and is associated with the development of parasympathetic head and neck paragangliomas in at least 79% of *SDHD* germline mutation carriers, however, tumors are frequently multifocal and adrenal and extra-adrenal tumors will also occur in more than 50% of patients expressing the disease [107]. *SDHD* mutations are maternally imprinted, therefore, disease will only occur in individuals who have inherited the mutated allele from their father [93].

SDHB germline mutations are inherited in an autosomal dominant manner and characterized by extra-adrenal sympathetic paraganglioma which have a high risk of malignant disease [46], although head and neck paragangliomas are reported to occur in 31% of *SDHB* germline mutation carriers [107]. Retrospective studies suggest that the risk of malignancy in a patient with an *SDHB* germline mutation is between 34 and 70% [45, 46]. *SDHB* mutations have an overall frequency of 1.7–6.7% in patients presenting with pheochromocytoma [108].

SDHC-associated disease is rare with an estimated frequency of less than 0.1%. SDHC-associated tumors occur almost exclusively as head and neck paragangliomas, however, *SDHC*-associated extra-adrenal abdominal pheochromocytoma have been reported [109]. Malignant pheochromocytoma/paraganglioma appears to be rare in *SDHD*- and *SDHC*-associated disease [107, 110].

The paraganglioma–GIST dyad (Carney–Stratakis syndrome) was originally thought to be a variant of the Carney triad but observed to have an autosomal dominant inheritance with variable penetrance. After the discovery of the *SDH* germline mutations as a cause for familial pheochromocytoma/paraganglioma, it was soon established that the paraganglioma–GIST dyad is associated with germline mutations of *SDHB, C,* and *D* and a separate entity to the Carney triad [97].

Carney Triad

Carney triad is a rare syndrome associated with the development of gastric stromal tumors (GISTs), pulmonary chondromas, and extra-adrenal paragangliomas. The occurrence of multifocal lesions in multiple organs is suggestive of an inherited disorder; however, Carney triad does not display a familial mode of inheritance. To date, no germline mutation has been identified although Carney triad-associated tumors frequently show allelic losses at chromosome 1p and 1q [111, 112].

Carney triad occurs predominantly in women (85%), with a mean age at first presentation of 20.2 years (range 7–48 years). GISTs are the most common tumor at presentation (73%), followed by pulmonary chondromas (15%) and paragangliomas (10%). Overall, approximately 47% of patients with Carney triad will develop paragangliomas at a mean age of 27.5 years (range 12–48 years). Both sympathetic and parasympathetic paragangliomas may occur. They are multifocal in 22% and malignant in 10% of patients. The location of paragangliomas appears to have an approximately equal distribution, with 1/3 of tumors occurring in the head and neck, 1/3 in the chest, and 1/3 in the abdomen and pelvis (of which 10% are adrenal pheochromocytomas) [112].

Genetic Testing

Guidelines from the First International Symposium on Pheochromocytoma (ISP2005) suggest genetic testing for any patient with a suggestive family history, age <35 years, multifocal, bilateral adrenal, extra-adrenal, or malignant disease [36]. However, regional differences in the frequency of germline mutations and local resources also need to be taken into consideration. The identification of a germline mutation should prompt screening for synchronous pheochromocytoma and life-long screening for metachronous pheochromocytomas and syndrome-related tumors. First degree relatives should also be offered genetic testing after appropriate counseling.

Pathogenesis

Genetic Mechanisms of Tumorigenesis

Identification of the susceptibility genes *VHL, RET, SDHD,* and *SDHB* in familial pheochromocytoma/paraganglioma syndromes has established some key genes that are involved in the development of familial tumors. However, somatic mutations of these genes are rarely present in sporadic pheochromocytomas or paragangliomas, and the mechanism of oncogenesis in sporadic tumors remains poorly understood. Mutations in well-recognized oncogenes such as *K-Ras, c-mos, N-myc, C-myc, Ernb,* and tumor suppressor genes such as *p53* and *p21* are not common in sporadic tumors although loss of *Rb* and over-expression of *mdm2, Bcl-2,* and *IGF-2* have been reported [113–115].

Several studies have used comparative genomic hybridization or loss of heterozygosity to characterize chromosomal alterations in pheochromocytoma and paraganglioma. Common chromosomal sites of deletion are 1p, 3p, 3q, 11p, 11q, and 22q with common sites of gain seen at 17q and chromosome 19. The chromosomal deletion at 1p appears as the earliest and most consistent site of gross loss and may be a site that harbors several tumor suppressor genes [116, 117]. Recently, mutations in the KIF1Bbeta gene located in this region were found to be present in neuroblastomas and pheochromocytomas suggesting its role as a potential tumor suppressor [118]. A cancer prone family with a *KIF1Bbeta* germline variant prone to neural and nonneural crest tumors has since been identified [95].

A recent gene expression profiling study on pheochromocytomas with a germline mutation has demonstrated that *VHL, SDHB,* and *SDHD* mutations are associated with a transcription signature characterized by genes related to hypoxia-driven transcription pathways. The signature of tumors with *RET* mutations, however, is consistent with increased activity of the *Ras*-mediated MAPK pathway [119]. Gene expression profiling studies have also identified a number of differentially expressed genes between benign and malignant tumors which could potentially be used as a prognostic tool, however, the studies to date have been small and further confirmatory studies are awaited [120, 121].

Succinate Dehydrogenase

SDH is an enzyme involved in both the citric acid cycle (also known as Krebs or tricarboxylic (TCA) cycle) and mitochondrial electron transport chain. The enzyme is a complex heterotetramer which consists of four subunits (SDHA, SDHB, SDHC, and SDHD) and catalyzes the oxidation of succinate to fumarate. The genes which code for the SDH subunits are highly conserved amongst species and are nuclear even though the enzyme is located within the inner mitochondrial membrane [122, 123].

The accumulation of succinate has been associated with tumor formation and mutations of the SDHB, C, and D subunits have recently been recognized to result in pheochromocytoma/paraganglioma familial syndromes. The SDHA subunit does not appear to demonstrate tumor suppressor behavior, however, bi-allelic mutations result in a degenerative neurological syndrome known as Leigh's syndrome [122].

HIF and EglN3/PHD Pathways

The observations that carotid body tumors occur at greater frequency at very high altitudes, play a central role in oxygen sensing and are highly vascular, led to the hypothesis that paraganglioma and pheochromocytoma oncogenesis was likely to involve a critical component of the oxygen sensing or signaling pathways.

The hypoxia inducible transcription factors HIF-1 and HIF-2 are key regulators of cellular oxygen homeostasis. Under normoxic conditions, HIF-1 is hydroxylated

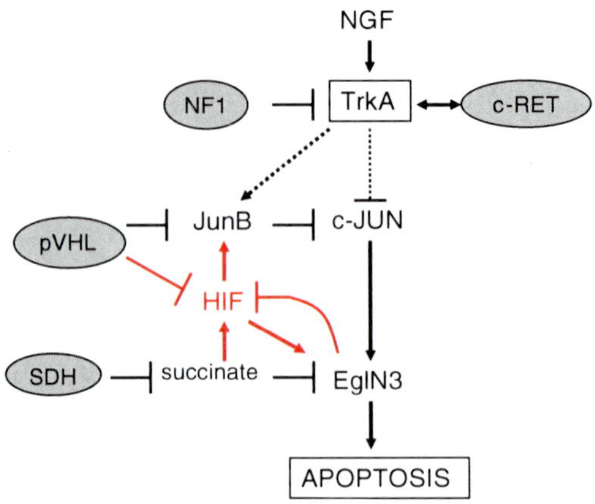

Fig. 9.4 As nerve growth factor (NGF) levels become limiting during development, mutations affecting *NF1*, *RET*, *VHL*, and SDH subunits decrease the apoptosis mediated by SM-20/EglN3/PHD3. Adapted from Lee et al. (2005) to show interactions with hypoxia inducible factor (HIF) (TrkA = NGF receptor) (Reprinted from PH Maxwell, Cancer Cell. 2005;8:91–3, modified from Lee et al. (2005) with permission from Elsevier)

by prolyl hydroxylase (PHD) with subsequent binding and ubiquitination by the pVHL–elonginB–elonginC/CUL2 complex thus targeting HIF-1 for proteasomal degradation. Under hypoxic conditions, increased expression of HIF-1 results in the activation of several hypoxia responsive genes including vascular endothelial growth factor, platelet-derived growth factor, endothelial growth factor receptor, glucose transporter protein 1, erythropoietin, and transforming growth factor-α. Mutations of the SDHB, C, and D subunits or the VHL protein can result in a pseudohypoxic state whereby a hypoxic cellular response will occur due to HIF-1 accumulation despite normal oxygen conditions, thereby promoting tumor growth by inducing angiogenesis, cellular survival, and proliferation [124].

Lee et al. provide evidence that mutations affecting *RET*, *NF1*, *VHL*, or SDH subunits result in dysregulation linked by a common apoptotic pathway involving JunB, c-Jun, and EglN3/PHD3 (Fig. 9.4). Dysregulation of this pathway results in defective apoptosis of neural crest cells during development which may explain the common phenotype seen with mutations in otherwise unrelated genes [125].

Conclusion

Significant improvements of the diagnosis, localization, pharmacological, and surgical management of pheochromocytomas in recent times have led to improved outcomes for patients with pheochromocytoma, with a current perioperative mortality of less than 2%. However, pheochromocytomas remain challenging tumors to manage and require multidisciplinary input for optimum outcomes. The recognition of familial pheochromocytoma susceptibility genes has given further insights into the pathogenesis of pheochromocytoma and has allowed the identification and screening of germline mutation carriers and affected family members. As a result of genetic testing and appropriate screening, germline mutation carriers will have improved outcomes due to the early detection and treatment of a pheochromocytoma or syndrome-associated tumor. The outcome of malignant pheochromocytoma remains poor, however, future development of effective novel treatment options or targeted gene therapy for malignant disease may become possible as our understanding of the pathogenesis and molecular events that occur with the development of pheochromocytoma and paraganglioma continues to improve.

References

1. Ronald A Delellis (2004) WHO histological classification of tumours of the adrenal gland. IARC Press, Lyon
2. Beard CM, Sheps SG, Kurland LT, Carney JA, Lie JT (1983) Occurrence of pheochromocytoma in Rochester, Minnesota, 1950 through 1979. Mayo Clin Proc 58(12):802–804
3. Fernandez-Calvet L, Garcia-Mayor RV (1994) Incidence of pheochromocytoma in South Galicia, Spain. J Intern Med 236(6):675–677
4. Stenstrom G, Svardsudd K (1986) Pheochromocytoma in Sweden 1958–1981. An analysis of the National Cancer Registry Data. Acta Med Scand 220(3):225–232
5. McNeil AR, Blok BH, Koelmeyer TD, Burke MP, Hilton JM (2000) Phaeochromocytomas discovered during coronial autopsies in Sydney, Melbourne and Auckland. Aust N Z J Med 30(6):648–652
6. Lo CY, Lam KY, Wat MS, Lam KS (2000) Adrenal pheochromocytoma remains a frequently overlooked diagnosis. Am J Surg 179(3):212–215
7. Ariton M, Juan CS, AvRuskin TW (2000) Pheochromocytoma: clinical observations from a Brooklyn tertiary hospital. Endocr Pract 6(3):249–252
8. Omura M, Saito J, Yamaguchi K, Kakuta Y, Nishikawa T (2004) Prospective study on the prevalence of secondary hypertension among hypertensive patients visiting a general outpatient clinic in Japan. Hypertens Res 27(3):193–202
9. Goldstein RE, O'Neill JA Jr, Holcomb GW, 3rd et al (1999) Clinical experience over 48 years with pheochromocytoma. Ann Surg 229(6):755–764; discussion 764–756
10. Kaufman BH, Telander RL, van Heerden JA, Zimmerman D, Sheps SG, Dawson B (1983) Pheochromocytoma in the pediatric age group: current status. J Pediatr Surg 18(6):879–884
11. Glibert SF (2000) Developmental Biology. In: Glibert SF (ed) Developmental Biology, 6th edn. Sinauer Associates Inc, Sunderland, Massachusetts
12. Lack E (1997) Tumors of the adrenal gland and extra-adrenal paraganglia. Atlas of tumor pathology, vol 3. Armed Forces Institute of Pathology, Washington, DC
13. Komminoth P, de Krijger R, Tischler A (2002) Paraganlia and the adrenal medulla. In: LiVolsi V, Asa S (eds) Endocrine pathology. Churchill Livingstone, Philadelphia, pp 149–169
14. McNicol AM, Young WF, Kawashima A, Komminoth P, Tischler AS (2004) Benign phaeochromocytoma. In: DeLellis RA, Lloyd RV, Heitz PU, Eng C (eds) WHO classification of tumours – pathology and genetics of tumours of endocrine organs. IARC Press, Lyon, pp 151–155
15. Demeure MJ (1993) Physiology of the APUD system. Semin Surg Oncol 9(5):362–367
16. Eisenhofer G, Walther MM, Huynh TT et al (2001) Pheochromocytomas in von Hippel-Lindau syndrome and multiple endocrine neoplasia type 2 display distinct biochemical and clinical phenotypes. J Clin Endocrinol Metab 86(5):1999–2008

17. Eisenhofer G, Keiser H, Friberg P et al (1998) Plasma metanephrines are markers of pheochromocytoma produced by catechol-O-methyltransferase within tumors. J Clin Endocrinol Metab 83(6):2175–2185
18. Grossman A, Pacak K, Sawka A et al (2006) Biochemical diagnosis and localization of pheochromocytoma: can we reach a consensus? Ann N Y Acad Sci 1073:332–347
19. Bravo EL, Tagle R (2003) Pheochromocytoma: state-of-the-art and future prospects. Endocr Rev 24(4):539–553
20. Adler JT, Meyer-Rochow GY, Chen H et al (2008) Pheochromocytoma: current approaches and future directions. Oncologist 13(7):779–793
21. Bravo EL (2002) Pheochromocytoma: an approach to antihypertensive management. Ann N Y Acad Sci 970:1–10
22. Lee JA, Zarnegar R, Shen WT, Kebebew E, Clark OH, Duh QY (2007) Adrenal incidentaloma, borderline elevations of urine or plasma metanephrine levels, and the "subclinical" pheochromocytoma. Arch Surg 142(9):870–873; discussion 873–874
23. Kasperlik-Zeluska AA, Roslonowska E, Slowinska-Srzednicka J et al (1997) Incidentally discovered adrenal mass (incidentaloma): investigation and management of 208 patients. Clin Endocrinol (Oxf) 46(1):29–37
24. Stein PP, Black HR (1991) A simplified diagnostic approach to pheochromocytoma. A review of the literature and report of one institution's experience. Medicine (Baltimore) 70(1):46–66
25. Bravo EL (2004) Pheochromocytoma: current perspectives in the pathogenesis, diagnosis, and management. Arq Bras Endocrinol Metabol 48(5):746–750
26. Eisenhofer G, Rivers G, Rosas AL, Quezado Z, Manger WM, Pacak K (2007) Adverse drug reactions in patients with phaeochromocytoma: incidence, prevention and management. Drug Saf 30(11):1031–1062
27. Taylor MJ, McIndoe A (2007) Unresponsive asystolic cardiac arrest responding to external cardiac pacing in a patient with phaeochromocytoma. Anaesthesia 62(8):838–841
28. Londe S (1978) Causes of hypertension in the young. Pediatr Clin North Am 25(1):55–65
29. De Krijger RR, Petri BJ, Van Nederveen FH et al (2006) Frequent genetic changes in childhood pheochromocytomas. Ann N Y Acad Sci 1073:166–176
30. Beltsevich DG, Kuznetsov NS, Kazaryan AM, Lysenko MA (2004) Pheochromocytoma surgery: epidemiologic peculiarities in children. World J Surg 28(6):592–596
31. Havekes B, Romijn JA, Eisenhofer G, Adams K, Pacak K (2009) Update on pediatric pheochromocytoma. Pediatr Nephrol 24(5):943–950
32. Whalen RK, Althausen AF, Daniels GH (1992) Extra-adrenal pheochromocytoma. J Urol 147(1):1–10
33. Neumann HP, Bausch B, McWhinney SR et al (2002) Germ-line mutations in nonsyndromic pheochromocytoma. N Engl J Med 346(19):1459–1466
34. Pomares FJ, Canas R, Rodriguez JM, Hernandez AM, Parrilla P, Tebar FJ (1998) Differences between sporadic and multiple endocrine neoplasia type 2A phaeochromocytoma. Clin Endocrinol (Oxf) 48(2):195–200
35. Walther MM, Reiter R, Keiser HR et al (1999) Clinical and genetic characterization of pheochromocytoma in von Hippel-Lindau families: comparison with sporadic pheochromocytoma gives insight into natural history of pheochromocytoma. J Urol 162(3 Pt 1):659–664
36. Bornstein SR, Gimenez-Roqueplo AP (2006) Genetic testing in pheochromocytoma: increasing importance for clinical decision making. Ann N Y Acad Sci 1073:94–103
37. Loh KC, Fitzgerald PA, Matthay KK, Yeo PP, Price DC (1997) The treatment of malignant pheochromocytoma with iodine-131 metaiodobenzylguanidine (131I-MIBG): a comprehensive review of 116 reported patients. J Endocrinol Invest 20(11):648–658
38. Plouin PF, Chatellier G, Fofol I, Corvol P (1997) Tumor recurrence and hypertension persistence after successful pheochromocytoma operation. Hypertension 29(5):1133–1139
39. Tischler AS (2008) Pheochromocytoma and extra-adrenal paraganglioma: updates. Arch Pathol Lab Med 132(8):1272–1284
40. Chrisoulidou A, Kaltsas G, Ilias I, Grossman AB (2007) The diagnosis and management of malignant phaeochromocytoma and paraganglioma. Endocr Relat Cancer 14(3):569–585

41. Shen WT, Sturgeon C, Clark OH, Duh QY, Kebebew E (2004) Should pheochromocytoma size influence surgical approach? A comparison of 90 malignant and 60 benign pheochromocytomas. Surgery 136(6):1129–1137
42. van der Harst E, de Herder WW, de Krijger RR et al (2002) The value of plasma markers for the clinical behaviour of phaeochromocytomas. Eur J Endocrinol 147(1):85–94
43. Helman LJ, Cohen PS, Averbuch SD, Cooper MJ, Keiser HR, Israel MA (1989) Neuropeptide Y expression distinguishes malignant from benign pheochromocytoma. J Clin Oncol 7(11):1720–1725
44. Linnoila RI, Keiser HR, Steinberg SM, Lack EE (1990) Histopathology of benign versus malignant sympathoadrenal paragangliomas: clinicopathologic study of 120 cases including unusual histologic features. Hum Pathol 21(11):1168–1180
45. Gimenez-Roqueplo AP, Favier J, Rustin P et al (2003) Mutations in the SDHB gene are associated with extra-adrenal and/or malignant phaeochromocytomas. Cancer Res 63(17):5615–5621
46. Brouwers FM, Eisenhofer G, Tao JJ et al (2006) High frequency of SDHB germline mutations in patients with malignant catecholamine-producing paragangliomas: implications for genetic testing. J Clin Endocrinol Metab 91(11):4505–4509
47. Eisenhofer G, Bornstein SR, Brouwers FM et al (2004) Malignant pheochromocytoma: current status and initiatives for future progress. Endocr Relat Cancer 11(3):423–436
48. Amar L, Bertherat J, Baudin E et al (2005) Genetic testing in pheochromocytoma or functional paraganglioma. J Clin Oncol 23(34):8812–8818
49. Thompson LD (2002) Pheochromocytoma of the Adrenal gland Scaled Score (PASS) to separate benign from malignant neoplasms: a clinicopathologic and immunophenotypic study of 100 cases. Am J Surg Pathol 26(5):551–566
50. Strong VE, Kennedy T, Al-Ahmadie H et al (2008) Prognostic indicators of malignancy in adrenal pheochromocytomas: clinical, histopathologic, and cell cycle/apoptosis gene expression analysis. Surgery 143(6):759–768
51. Brouwers FM, Petricoin EF 3rd, Ksinantova L et al (2005) Low molecular weight proteomic information distinguishes metastatic from benign pheochromocytoma. Endocr Relat Cancer 12(2):263–272
52. John H, Ziegler WH, Hauri D, Jaeger P (1999) Pheochromocytomas: can malignant potential be predicted? Urology 53(4):679–683
53. Sisson JC, Shulkin BL, Esfandiari NH (2006) Courses of malignant pheochromocytoma: implications for therapy. Ann N Y Acad Sci 1073:505–511
54. Eisenhofer G, Siegert G, Kotzerke J, Bornstein SR, Pacak K (2008) Current progress and future challenges in the biochemical diagnosis and treatment of pheochromocytomas and paragangliomas. Horm Metab Res 40(5):329–337
55. Lenders JW, Eisenhofer G, Mannelli M, Pacak K (2005) Phaeochromocytoma. Lancet 366(9486):665–675
56. Abe M, Orita Y, Nakashima Y, Nakamura M (1984) Hypertensive crisis induced by metoclopramide in patient with pheochromocytoma. Angiology 35(2):122–128
57. Lawrence AM (1967) Glucagon provocative test for pheochromocytoma. Ann Intern Med 66(6):1091–1096
58. Eisenhofer G, Goldstein DS, Walther MM et al (2003) Biochemical diagnosis of pheochromocytoma: how to distinguish true- from false-positive test results. J Clin Endocrinol Metab 88(6):2656–2666
59. Sjoberg RJ, Simcic KJ, Kidd GS (1992) The clonidine suppression test for pheochromocytoma. A review of its utility and pitfalls. Arch Intern Med 152(6):1193–1197
60. Ilias I, Pacak K (2004) Current approaches and recommended algorithm for the diagnostic localization of pheochromocytoma. J Clin Endocrinol Metab 89(2):479–491
61. Maurea S, Cuocolo A, Reynolds JC, Neumann RD, Salvatore M (1996) Diagnostic imaging in patients with paragangliomas. Computed tomography, magnetic resonance and MIBG scintigraphy comparison. Q J Nucl Med 40(4):365–371
62. Sahdev A, Sohaib A, Monson JP, Grossman AB, Chew SL, Reznek RH (2005) CT and MR imaging of unusual locations of extra-adrenal paragangliomas (pheochromocytomas). Eur Radiol 15(1):85–92

63. Van Der Horst-Schrivers AN, Jager PL, Boezen HM, Schouten JP, Kema IP, Links TP (2006) Iodine-123 metaiodobenzylguanidine scintigraphy in localising phaeochromocytomas – experience and meta-analysis. Anticancer Res 26(2B):1599–1604
64. Ilias I, Yu J, Carrasquillo JA et al (2003) Superiority of 6-[18F]-fluorodopamine positron emission tomography versus [131I]-metaiodobenzylguanidine scintigraphy in the localization of metastatic pheochromocytoma. J Clin Endocrinol Metab 88(9):4083–4087
65. Shapiro B, Sisson JC, Shulkin BL, Gross MD, Zempel S (1995) The current status of meta-iodobenzylguanidine and related agents for the diagnosis of neuro-endocrine tumors. Q J Nucl Med 39(4 Suppl 1):3–8
66. Esfandiari NH, Shulkin BL, Bui C, Jaffe CA (2006) Multimodality imaging of malignant pheochromocytoma. Clin Nucl Med 31(12):822–825
67. Khorram-Manesh A, Ahlman H, Nilsson O et al (2005) Long-term outcome of a large series of patients surgically treated for pheochromocytoma. J Intern Med 258(1):55–66
68. Modlin IM, Farndon JR, Shepherd A et al (1979) Phaeochromocytomas in 72 patients: clinical and diagnostic features, treatment and long term results. Br J Surg 66(7):456–465
69. Schuttler J, Westhofen P, Kania U, Ihmsen H, Kammerecker S, Hirner A (1995) Quantitative assessment of catecholamine secretion as a rational principle of anesthesia management in pheochromocytoma surgery. Anasthesiol Intensivmed Notfallmed Schmerzther 30(6):341–349
70. Lebuffe G, Dosseh ED, Tek G et al (2005) The effect of calcium channel blockers on outcome following the surgical treatment of phaeochromocytomas and paragangliomas. Anaesthesia 60(5):439–444
71. Prys-Roberts C (2000) Phaeochromocytoma – recent progress in its management. Br J Anaesth 85(1):44–57
72. Steinsapir J, Carr AA, Prisant LM, Bransome ED Jr (1997) Metyrosine and pheochromocytoma. Arch Intern Med 157(8):901–906
73. Elliott HL, Meredith PA, Vincent J, Reid JL (1986) Clinical pharmacological studies with doxazosin. Br J Clin Pharmacol 21(Suppl 1):27S–31S
74. Bravo EL (1997) Pheochromocytoma. Curr Ther Endocrinol Metab 6:195–197
75. Mannelli M (2006) Management and treatment of pheochromocytomas and paragangliomas. Ann N Y Acad Sci 1073:405–416
76. Pacak K (2007) Preoperative management of the pheochromocytoma patient. J Clin Endocrinol Metab 92(11):4069–4079
77. Kinney MA, Narr BJ, Warner MA (2002) Perioperative management of pheochromocytoma. J Cardiothorac Vasc Anesth 16(3):359–369
78. Kanto JH (1985) Current status of labetalol, the first alpha- and beta-blocking agent. Int J Clin Pharmacol Ther Toxicol 23(11):617–628
79. Thompson GB, Grant CS, van Heerden JA et al (1997) Laparoscopic versus open posterior adrenalectomy: a case-control study of 100 patients. Surgery 122(6):1132–1136
80. Ippolito G, Palazzo FF, Sebag F, Thakur A, Cherenko M, Henry JF (2008) Safety of laparoscopic adrenalectomy in patients with large pheochromocytomas: a single institution review. World J Surg 32(5):840–844
81. Soon PS, Yeh MW, Delbridge LW et al (2008) Laparoscopic surgery is safe for large adrenal lesions. Eur J Surg Oncol 34(1):67–70
82. Jansson S, Khorram-Manesh A, Nilsson O et al (2006) Treatment of bilateral pheochromocytoma and adrenal medullary hyperplasia. Ann N Y Acad Sci 1073:429–435
83. Yip L, Lee JE, Shapiro SE et al (2004) Surgical management of hereditary pheochromocytoma. J Am Coll Surg 198(4):525–534; discussion 534–525
84. Amar L, Servais A, Gimenez-Roqueplo AP, Zinzindohoue F, Chatellier G, Plouin PF (2005) Year of diagnosis, features at presentation, and risk of recurrence in patients with pheochromocytoma or secreting paraganglioma. J Clin Endocrinol Metab 90(4):2110–2116
85. Huang H, Abraham J, Hung E et al (2008) Treatment of malignant pheochromocytoma/paraganglioma with cyclophosphamide, vincristine, and dacarbazine: recommendation from a 22-year follow-up of 18 patients. Cancer 113(8):2020–2028

86. Gedik GK, Hoefnagel CA, Bais E, Valdes Olmos RA (2008) (131)I-MIBG therapy in metastatic phaeochromocytoma and paraganglioma. Eur J Nucl Med Mol Imaging 35(4):725–733
87. Scholz T, Eisenhofer G, Pacak K, Dralle H, Lehnert H (2007) Clinical review: current treatment of malignant pheochromocytoma. J Clin Endocrinol Metab 92(4):1217–1225
88. Fitzgerald PA, Goldsby RE, Huberty JP et al (2006) Malignant pheochromocytomas and paragangliomas: a phase II study of therapy with high-dose 131I-metaiodobenzylguanidine (131I-MIBG). Ann N Y Acad Sci 1073:465–490
89. Yu L, Fleckman AM, Chadha M, Sacks E, Levetan C, Vikram B (1996) Radiation therapy of metastatic pheochromocytoma: case report and review of the literature. Am J Clin Oncol 19(4):389–393
90. Forrer F, Riedweg I, Maecke HR, Mueller-Brand J (2008) Radiolabeled DOTATOC in patients with advanced paraganglioma and pheochromocytoma. Q J Nucl Med Mol Imaging 52(4):334–340
91. Astuti D, Latif F, Dallol A et al (2001) Gene mutations in the succinate dehydrogenase subunit SDHB cause susceptibility to familial pheochromocytoma and to familial paraganglioma. Am J Hum Genet 69(1):49–54
92. Niemann S, Muller U (2000) Mutations in SDHC cause autosomal dominant paraganglioma, type 3. Nat Genet 26(3):268–270
93. Baysal BE, Ferrell RE, Willett-Brozick JE et al (2000) Mutations in SDHD, a mitochondrial complex II gene, in hereditary paraganglioma. Science 287(5454):848–851
94. Mannelli M, Simi L, Gagliano MS et al (2007) Genetics and biology of pheochromocytoma. Exp Clin Endocrinol Diabetes 115(3):160–165
95. Yeh IT, Lenci RE, Qin Y et al (2008) A germline mutation of the KIF1B beta gene on 1p36 in a family with neural and nonneural tumors. Hum Genet 124(3):279–285
96. Carney JA, Stratakis CA (2002) Familial paraganglioma and gastric stromal sarcoma: a new syndrome distinct from the Carney triad. Am J Med Genet 108(2):132–139
97. Pasini B, McWhinney SR, Bei T et al (2008) Clinical and molecular genetics of patients with the Carney-Stratakis syndrome and germline mutations of the genes coding for the succinate dehydrogenase subunits SDHB, SDHC, and SDHD. Eur J Hum Genet 16(1):79–88
98. Maher ER, Yates JR, Harries R et al (1990) Clinical features and natural history of von Hippel-Lindau disease. Q J Med 77(283):1151–1163
99. Friedrich CA (1999) Von Hippel-Lindau syndrome. A pleomorphic condition. Cancer 86(11 Suppl):2478–2482
100. Lonser RR, Glenn GM, Walther M et al (2003) von Hippel-Lindau disease. Lancet 361(9374):2059–2067
101. Maher ER, Kaelin WG Jr (1997) von Hippel-Lindau disease. Medicine (Baltimore) 76(6):381–391
102. Gagel RF, Tashjian AH Jr, Cummings T et al (1988) The clinical outcome of prospective screening for multiple endocrine neoplasia type 2a. An 18-year experience. N Engl J Med 318(8):478–484
103. Modigliani E, Vasen HM, Raue K et al (1995) Pheochromocytoma in multiple endocrine neoplasia type 2: European study. The Euromen Study Group. J Intern Med 238(4):363–367
104. Chevinsky AH, Minton JP, Falko JM (1990) Metastatic pheochromocytoma associated with multiple endocrine neoplasia syndrome type II. Arch Surg 125(7):935–938
105. Karagiannis A, Mikhailidis DP, Athyros VG, Harsoulis F (2007) Pheochromocytoma: an update on genetics and management. Endocr Relat Cancer 14(4):935–956
106. Gutmann DH, Aylsworth A, Carey JC et al (1997) The diagnostic evaluation and multidisciplinary management of neurofibromatosis 1 and neurofibromatosis 2. JAMA 278(1):51–57
107. Neumann HP, Pawlu C, Peczkowska M et al (2004) Distinct clinical features of paraganglioma syndromes associated with SDHB and SDHD gene mutations. JAMA 292(8):943–951
108. Gimenez-Roqueplo AP, Lehnert H, Mannelli M et al (2006) Phaeochromocytoma, new genes and screening strategies. Clin Endocrinol (Oxf) 65(6):699–705

109. Mannelli M, Ercolino T, Giache V, Simi L, Cirami C, Parenti G (2007) Genetic screening for pheochromocytoma: should SDHC gene analysis be included? J Med Genet 44(9):586–587
110. Benn DE, Richardson AL, Marsh DJ, Robinson BG (2006) Genetic testing in pheochromocytoma- and paraganglioma-associated syndromes. Ann N Y Acad Sci 1073:104–111
111. Matyakhina L, Bei TA, McWhinney SR et al (2007) Genetics of carney triad: recurrent losses at chromosome 1 but lack of germline mutations in genes associated with paragangliomas and gastrointestinal stromal tumors. J Clin Endocrinol Metab 92(8):2938–2943
112. Carney JA (1999) Gastric stromal sarcoma, pulmonary chondroma, and extra-adrenal paraganglioma (Carney Triad): natural history, adrenocortical component, and possible familial occurrence. Mayo Clin Proc 74(6):543–552
113. Gelato MC, Vassalotti J (1990) Insulin-like growth factor-II: possible local growth factor in pheochromocytoma. J Clin Endocrinol Metab 71(5):1168–1174
114. Lam KY, Lo CY, Wat NM, Luk JM, Lam KS (2001) The clinicopathological features and importance of p53, Rb, and mdm2 expression in phaeochromocytomas and paragangliomas. J Clin Pathol 54(6):443–448
115. Clarke MR, Weyant RJ, Watson CG, Carty SE (1998) Prognostic markers in pheochromocytoma. Hum Pathol 29(5):522–526
116. Geli J, Nord B, Frisk T et al (2005) Deletions and altered expression of the RIZ1 tumour suppressor gene in 1p36 in pheochromocytomas and abdominal paragangliomas. Int J Oncol 26(5):1385–1391
117. Benn DE, Dwight T, Richardson AL et al (2000) Sporadic and familial pheochromocytomas are associated with loss of at least two discrete intervals on chromosome 1p. Cancer Res 60(24):7048–7051
118. Schlisio S, Kenchappa RS, Vredeveld LC et al (2008) The kinesin KIF1Bbeta acts downstream from EglN3 to induce apoptosis and is a potential 1p36 tumor suppressor. Genes Dev 22(7):884–893
119. Dahia PL (2006) Transcription association of VHL and SDH mutations link hypoxia and oxidoreductase signals in pheochromocytomas. Ann N Y Acad Sci 1073:208–220
120. Thouennon E, Elkahloun AG, Guillemot J et al (2007) Identification of potential gene markers and insights into the pathophysiology of pheochromocytoma malignancy. J Clin Endocrinol Metab 92(12):4865–4872
121. Brouwers FM, Elkahloun AG, Munson PJ et al (2006) Gene expression profiling of benign and malignant pheochromocytoma. Ann N Y Acad Sci 1073:541–556
122. Favier J, Briere JJ, Strompf L et al (2005) Hereditary paraganglioma/pheochromocytoma and inherited succinate dehydrogenase deficiency. Horm Res 63(4):171–179
123. Rustin P, Munnich A, Rotig A (2002) Succinate dehydrogenase and human diseases: new insights into a well-known enzyme. Eur J Hum Genet 10(5):289–291
124. Semenza GL (2007) Hypoxia-inducible factor 1 (HIF-1) pathway. Sci STKE 2007(407):cm8
125. Lee S, Nakamura E, Yang H et al (2005) Neuronal apoptosis linked to EglN3 prolyl hydroxylase and familial pheochromocytoma genes: developmental culling and cancer. Cancer Cell 8(2):155–167

Chapter 10
Functional Cortical Neoplasms

Ali Zarrinpar and Michael W. Yeh

Introduction

Adrenocortical neoplasms affect men and women equally. While they do not spare children [1], the prevalence of these tumors does increase with age, up to 7% in adults older than 50 [2, 3]. Many are found incidentally at autopsy [4] or by imaging done for other purposes. They may be detected because of symptoms or signs related to hormone production [5, 6] or size [5]. Some even appear outside of the actual adrenal gland [7].

Tumors of the adrenal cortex are classified according to function and malignancy. Functional adrenocortical tumors hypersecrete hormones that reflect their cells of origin. Tumors that produce aldosterone, cortisol, and sex steroids correspond to the zona glomerulosa, zona fasciculata, and zona reticularis, respectively. The fraction of detected adrenocortical tumors that are functional has increased from 50 to 79% in recent series [3, 8, 9]. Interestingly, acquired hyperplasia and adenomas may start out as nonfunctional processes and only later result in clinical manifestations of hormonal excess [10].

Adrenocortical carcinomas also frequently elaborate multiple hormones; however, these aggressive neoplasms will be specifically addressed in depth in Chap. 11. This chapter will cover the usually benign variants of functional tumors of the adrenal cortex. These tumors may cause hyperaldosteronism (Conn's syndrome), hypercortisolism (Cushing's syndrome), and, less commonly, virilizing or feminizing syndromes due to sex steroid excess. It is important to note that the distinction between benign and malignant adrenocortical tumors may be difficult to establish preoperatively, intraoperatively, and even on histopathology. Surgical specimens should be analyzed by pathologists experienced in using the microscopic criteria for malignancy, such as the Weiss revisited index (WRI) or the van Slooten index (VSI) [11–13]. Although routine use is currently not recommended, there are molecular markers such as IGF-II overexpression and allelic losses at 17p13 with immunohistochemistry

M.W. Yeh (✉)
David Geffen School of Medicine, University of California, Los Angeles, CA, USA
e-mail: myeh@mednet.ucla.edu

C. Sturgeon (ed.), *Endocrine Neoplasia*, Cancer Treatment and Research, vol 153,
DOI 10.1007/978-1-4419-0857-5_10, © Springer Science+Business Media, LLC 2010

of Cyclin E or Ki-67 that are being used experimentally to assess malignancy [3]. Ultimately, the diagnosis of adrenal malignancy is based on clinical behavior, i.e., local invasion, recurrence, or development of distant metastases over time. Thus, the histopathologic diagnosis of atypical adenoma mandates serial surveillance cross-sectional imaging to screen for the possibility of metastatic disease.

Genetic alterations found in familial cases of adrenocortical tumors include TP53 (17q13) in Li-Fraumeni syndrome, menin (11q13) in multiple endocrine neoplasia type 1, PRKARIA (17q22-24) in Carney complex, and p57kip2 (CDKN1C), KCNQ10T, H19, and IGF-II overexpression in Beckwith–Wiedemann syndrome. Mutations in menin, TP53, and CYP21 are also found in sporadic adrenocortical tumors.

Treatment, in general, consists of adrenalectomy for all functional adenomas. Laparoscopic adrenalectomy is the preferred approach in almost all cases. Laparoscopic resection is relatively contraindicated in tumors larger than 10 or 12 cm, in those that are locally invasive, and in known carcinomas [14]. Some surgeons will approach considerably smaller tumors with a conventional open technique based on concerns over safety and malignant potential.

Primary Hyperaldosteronism and Aldosteronoma

Hyperaldosteronism results in loss of potassium in the urine, retention of sodium, and hypertension [15, 16]. The hypertension can be moderate to severe and resistant to medication. The hypersecretion of aldosterone due to renal artery stenosis, or low-flow states such as congestive heart failure and cirrhosis, is considered secondary hyperaldosteronism. In these cases, high levels of aldosterone are the result of high renin levels, and the underlying causes need to be addressed. Primary hyperaldosteronism, on the other hand, is due to autonomous aldosterone oversecretion, which leads to suppression of renin levels via negative feedback on the juxtaglomerular apparatus.

Primary hyperaldosteronism predominantly occurs in people between the ages of 30 and 50 years and has a slight male predilection. According to most reports, it accounts for approximately 1% of cases of hypertension [17]. Studies examining widespread screening of hypertensive populations reported a 10–40% prevalence of primary hyperaldosteronism [18], though these elevated figures are generally thought to reflect strong referral bias. The current consensus is that the actual prevalence of primary hyperaldosteronism in unselected hypertensive patients is approximately 5–13% [19]. The use of the plasma aldosterone concentration to plasma renin activity ratio (PAC/PRA) to screen hypertensive patients for primary hyperaldosteronism has been shown to increase the absolute number of unilateral adrenal-producing adenomas identified; however, the PAC/PRA ratio is nonspecific for this tumor because it is also positive in cases of primary hyperaldosteronism due to bilateral adrenal hyperplasia [20].

Studies comparing subjects biochemically confirmed to have primary hyperaldosteronism with controls matched for age and systolic blood pressure have demonstrated that primary hyperaldosteronism is independently associated with a significantly increased risk of stroke, myocardial infarction, atrial fibrillation, arterial wall stiffness, urinary albumin excretion, and left ventricular hypertrophy [21]. Much of this comorbid disease appears to improve 1 year after resection of an aldosterone-producing adenoma.

Primary hyperaldosteronism may be due to a solitary aldosterone-producing adenoma as in the classic Conn's syndrome (constituting about 60% of cases), bilateral idiopathic hyperplasia (35%), unilateral adrenal hyperplasia (~2%), adrenocortical carcinoma (<1%), familial hyperaldosteronism (<1%), and ectopic aldosterone producing tumors (very rare). Aldosteronoma are usually unilateral, solitary, and small (<2 cm in diameter) [22]. The fraction of primary hyperaldosteronism cases due to bilateral idiopathic hyperplasia may be increasing as a result of increased detection. A few groups report that these two entities can be distinguished from one another through a combination of clinical and lab parameters including PAC to PRA ratio [23, 24]. This is not certain, however, as there appears to be some overlap among the biochemical features of the two processes [25, 26].

Symptoms and Signs

Patients with primary hyperaldosteronism characteristically present with resistant hypertension, hypokalemia, and normal cortisol excretion [27]. In patients with marked hypokalemia, muscle weakness, paresthesias, fatigue, cramping, headaches, palpitations, polyuria, polydipsia, or nocturia can be common. Symptoms of weakness and fatigue are associated with hypokalemia. However, there is accumulating evidence that the majority of patients may actually be normokalemic, depending on the population screened. One study found that up to 40% of patients with a confirmed aldosteronoma were normokalemic preoperatively [28]. Hypokalemia seems to be a manifestation of severe or late-stage disease. Typically, patients have moderate to severe hypertension for an average of 7–11 years prior to diagnosis, despite treatment with two to four antihypertensive drugs. Hypertension is generally responsive to spironolactone and this may be predictive of a good response to surgical treatment [29]. A subset of patients with primary hyperaldosteronism will also have superimposed essential hypertension. These patients, who tend to be older, male, and who often have several first degree relatives with essential hypertension, appear to have less blood pressure response from adrenalectomy.

Laboratory Studies

The diagnostic process can be divided into three steps: screening, confirmation, and localization (Fig. 10.1). The first two steps are done biochemically. Screening for primary hyperaldosteronism should be considered in patients with (1) unexplained

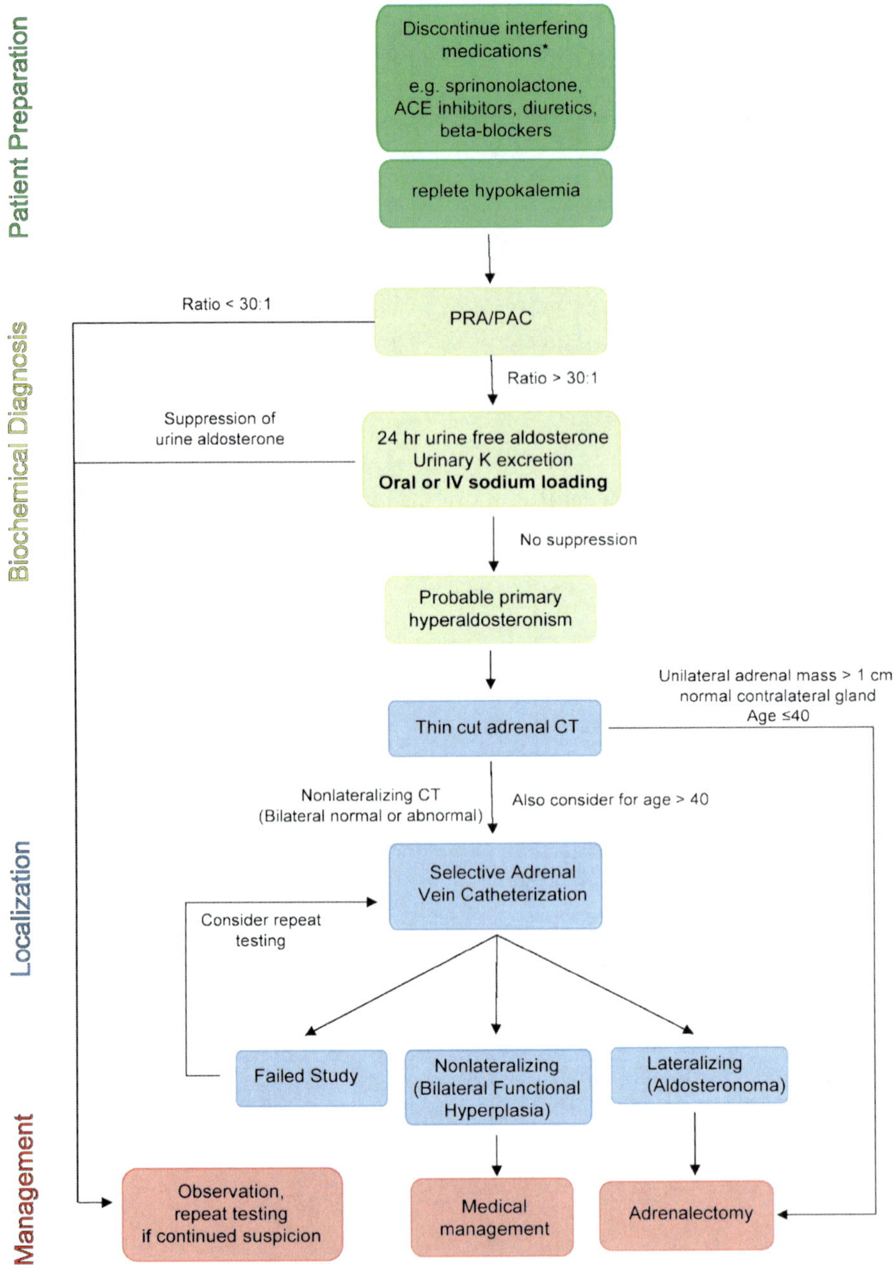

Fig. 10.1 Evaluation and treatment of hyperaldosteronism

hypokalemia, (2) medication-resistant hypertension, (3) hypertension in the setting of an adrenal incidentaloma, (4) early onset hypertension and/or stroke (<50 years), (5) severe hypertension (systolic blood pressure >160 mm Hg or diastolic blood pressure >100 mm Hg), (6) evidence of end organ damage disproportionate to severity of hypertension, (7) diabetes and resistant hypertension (still controversial), or (8) a first degree relative with hyperaldosteronism.

The screening test of choice is a morning paired plasma aldosterone concentration (PAC) and plasma renin activity (PRA). This test is most useful with appropriate patient preparation [30]. All patients being evaluated for hyperaldosteronism should be sodium and potassium replete. To maximize the accuracy of screening tests, the antihypertensive regimen needs to be carefully scrutinized and often modified (if it is safe to do so). The mineralocorticoid antagonists spironolactone and eplerenone or high-dose amiloride should be discontinued for at least 6 weeks. Diuretics, ACE inhibitors, and angiotensin II receptor blockers can falsely elevate the PRA and should be discontinued for 2–3 weeks. Calcium channel blockers can cause a falsely low PAC. Adrenergic inhibitors such as β-blockers and central α_2-agonists suppress renin secretion, but they also inhibit aldosterone secretion, and thus do not appear to affect the screening test significantly. Beta blockers can cause a low PRA and false positive PAC/PRA ratio, however. Other drugs that do not appear to substantially interfere with plasma aldosterone include verapamil slow release, hydralazine, prazosin, doxazosin, and terazosin [31]. Caution should be used when adjusting antihypertensive regimens in these patients, and frequent monitoring is required.

A PAC >15 ng/dL by itself has a high specificity for primary hyperaldosteronism. When divided by PRA, a ratio greater than 25 to 30:1 is a very sensitive test for primary hyperaldosteronism. False-positive results can occur, particularly in patients with chronic renal failure [32]. One should also keep in mind that patients who test positive and are under the age of 30 should be genetically screened for familial glucocorticoid-suppressible aldosteronism, especially if they have a family history of early onset hypertension.

Recently published clinical guidelines recommend that the PAC/PRA ratio only be used as a case-finding test [31]. Confirmation of the diagnosis can be achieved by any one of four additional tests: oral sodium loading, saline infusion, fludrocortisone suppression, and captopril challenge [31].

A commonly used method of confirmation is demonstrating the failure to suppress aldosterone levels despite sodium loading [15, 33]. The initial goal is to create a state of hypervolemia and sodium excess either by oral sodium intake or intravenous saline infusion. In this state, along with measuring the PAC and PRA, a 24-h urine collection is conducted to assess the amount of excreted urinary cortisol, creatinine, sodium, and aldosterone. Oral sodium loading is done by 3 days of a high-sodium diet (5 g NaCl/24 h). As the high sodium diet can lead to worsening urinary potassium excretion and thus hypokalemia, potassium levels need to be checked and repleted daily. To ensure adequate sodium loading, the 24-h urine sodium excretion should exceed 200 mEq. A 24-h urine aldosterone level less than 12 μg after saline loading essentially rules out primary hyperaldosteronism. Some centers have concurrently administered high-dose fludrocortisone (0.1 mg every 6 h) during the oral salt loading to increase the specificity of suppression testing, but this method has not been widely adopted. An alternative method involves loading patients with 2–3 L of normal saline while in supine position over 4–6 h, 2–3 days after being on a low-sodium diet [34]. PAC is normally less than 6 ng/dL in normal subjects and above 10 ng/dL in primary hyperaldosteronism.

Pathology

Aldosteronomas are usually completely encapsulated and small, less than 2 cm in diameter and 50 g [35]. The cut surfaces usually is solid, homogeneous, golden yellow or yellow-brown (except for black adenomas) [36], and without hemorrhage or necrosis [12, 37] (Fig. 10.2). Likewise, microscopically, adrenal cortical tumors can recapitulate the appearance of the zona fasciculata, the zona glomerulosa, or a combination of both (Fig. 10.3). Mitoses are exceptionally rare [38], but they are more frequent in pediatric tumors. There are a number of morphological variants of adrenocortical neoplasms, ranging from those with foci of myelolipoma [39], to black adenomas [40, 41] with either lipofuscin [42] or neuromelanin [43], to corticomedullary mixed tumors with both adrenocortical and adrenomedullary differentiation [44]. Other more rare variants include oncocytomas [45, 46], myxoid neoplasms [47], and lipoadenomas [48].

Radiologic Studies

The treatment of primary hyperaldosteronism relies entirely on finding the cause, be it unilateral, bilateral, or extra-adrenal. Identifying adrenal adenomas can be difficult because most are smaller than 15 mm in maximum dimension. A number of different techniques have been employed, including ultrasound, CT, MRI, selective venous sampling, and scintigraphy. Though adrenal tumors are sometimes found incidentally by ultrasound, with reportedly high sensitivity (up to 96% for tumors smaller than 2 cm) [49], the need for thorough characterization of the tumor and the remainder of

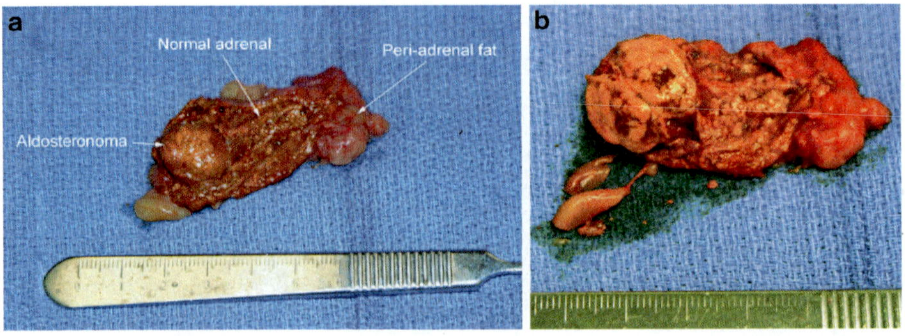

Fig. 10.2 Aldosteronoma (**a**) surgical specimen, (**b**) bisected

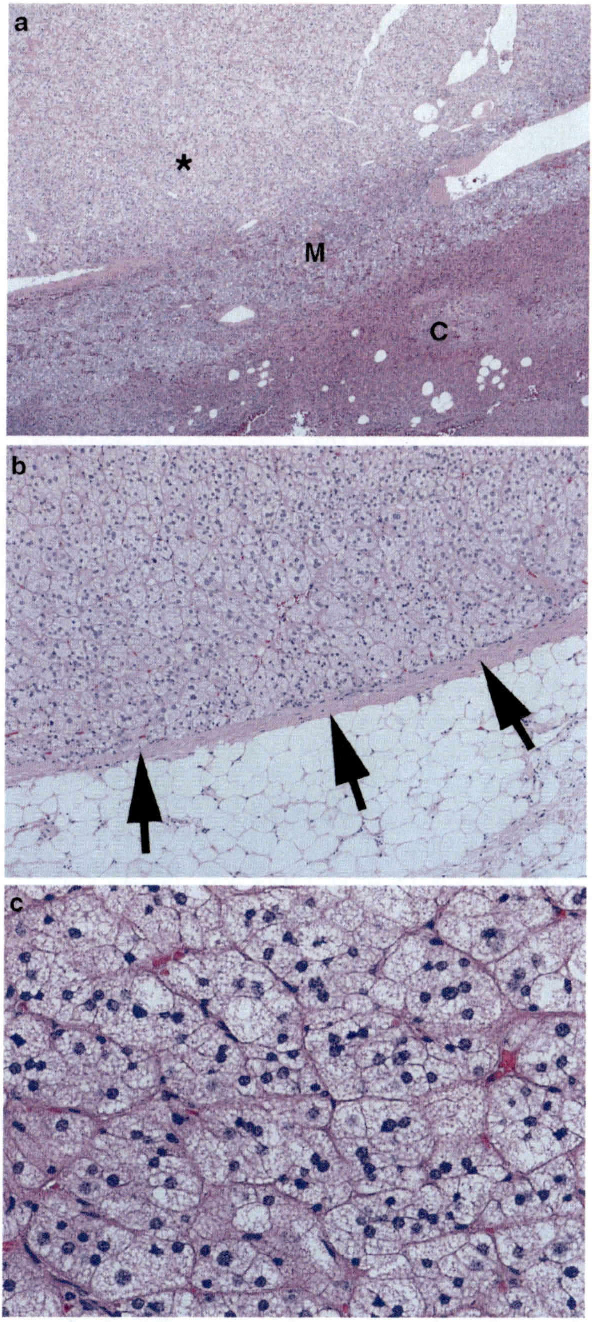

Fig. 10.3 (**a**) An adrenal cortical adenoma (*) is seen compressing adjacent normal adrenal medulla (M) and cortex (C). Often, the tumor is only well delineated from the surrounding cortex rather than being encapsulated (H&E stain, 40×). (**b**) If a capsule (*arrows*) is present, it tends to be thinner and less well-developed than that of an adrenocortical carcinoma (H&E stain, 100×). (**c**) The tumor cells are arranged in cords and nests and have foamy, microvesicular cytoplasm with fairly small, round nuclei and relatively inconspicuous nucleoli (H&E stain, 400×)

the abdomen requires cross-sectional imaging. Computed tomography (CT) is usually the most useful technique for the detection, pretreatment staging, and determination of resectability of these tumors [50] (Fig. 10.4a). It is critical to make the distinction between unilateral and bilateral disease. CT is reasonably reliable for this purpose [51]. It should be performed with thin cuts (3 mm) of the adrenal to achieve a sensitivity of 90%. Usually adenomas appear as unilateral 0.5- to 2-cm adrenal tumors with a normal-appearing contralateral gland, thus confirming an aldosteronoma in the context of appropriate biochemical parameters [52]. CT is also useful in distinguishing adenomas from nonadenomas using contrast washout [53]. Furthermore, adenomas are usually smaller, more homogeneous, and better defined than metastases. Necrosis, hemorrhage, or calcifications are suggestive of malignancy.

MRI is less sensitive but more specific than CT [54](Fig. 10.4b). It also has increased utility in pregnant patients and in patients unable to receive iodinated radiocontrast agents. Adenomas appear homogeneous on MRI.

Cases with equivocal results from cross-sectional imaging may benefit from selective adrenal vein catheterization. Patients with normal adrenal imaging studies and those with bilateral adrenal masses should undergo selective venous catheterization. While many of these patients likely suffer from bilateral hyperplasia, those with more severe hypertension, hypokalemia, higher levels of aldosterone, and those of a younger age at diagnosis should be regarded as having a high probability of unilateral disease. These patients, in addition to those over the age of 40 with a unilateral finding on CT, should undergo adrenal venous sampling. This technique is 95% sensitive and 90% specific in localizing aldosteronomas. The success rate of this technically challenging study is highly operator-dependent. Blood samples are obtained from the vena cava and both adrenal veins. Many institutions use adrenocorticotropic hormone (ACTH) infusion before and during the procedure, but there are reports of falsely increased diagnoses of bilateral disease with the use of ACTH [55]. Blood samples are then assayed for aldosterone and cortisol [56]. It is essential to measure cortisol levels to confirm the proper placement of the catheters in the adrenal veins; the positive

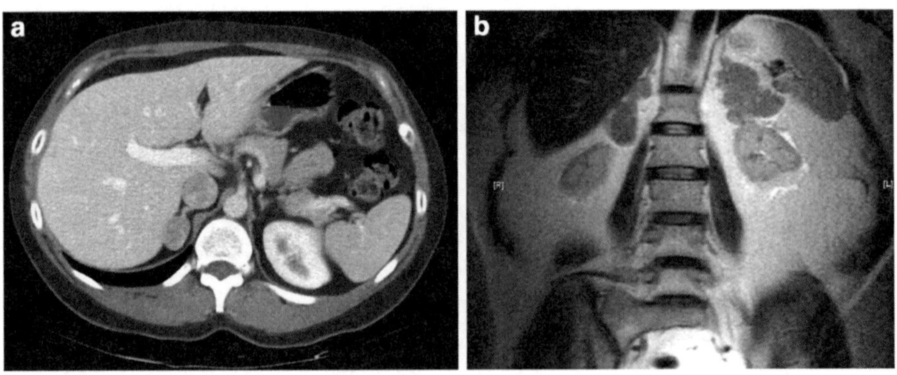

Fig. 10.4 CT and MRI of the adrenal glands. (**a**) CT of right benign adrenal adenoma. (**b**) MRI of bilateral macronodular hyperplasia

control indicating successful cannulation of an adrenal vein is greater than a fivefold increase of the cortisol concentration in a sample relative to peripheral blood. The presence of a unilateral tumor is confirmed by a greater than fourfold difference in the aldosterone/cortisol ratios between the adrenal veins.

Two to ten percent of CT scans demonstrating a unilateral adrenal mass will represent false-positive localization. As a result of this, some advocate the routine use of selective venous catheterization [57]. In cases of false positive imaging, persistent hyperaldosteronism may be due to the simultaneous presence of a nonfunctioning cortical adenoma and either a contralateral microaldosteronoma or bilateral adrenal hyperplasia. This is especially true in patients 40 years of age or older. Some clinicians believe that due to improved imaging resolution and experience, that the routine use of adrenal venous sampling is not necessary to achieve high cure rates for aldosteronomas. The authors believe that in patients less than 40 years of age, a high resolution CT scan revealing the presence of a solitary adrenal mass 1 cm or greater in size and a normal contralateral adrenal gland is probably sufficient for localization of aldosteronoma. Ninety-five percent of such cases will meet with successful clinical outcomes after unilateral adrenalectomy [58].

Certainly there are distinct disadvantages to routine selective venous catheterization. This procedure is invasive, it requires an experienced interventional radiologist, and it can lead to adrenal vein rupture in approximately 1–2.5% of cases. Even in experienced hands there is a low success rate (40–80%), usually due to incomplete adrenal venous sampling because of the inability to cannulate the right adrenal vein. Variations in venous anatomy, such as aberrant or accessory veins, contribute to the already difficult geometry of the right adrenal vein. Therefore, most groups advocate the selective use of venous catheterization only in ambiguous cases, for example, patients with nonlocalized tumors and patients with bilateral adrenal enlargement, in order to distinguish between unilateral and bilateral increases of aldosterone secretion. Even if the study is not successful at catheterizing both sides, sufficient information can often be obtained to guide surgical treatment [59].

One other method to localize aldosteronomas is scintigraphy with ^{131}I-6β-iodomethyl noriodocholesterol (NP-59). This cholesterol-like compound is taken up by the adrenal cortex, but it remains in the gland without undergoing further metabolism. Solitary adrenal adenomas appear "hot" with suppressed uptake on the other side; hyperplastic glands or bilateral adenomas show increased uptake on both sides. NP-59 scanning has low sensitivity in small tumors. Since aldosteronomas that cannot be localized by CT scans are usually quite small, NP-59 scanning generally does not add much information to the management of primary hyperaldosteronism.

Treatment

Preoperative treatment of hyperaldosteronism must start with controlling hypertension and supplementing potassium adequately to keep the serum potassium level greater than 3.5 mmol/L. High blood pressure can be treated by aldosterone antagonists (spironolactone or eplerenone), potassium-sparing diuretics that block sodium channels in the distal nephron (amiloride or triamterene), calcium channel blockers, or ACE inhibitors.

Aldosteronomas are best managed surgically, either by a laparoscopic adrenalectomy [14, 60] or via a posterior open approach. Since almost all aldosteronomas are small and benign, larger lesions or those with mixed hormone secretion should be considered malignant. For larger tumors, an anterior transabdominal approach is necessary to allow adequate visualization of local invasion and distant metastases, and to allow en-bloc resection if necessary.

Patients with bilateral tumors are less amenable to surgical management. Only 20–30% of patients with hyperaldosteronism with bilateral tumors benefit from surgery. These patients require selective venous catheterization to predict their response. For patients without a lateralized hypersecreting gland, medical therapy is the best option. Bilateral adrenalectomy obligates lifelong pharmacologic glucocorticoid and mineralocorticoid replacement and subjects patients to the risk of hypoadrenal crisis. Hence, it is almost never performed for hyperaldosteronism. Medical therapy for patients with bilateral hyperplasia is generally achieved with spironolactone. The selective mineralocorticoid receptor antagonist eplerenone has also been used. Reportedly, there is less breast tenderness and gynecomastia in men. This advantage must be weighed against the agent's high cost. Patients with glucocorticoid-suppressible hyperaldosteronism are best treated by administration of 0.5–1 mg of dexamethasone daily.

Postoperative care following aldosteronoma resection may last months, as some patients may require mineralocorticoids for up to 3 months as a result of a transient hypoaldosteronism. All patients should have PAC levels measured on postoperative day one or two to assess biochemical cure. They may suffer from temporary hyperkalemia and hyponatremia because of hypoaldosteronism due to suppression of their renin-angiotensin-aldosterone axis. β-blockers may exacerbate postoperative hyperkalemia. Serum potassium levels should be monitored weekly for 4 weeks. These patients may require a few days or weeks of a high salt diet. Five percent of patients will require short-term mineralocorticoid therapy with daily fludrocortisone. Acute hypoadrenalism occurs rarely, typically 2–3 days after unilateral adrenalectomy. It should be noted that Addisonian crisis can occur intraoperatively [61], postoperatively, months later, or as a result of other factors [62, 63]. It is usually safest to stop all antihypertensive medications immediately postoperatively, with the exception of β-blockers, which must be tapered to avoid rebound tachycardia and hypertension. In the following few days to weeks, antihypertensives can gradually be added back, if necessary.

Adrenalectomy is more than 90% successful in improving hypokalemia, more than 80% successful in reducing blood pressure medication requirements, and even up to 70% successful in correcting the hypertension entirely. These are long-term results; depending on the degree of preoperative sodium overload, it may take several weeks to stabilize at the new levels. The patients most likely to experience improvement in their hypertension are those who preoperatively respond to spironolactone therapy and those with the shortest duration of hypertension resulting in the least amount of end-organ damage. Those least likely to benefit from surgery are male, older than 45–50 years of age, nonresponsive to spironolactone, with a family history of hypertension, a long-standing personal history of hypertension, and multiple adrenal nodules [58]. Patients who are not surgical candidates should be treated medically. The cornerstone of treatment is either spironolactone or eplerenone, supplemented by sodium-restriction, maintenance of ideal body weight, nonsmoking, and regular exercise.

Cushing's Syndrome and Cortisol Producing Adrenal Tumors

Cushing's syndrome is defined as a complex of symptoms and signs resulting from excessive amounts of serum cortisol, regardless of etiology [64]. Patients with Cushing's syndrome usually present with weight gain, easy bruisability, abdominal striae, and manifestations of the metabolic syndrome (Fig. 10.5). Classic features include rounding of the face ("moon facies"), and fat deposition in the supraclavicular or posterior cervical areas ("buffalo hump"). There is an associated four- to fivefold increase in mortality, usually due to cardiovascular complications of chronic hypertension and obesity [65]. For this reason, physicians should adopt an aggressive stance in diagnosing and treating Cushing's syndrome. Endogenous Cushing's syndrome is rare, affecting 5–10 in 1 million individuals. It is more common in adults, but about 20% of cases occur before puberty. Women are affected eight times more frequently than men. While most individuals have sporadic disease, this syndrome can sometimes be found in MEN1 families.

The great majority of Cushing's syndrome cases arise from the exogenous administration of glucocorticoids for inflammatory conditions. Among endogenous causes of Cushing's syndrome, ACTH-secreting pituitary adenomas (termed Cushing's disease) are the most common, accounting for 75% of cases. Primary adrenal processes (adenoma, hyperplasia, and carcinoma) comprise about 20% of cases [66], and most of the remaining cases arise from ectopic (nonpituitary) sources of ACTH. Ectopic sources of ACTH include carcinoid tumors (more common in men) of the lung, thymus, intestines, pancreas, and ovary; bronchial adenomas (more common in women); and other neoplasms such as small-cell lung cancers, pancreatic islet cell tumors, medullary thyroid cancers, and pheochromocytomas. Rarely (in less than 1% of cases) corticotropin-releasing hormone (CRH) may be secreted ectopically in bronchial carcinoid tumors, pheochromocytomas, and other tumors, making these patients difficult to distinguish from those with ectopic ACTH production. Measuring CRH levels can make the distinction [67].

Adrenal hyperplasia almost always presents bilaterally. Most of these cases of diffuse cortical hyperplasia are ACTH dependent, whether from Cushing's disease or a nonpituitary source. Hyperplasia is usually macronodular, with nodules of about 3 cm in diameter. The exceptions are pigmented micronodular hyperplasia (with black nodules smaller than 5 mm), gastric inhibitory peptide-sensitive macronodular hyperplasia [68–71], and Carney's syndrome (atrial myxomas, schwannomas, and pigmented nevi) with pigmented nodules [72].

Ten to fifteen percent of primary adrenal Cushing's cases are adenomas, almost all are unilateral, but bilateral cases have been reported [73]. Five to ten percent of

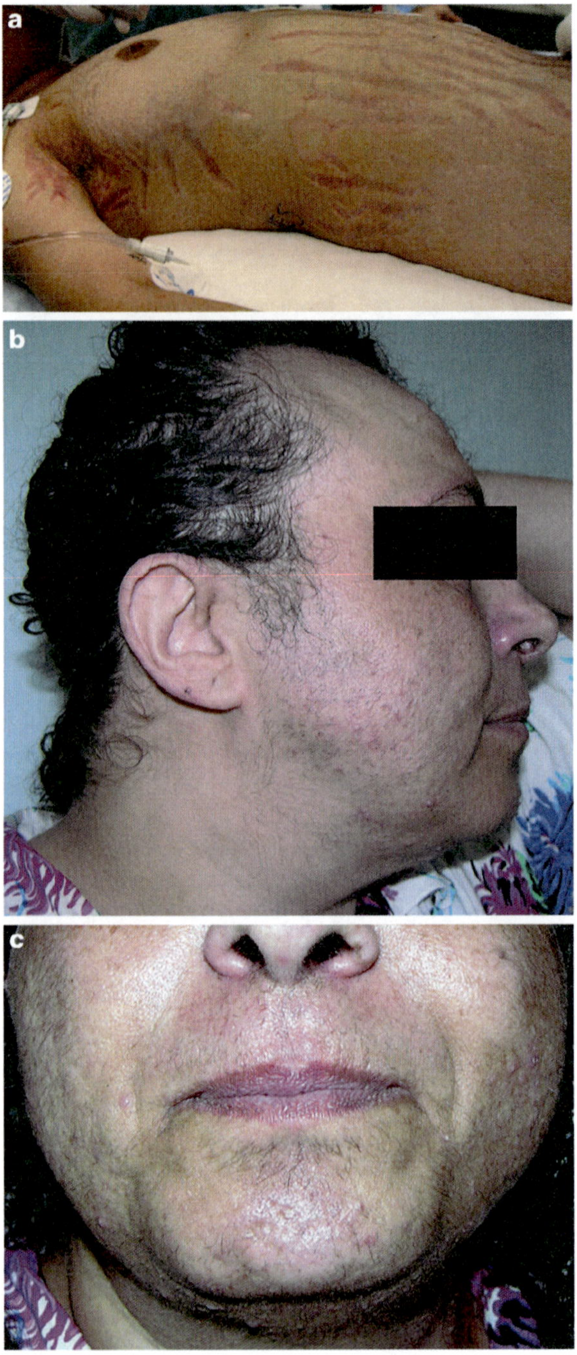

Fig. 10.5 Characteristic clinical features of a patient with Cushing's syndrome. Note the (**a**) central obesity, the wide, purple striae, (**b**) cervical fat pad, temporal balding, (**c**) acne, and hirsutism

cases result from carcinomas [74–77]. Cushing's syndrome is present in 30–40% of adrenocortical carcinomas [3]. There are rare cases of Cushing's syndrome associated with pheochromocytomas [78]. It is important to note that patients with major depression, alcoholism, pregnancy, chronic renal failure, or stress can also have elevated cortisol levels and symptoms of hypercortisolism. Such cases of pseudo-Cushing's syndrome resolve with treatment of the underlying problem.

Symptoms and Signs

The clinical diagnosis of Cushing's syndrome, especially in the early stages, requires knowledge of the manifestations of the disease and a high clinical suspicion. In some patients, symptoms are less pronounced and may be more difficult to recognize, particularly given the diversity of symptoms and the absence of a single defining symptom or sign. The most common symptom is progressive truncal obesity, occurring in up to 95% of patients. This fat distribution is the result of the central lipogenic action of excessive corticosteroids and peripheral catabolic effects, in conjunction with peripheral muscle wasting.

Fat deposition occurs in distinctive sites, like the supraclavicular space and posterior neck region. Wide purple striae on a protuberant abdomen and proximal extremities, rounding of the face because of the thickening of the facial fat, and the thinning of subcutaneous tissue leading to plethora all contribute to the characteristic body morphology. Other endocrine abnormalities include glucose intolerance, amenorrhea, and decreased libido or impotence. Children manifest the disease through obesity and stunted growth curves. Hyperpigmentation of the skin, if present, is associated with the presence of proopiomelanocortin (POMC), the peptide precursor of ACTH, suggesting an ectopic ACTH-producing tumor with high levels of circulating hormone. Other manifestations include acne, ecchymoses, hypertension, generalized weakness, osteopenia, emotional lability, psychosis, depression, hyperlipidemia, polyuria, and renal stones.

A Task Force of The Endocrine Society recommends screening tests only after a thorough drug history excluding exogenous glucocorticoid exposure. Only patients with (1) clinical features unusual for their age, (2) multiple and progressive features described above, (3) or adrenal incidentalomas compatible with adenoma, and (4) children with decreasing height percentile and increasing weight should be tested for Cushing's syndrome [79].

Laboratory Studies

A single measurement of the plasma cortisol level is unreliable, because secretion of cortisol is episodic and has a diurnal variation. In normal individuals, cortisol secretion follows a predictable circadian rhythm: it has a peak approximately 1 h after waking and a trough around midnight. The diagnosis of Cushing's syndrome is established by demonstrating nonsuppressibility of elevated glucocorticoid levels and/or the loss of normal diurnal variation. (Fig. 10.6) The two most commonly used screening tests are measurement of 24-h urine free cortisol and the overnight low-dose dexamethasone suppression test. 24-h urine measurements are useful because they reflect the integral of serum hormone levels throughout the day, thus avoiding potential diagnostic errors that may result from episodic hormone secretion. Greater than threefold elevations in a 24-h urinary cortisol above normal are virtually diagnostic of Cushing's syndrome, whereas a level of lesser than 100 μg/24 h effectively rules out hypercortisolism.

The overnight low-dose dexamethasone suppression test is performed by giving the patient 1 mg of a synthetic glucocorticoid (preferably dexamethasone because it does not cross-react with biochemical assays for cortisol) at 11 PM and then measuring the plasma cortisol levels at 8 AM the following morning. In physiologically normal adults cortisol levels should be suppressed to less than 3 μg/dL. In some patients with mild disease, cortisol levels may also drop to less than 3 μg/dL; therefore recent clinical guidelines advocate increasing the sensitivity by making the cut-off value 1.8 μg/dL [79]. Chronic renal failure, depression, and medications that enhance dexamethasone metabolism can cause false-positive results in up to 3% of patients. Fifty percent of women taking oral contraceptive pills who undergo the dexamethasone suppression test will test positive because estrogens increase the cortisol-binding globulin and thus the circulating amount of cortisol. By the same token, critically ill patients and other protein deficient patients, such as those with nephrotic syndrome or cirrhosis, can have decreased serum cortisol levels.

In patients with a high clinical suspicion but a negative overnight test, a more sensitive, standard (3 day) low-dose dexamethasone suppression test is performed. Urine is collected for three consecutive days. On the second day, dexamethasone (0.5 mg every 6 h for 48 h) is given. The detection of elevated 24-h urinary cortisol levels in this setting is a very sensitive (95–100%) and specific (98%) way to diagnose Cushing's syndrome. The test is particularly useful in identifying patients with pseudo-Cushing's syndrome (who do not have true cortisol excess), but not as useful in patients with hypercortisolism arising from non-neoplastic causes, such as those with depression, anxiety, obsessive compulsive disorder, morbid obesity, or alcoholism.

Patients with borderline or equivocal urine and serum results may be further evaluated by measurement of late-night salivary cortisol levels. A high cutoff value of 550 ng/dL had a sensitivity of 93% and specificity of 100% for the detection of Cushing's syndrome in one study [80]. Due to the normal diurnal variation in cortisol levels, most normal subjects have a midnight salivary cortisol level less than 145 ng/dL [79]. The test may be performed using commercially available kits. Because of its convenience, some experts have advocated late-night salivary cortisol measurement as a screening test. It has demonstrated good sensitivity in diagnosing Cushing's syndrome [81], as unbound cortisol diffuses freely into saliva and achieves concentrations that are independent of the salivary flow rate. To rule out

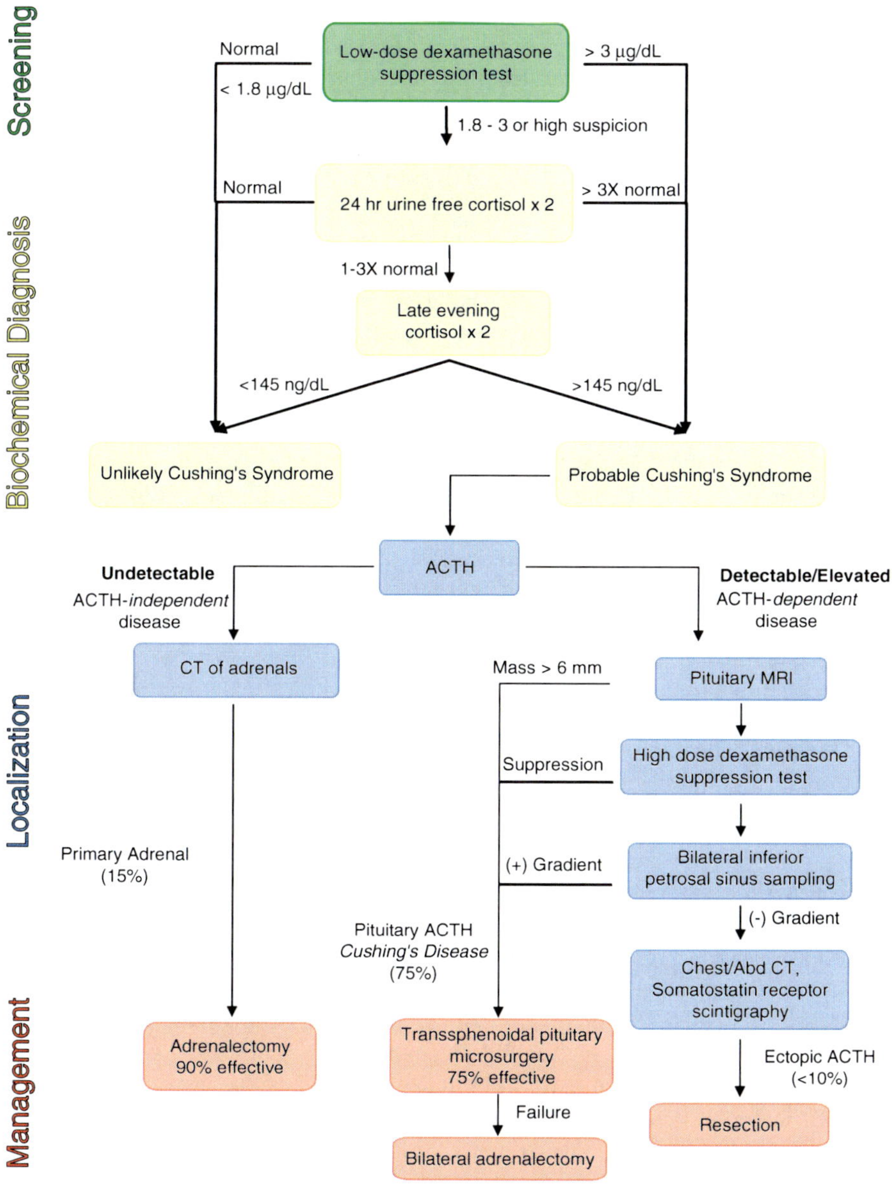

Fig. 10.6 Evaluation and treatment of hypercortisolism

Cushing's syndrome, two late-night measurements are recommended with a value of less than 145 ng/dL (4 nmol/L) expected in normal individuals [79].

After the biochemical diagnosis of Cushing's syndrome has been established, measurement of the serum ACTH level allows segregation of the disease into

ACTH-dependent and ACTH-independent causes. Elevated ACTH levels of 15–500 pg/mL are found in patients with ACTH-dependent adrenal hyperplasia resulting from Cushing's disease (pituitary corticotroph adenoma) and those with CRH-secreting tumors. The highest levels are found in patients with ectopic sources of ACTH (>1,000 pg/mL). Conversely, ACTH levels are characteristically suppressed or undetectable (<5 pg/mL) in patients with primary cortisol-secreting adrenal tumors. As ectopic sources of ACTH are typically very difficult to suppress, the high-dose dexamethasone suppression test is used to distinguish an ectopic from the pituitary source. The standard test (2 mg dexamethasone every 6 h for 48 h) or an overnight test (8 mg) may be used, with 24-h urine collections for cortisol and 17-hydroxy steroids performed over the next day. The failure to suppress urinary cortisol by 50% confirms the diagnosis of an ectopic ACTH-producing tumor. Patients suspected of having ectopic tumors should also have serum calcitonin and urine catecholamines levels checked to rule out medullary thyroid cancer and MEN syndromes. Bilateral petrosal vein sampling is helpful in determining whether the patient has Cushing's disease or ectopic Cushing's syndrome.

Another useful test in determining the etiology of Cushing's syndrome is the CRH test. In this test, CRH (1 μg/kg) is administered intravenously. Then at 15-min intervals for 1 h, ACTH and cortisol levels are measured. ACTH-independent (primary adrenal) causes of hypercortisolism are associated with a blunted response (ACTH peak <10 pg/mL), whereas those with ACTH-dependent disease demonstrate a higher elevation of ACTH (>30 pg/mL). Furthermore, patients with pituitary tumors have a higher peak ACTH than those with ectopic ACTH-producing tumors. CRH stimulation can also enhance the sensitivity of petrosal vein sampling.

Radiologic Studies

If an ACTH-independent, endogenous cause of Cushing's syndrome is suspected after biochemical evaluation, cross-sectional imaging of the adrenal glands with CT or MRI should be performed. Nearly all cortisol-producing adrenal lesions, except micronodular hyperplasia, are readily apparent on CT scan [82], as most cortisol-producing neoplasms are at least 3 cm in diameter. It is frequently difficult to distinguish benign from malignant cortisol-producing tumors radiographically. Special attention should be paid to any evidence of local invasion or metastasis when primary tumors exceed 6 cm in diameter. Radioscintigraphic imaging of the adrenals using NP-59 also can be used to distinguish adenoma from hyperplasia. Adenomas usually show increased uptake of NP-59 with suppression of uptake in the contralateral gland; hyperplastic glands take up the molecule bilaterally. However, there are reports suggesting that "cold" adrenal nodules are more likely to be cancerous. In the setting of ectopic ACTH, imaging studies should first be performed of the chest and anterior mediastinum and if negative, imaging of the neck, abdomen, and pelvis should follow.

Treatment

Treatment of adrenocortical Cushing's syndrome is usually surgical. Unilateral laparoscopic adrenalectomy is the preferred procedure for patients with small benign adrenal adenomas, as it is more than 90% effective in the treatment of primary adrenal Cushing's syndrome. Recurrence or persistence may be the result of local recurrence, or distant tumor in the case of malignant disease. Therefore, open adrenalectomy is indicated for large tumors (≥6 cm has been recommended by some experts) or those suspected to be adrenocortical cancers either clinically or radiographically.

Patients with ectopic sources of ACTH need treatment of their primary tumors, including recurrences, if possible. In some cases, the source cannot be identified. Patients with unresectable disease are usually palliated by medical adrenalectomy with metyrapone, aminoglutethimide, and mitotane. Bilateral laparoscopic adrenalectomy has also been shown to be safe and effective in the management of patients with Cushing's syndrome whose ectopic ACTH-secreting tumor cannot be localized. Anadrenal patients must, of course, be maintained on lifelong glucocorticoid and mineralocorticoid replacement, and receive education regarding scenarios in which additional glucocorticoids may be necessary (trauma, burn, or severe infection).

A fraction of patients with cortisol-producing adrenal tumors present with subclinical Cushing's syndrome. These tumors are generally discovered incidentally, when cross-sectional abdominal imaging is performed for unrelated reasons. Biochemical evidence of cortisol hypersecretion, frequently mild, is then demonstrated, but the overt signs or symptoms of Cushing's syndrome are not usually present. Hypertension, dyslipidemia, obesity, and impaired glucose tolerance are highly prevalent among these individuals [83, 84]. Although there is no consensus on the appropriate therapy for this condition, adrenalectomy has been shown to improve clinical and metabolic parameters in some patients with subclinical Cushing's syndrome [85].

Perioperative care for patients undergoing surgery for primary adrenal causes of Cushing's syndrome must include preoperative and postoperative steroids. This is due to the chronic suppression of the hypothalamic–pituitary–adrenal (HPA) axis. Perioperative "stress dose" glucocorticoids (hydrocortisone 100 mg IV q8 h for 24 h) are recommended. Generally, these can be rapidly tapered to physiologic replacement levels over the course of days to weeks. In some institutions, the practice is to withhold glucocorticoids during the immediate postoperative period to allow the identification of early remission [86]. Finding a subnormal morning cortisol level on the first or second postoperative day indicates an adequate resection.

Patients with less severe or subclinical Cushing's syndrome can usually tolerate the mild symptoms of glucocorticoid withdrawal and are given only 20 mg hydrocortisone (12–15 mg/m^2) in the early morning until their normal morning endogenous cortisol levels and their response to exogenous ACTH are restored.

However, all patients should wear a medical bracelet and be instructed to increase their hydrocortisone intake during episodes of physiologic stress until the HPA axis has regained function. The duration of HPA axis suppression is related to the severity and duration of prior cortisol excess. Periodic assessment with ACTH stimulation testing may facilitate the timely withdrawal of pharmacologic glucocorticoid replacement. In patients with long term or severe Cushing's syndrome, exogenous steroids may be needed for up to 2 years.

Patients with Cushing's syndrome have an increased risk of infectious and thromboembolic complications. The myriad immunosuppressive effects of glucocorticoids have been described elsewhere. Despite the routine administration of perioperative antibiotics for 24 h in patients undergoing adrenalectomy for Cushing's syndrome, approximately 5% still develop wound infections. The increased risk of thromboembolism is reportedly due to a hypercoagulable state resulting from an increase in clotting factor levels, such as factor VIII and von Willebrand factor complex, and by impaired fibrinolysis.

Virilizing and Feminizing Adrenal Tumors

The last of the three types of hormones made in the adrenal cortex are the sex steroids. Tumors producing these hormones can be virilizing or feminizing. Virilizing syndromes comprise the most common presentation of adrenocortical tumors in children [87, 88]. Adult patients, 80% of whom are female [89], can develop hirsutism, amenorrhea, infertility, and other signs of virilization, such as increased muscle mass, deepened voice, and temporal balding. Sex steroid-producing adrenal tumors can secrete testosterone, androstenedione, dehydroepiandrosterone (DHEA) and DHEA sulfate, with up to 56% of patients having elevations of all three [90] (Fig. 10.7). Seventy percent of virilizing tumors are malignant, and most of these are metastatic at the time of diagnosis. The proportion of malignancy is even higher if sex steroid production is accompanied by Cushing's syndrome [91, 92]. Because of this high risk for malignancy, long-term postoperative surveillance of patients with androgen secreting adrenal tumors is mandatory, even in the absence of initial evidence of tumor dissemination.

Clinical evidence of androgen excess may be difficult to identify in men, who, as a consequence, usually present with advanced malignancies [93]. Children with virilizing tumors typically present with accelerated growth, premature development of facial and pubic hair, acne, genital enlargement, and deepening of the voice [94, 95].

Feminizing adrenal tumors are much less common and are almost always malignant. Most occur in men in their third to fifth decades of life, whose symptoms commonly include gynecomastia, impotence, and testicular atrophy. Women with feminizing tumors develop irregular menses and dysfunctional uterine bleeding, whereas girls experience precocious puberty with breast enlargement and early menarche.

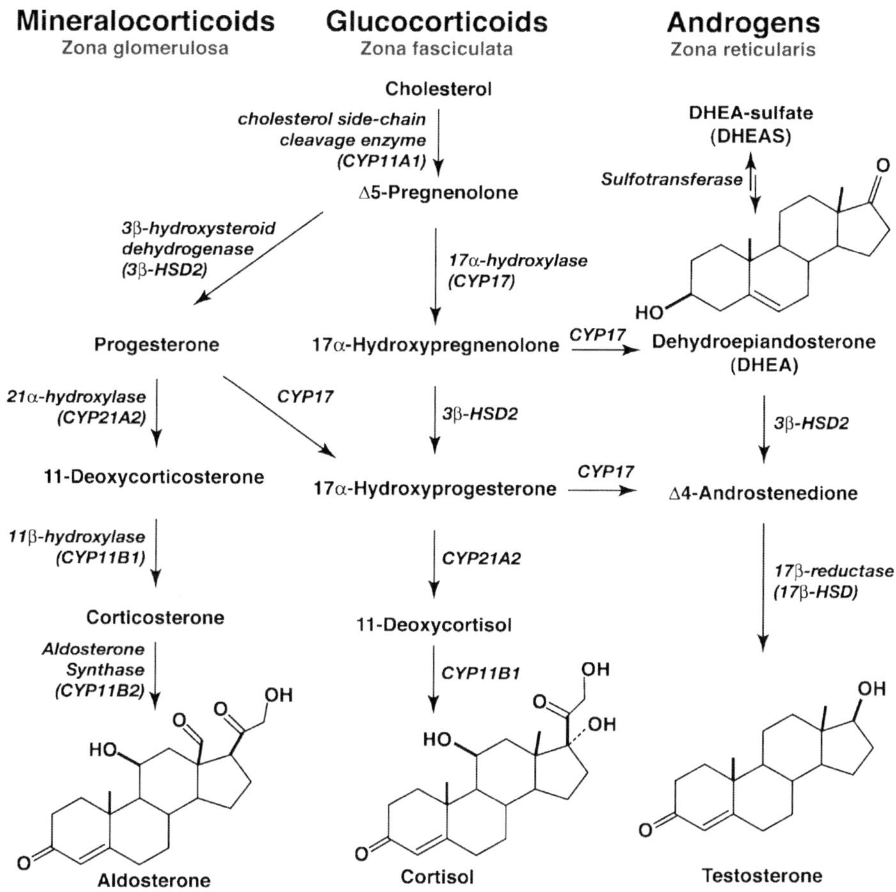

Fig. 10.7 Steroid hormone biosynthetic pathways

Diagnostic Tests

In addition to localization studies pointing to the presence of a functional adrenocortical neoplasm, the confirming test for an adrenocortical virilizing tumor is to measure the amounts of testosterone, DHEA, and DHEA-sulfate. DHEA can be measured in the serum or as a 24 h urine collection for 17-ketosteroids. The production of DHEA is often associated with production of other hormones such as glucocorticoids. New reports implicate high levels of 11-deoxycortisol (compound S, >7 ng/mL) to be a sensitive and specific test for androgen secreting adrenocortical tumors [90]. Feminizing tumors can be worked up by looking for elevated urine or serum 17-ketosteroids and estrogen levels.

Treatment

Sex steroid-producing tumors should be surgically removed whenever possible. Malignancy is difficult to diagnose histologically. It may be suggested by the presence of local invasion, recurrence, or distant metastases. Patients who are not acceptable surgical candidates can have chemical adrenolysis, using drugs such as mitotane, aminoglutethimide, ketoconazole, and flutamide. These agents may also be useful achieving palliation in patients with metastatic disease [96].

References

1. Bergada I, Venara M, Maglio S et al (1996) Functional adrenal cortical tumors in pediatric patients: a clinicopathologic and immunohistochemical study of a long term follow-up series. Cancer 77:771–777
2. Latronico AC, Chrousos GP (1997) Extensive personal experience: adrenocortical tumors. J Clin Endocrinol Metab 82:1317–1324
3. Libe R, Fratticci A, Bertherat J (2007) Adrenocortical cancer: pathophysiology and clinical management. Endocr Relat Cancer 14:13–28
4. Saeger W, Reinhard K, Reinhard C (1998) Hyperplastic and tumorous lesions of the adrenals in an unselected autopsy series. Endocr Pathol 9:235–239
5. Hensen J, Buhl M, Oelkers W (1993) The functional spectrum of adrenocortical adenomas. Med Hypotheses 40:217–222
6. Icard P, Goudet P, Charpenay C et al (2001) Adrenocortical carcinomas: surgical trends and results of a 253-patient series from the French Association of Endocrine Surgeons study group. World J Surg 25:891–897
7. Cassarino DS, Santi M, Arruda A et al (2004) Spinal adrenal cortical adenoma with oncocytic features: report of the first intramedullary case and review of the literature. Int J Surg Pathol 12:259–264
8. Henley DJ, van Heerden JA, Grant CS, Carney JA, Carpenter PC (1983) Adrenal cortical carcinoma – a continuing challenge. Surgery 94:926–931
9. Roman S (2006) Adrenocortical carcinoma. Curr Opin Oncol 18:36–42
10. Grunberg SM (1982) Development of Cushing's syndrome and virilization after presentation of a nonfunctioning adrenocortical carcinoma. Cancer 50:815–816
11. Weiss LM, Medeiros LJ, Vickery AL Jr (1989) Pathologic features of prognostic significance in adrenocortical carcinoma. Am J Surg Pathol 13:202–206
12. van Slooten H, Schaberg A, Smeenk D, Moolenaar AJ (1985) Morphologic characteristics of benign and malignant adrenocortical tumors. Cancer 55:766–773
13. Van't Sant HP, Bouvy ND, Kazemier G et al (2007) The prognostic value of two different histopathological scoring systems for adrenocortical carcinomas. Histopathology 51:239–245
14. Gumbs AA, Gagner M (2006) Laparoscopic adrenalectomy. Best Pract Res Clin Endocrinol Metab 20:483–499
15. Ganguly A (1998) Primary aldosteronism. N Engl J Med 339:1828–1834
16. White PC (1994) Disorders of aldosterone biosynthesis and action. N Engl J Med 331:250–258
17. Auchus RJ (2003) Aldo is back: recent advances and unresolved controversies in hyperaldosteronism. Curr Opin Nephrol Hypertens 12:153–158
18. Kaplan NM (2004) The current epidemic of primary aldosteronism: causes and consequences. J Hypertens 22:863–869

19. Fogari R, Preti P, Zoppi A, Rinaldi A, Fogari E, Mugellini A (2007) Prevalence of primary aldosteronism among unselected hypertensive patients: a prospective study based on the use of an aldosterone/renin ratio above 25 as a screening test. Hypertens Res 30:111–117
20. Mulatero P, Stowasser M, Loh KC et al (2004) Increased diagnosis of primary aldosteronism, including surgically correctable forms, in centers from five continents. J Clin Endocrinol Metab 89:1045–1050
21. Milliez P, Girerd X, Plouin PF, Blacher J, Safar ME, Mourad JJ (2005) Evidence for an increased rate of cardiovascular events in patients with primary aldosteronism. J Am Coll Cardiol 45:1243–1248
22. Neville AM, Symington T (1966) Pathology of primary aldosteronism. Cancer 19:1854–1868
23. Gleason PE, Weinberger MH, Pratt JH et al (1993) Evaluation of diagnostic tests in the differential diagnosis of primary aldosteronism: unilateral adenoma versus bilateral micronodular hyperplasia. J Urol 150:1365–1368
24. Weinberger MH, Fineberg NS (1993) The diagnosis of primary aldosteronism and separation of two major subtypes. Arch Intern Med 153:2125–2129
25. Banks WA, Kastin AJ, Biglieri EG, Ruiz AE (1984) Primary adrenal hyperplasia: a new subset of primary hyperaldosteronism. J Clin Endocrinol Metab 58:783–785
26. Imai T, Seo H, Murata Y et al (1991) Dexamethasone-nonsuppressible cortisol in two cases with aldosterone-producing adenoma. J Clin Endocrinol Metab 72:575–581
27. Young WF Jr, Hogan MJ, Klee GG, Grant CS, van Heerden JA (1990) Primary aldosteronism: diagnosis and treatment. Mayo Clin Proc 65:96–110
28. Stewart PM (1999) Mineralocorticoid hypertension. Lancet 353:1341–1347
29. Zarnegar R, Lee J, Brunaud L et al (2007) Good blood pressure control on antihypertensives, not only response to spironolactone, predicts improved outcome after adrenalectomy for aldosteronoma. Surgery 142:921–929; discussion 9
30. Jackson RV, Lafferty A, Torpy DJ, Stratakis C (2002) New genetic insights in familial hyperaldosteronism. Ann N Y Acad Sci 970:77–88
31. Funder JW, Carey RM, Fardella C et al (2008) Case detection, diagnosis, and treatment of patients with primary aldosteronism: an endocrine society clinical practice guideline. J Clin Endocrinol Metab 93:3266–3281
32. Doi SA, Abalkhail S, Al-Qudhaiby MM, Al-Humood K, Hafez MF, Al-Shoumer KA (2006) Optimal use and interpretation of the aldosterone renin ratio to detect aldosterone excess in hypertension. J Hum Hypertens 20:482–489
33. Kem DC, Weinberger MH, Mayes DM, Nugent CA (1971) Saline suppression of plasma aldosterone in hypertension. Arch Intern Med 128:380–386
34. Holland OB, Brown H, Kuhnert L, Fairchild C, Risk M, Gomez-Sanchez CE (1984) Further evaluation of saline infusion for the diagnosis of primary aldosteronism. Hypertension 6:717–723
35. Gandour MJ, Grizzle WE (1986) A small adrenocortical carcinoma with aggressive behavior. An evaluation of criteria for malignancy. Arch Pathol Lab Med 110:1076–9
36. Cohen RJ, Brits R, Phillips JI, Botha JR (1991) Primary hyperaldosteronism due to a functional black (pigmented) adenoma of the adrenal cortex. Arch Pathol Lab Med 115:813–815
37. Bugg MF, Ribeiro RC, Roberson PK et al (1994) Correlation of pathologic features with clinical outcome in pediatric adrenocortical neoplasia. A study of a Brazilian population. Brazilian Group for Treatment of Childhood Adrenocortical Tumors. Am J Clin Pathol 101:625–629
38. Evans HL, Vassilopoulou-Sellin R (1996) Adrenal cortical neoplasms. A study of 56 cases. Am J Clin Pathol 105:76–86
39. Vyberg M, Sestoft L (1986) Combined adrenal myelolipoma and adenoma associated with Cushing's syndrome. Am J Clin Pathol 86:541–545
40. Sienkowski IK, Watkins RM, Anderson VE (1984) Primary tumorous aldosteronism due to a black adrenal adenoma: a light and electron microscopic study. J Clin Pathol 37:143–149
41. Komiya I, Takasu N, Aizawa T et al (1985) Black (or brown) adrenal cortical adenoma: its characteristic features on computed tomography and endocrine data. J Clin Endocrinol Metab 61:711–717

42. Macadam RF (1971) Black adenoma of the human adrenal cortex. Cancer 27:116–119
43. Damron TA, Schelper RL, Sorensen L (1987) Cytochemical demonstration of neuromelanin in black pigmented adrenal nodules. Am J Clin Pathol 87:334–341
44. Ivsic T, Komorowski RA, Sudakoff GS, Wilson SD, Datta MW (2002) Adrenal cortical adenoma with adrenalin-type neurosecretory granules clinically mimicking a pheochromocytoma. Arch Pathol Lab Med 126:1530–1533
45. Hoang MP, Ayala AG, Albores-Saavedra J (2002) Oncocytic adrenocortical carcinoma: a morphologic, immunohistochemical and ultrastructural study of four cases. Mod Pathol 15:973–978
46. Lin BT, Bonsib SM, Mierau GW, Weiss LM, Medeiros LJ (1998) Oncocytic adrenocortical neoplasms: a report of seven cases and review of the literature. Am J Surg Pathol 22:603–614
47. Brown FM, Gaffey TA, Wold LE, Lloyd RV (2000) Myxoid neoplasms of the adrenal cortex: a rare histologic variant. Am J Surg Pathol 24:396–401
48. Feldberg E, Guy M, Eisenkraft S, Czernobilsky B (1996) Adrenal cortical adenoma with extensive fat cell metaplasia. Pathol Res Pract 192:62–65; discussion 6
49. Trojan J, Schwarz W, Sarrazin C, Thalhammer A, Vogl TJ, Dietrich CF (2002) Role of ultrasonography in the detection of small adrenal masses. Ultraschall Med 23:96–100
50. McClennan BL (1991) Oncologic imaging. Staging and follow-up of renal and adrenal carcinoma. Cancer 67:1199–208
51. Doppman JL, Gill JR Jr, Miller DL et al (1992) Distinction between hyperaldosteronism due to bilateral hyperplasia and unilateral aldosteronoma: reliability of CT. Radiology 184:677–682
52. Mayo-Smith WW, Boland GW, Noto RB, Lee MJ (2001) State-of-the-art adrenal imaging. Radiographics 21:995–1012
53. Szolar DH, Korobkin M, Reittner P et al (2005) Adrenocortical carcinomas and adrenal pheochromocytomas: mass and enhancement loss evaluation at delayed contrast-enhanced CT. Radiology 234:479–485
54. Ilias I, Sahdev A, Reznek RH, Grossman AB, Pacak K (2007) The optimal imaging of adrenal tumours: a comparison of different methods. Endocr Relat Cancer 14:587–599
55. Daunt N (2005) Adrenal vein sampling: how to make it quick, easy, and successful. Radiographics 25(Suppl 1):S143–S158
56. Espiner EA, Ross DG, Yandle TG, Richards AM, Hunt PJ (2003) Predicting surgically remedial primary aldosteronism: role of adrenal scanning, posture testing, and adrenal vein sampling. J Clin Endocrinol Metab 88:3637–3644
57. Young WF, Stanson AW, Thompson GB, Grant CS, Farley DR, van Heerden JA (2004) Role for adrenal venous sampling in primary aldosteronism. Surgery 136:1227–1235
58. Tan YY, Ogilvie JB, Triponez F et al (2006) Selective use of adrenal venous sampling in the lateralization of aldosterone-producing adenomas. World J Surg 30:879–885; discussion 86–87
59. Harvey A, Kline G, Pasieka JL (2006) Adrenal venous sampling in primary hyperaldosteronism: comparison of radiographic with biochemical success and the clinical decision-making with "less than ideal" testing. Surgery 140:847–853; discussion 53–55
60. Lal G, Duh QY (2003) Laparoscopic adrenalectomy – indications and technique. Surg Oncol 12:105–123
61. Mohler JL, Flueck JA, McRoberts JW (1986) Adrenal insufficiency following unilateral adrenalectomy: a case report. J Urol 135:554–556
62. Nagai Y, Ohsawa K, Hayakawa T et al (1994) Acute adrenal insufficiency after unilateral adrenalectomy in Cushing's syndrome: precipitation by lithium-induced thyrotoxicosis during cortisol replacement. Endocr J 41:177–182
63. Kazama I, Komatsu Y, Ohiwa T, Sanayama K, Nagata M (2005) Delayed adrenal insufficiency long after unilateral adrenalectomy: prolonged glucocorticoid therapy reduced reserved secretory capacity of cortisol. Int J Urol 12:574–577

64. Orth DN (1995) Cushing's syndrome. N Engl J Med 332:791–803
65. Lindholm J, Juul S, Jorgensen JO et al (2001) Incidence and late prognosis of cushing's syndrome: a population-based study. J Clin Endocrinol Metab 86:117–123
66. Perry RR, Nieman LK, Cutler GB Jr et al (1989) Primary adrenal causes of Cushing's syndrome. Diagnosis and surgical management. Ann Surg 210:59–68
67. Raff H, Findling JW (2003) A physiologic approach to diagnosis of the Cushing syndrome. Ann Intern Med 138:980–991
68. Aiba M, Hirayama A, Iri H et al (1991) Adrenocorticotropic hormone-independent bilateral adrenocortical macronodular hyperplasia as a distinct subtype of Cushing's syndrome. Enzyme histochemical and ultrastructural study of four cases with a review of the literature. Am J Clin Pathol 96:334–340
69. Joffe SN, Brown C (1983) Nodular adrenal hyperplasia and Cushing's syndrome. Surgery 94:919–925
70. Smals AG, Pieters GF, van Haelst UJ, Kloppenborg PW (1984) Macronodular adrenocortical hyperplasia in long-standing Cushing's disease. J Clin Endocrinol Metab 58:25–31
71. Zeiger MA, Nieman LK, Cutler GB et al (1991) Primary bilateral adrenocortical causes of Cushing's syndrome. Surgery 110:1106–1115
72. Young WF Jr, Carney JA, Musa BU, Wulffraat NM, Lens JW, Drexhage HA (1989) Familial Cushing's syndrome due to primary pigmented nodular adrenocortical disease. Reinvestigation 50 years later. N Engl J Med 321:1659–1664
73. Aiba M, Kawakami M, Ito Y, Fujimoto Y, Suda T, Demura H (1992) Bilateral adrenocortical adenomas causing Cushing's syndrome. Report of two cases with enzyme histochemical and ultrastructural studies and a review of the literature. Arch Pathol Lab Med 116:146–150
74. Newell-Price J, Bertagna X, Grossman AB, Nieman LK (2006) Cushing's syndrome. Lancet 367:1605–1617
75. Gilbert MG, Cleveland WW (1970) Cushing's syndrome in infancy. Pediatrics 46:217–229
76. Neville AM, Symington T (1972) Bilateral adrenocortical hyperplasia in children with Cushing's syndrome. J Pathol 107:95–106
77. Thomas CG Jr, Smith AT, Griffith JM, Askin FB (1984) Hyperadrenalism in childhood and adolescence. Ann Surg 199:538–548
78. Hartmann CA, Gross U, Stein H (1992) Cushing syndrome-associated pheochromocytoma and adrenal carcinoma. An immunohistological investigation. Pathol Res Pract 188:287–295
79. Nieman LK, Biller BM, Findling JW et al (2008) The diagnosis of Cushing's syndrome: an endocrine society clinical practice guideline. J Clin Endocrinol Metab 93:1526–1540
80. Papanicolaou DA, Mullen N, Kyrou I, Nieman LK (2002) Nighttime salivary cortisol: a useful test for the diagnosis of Cushing's syndrome. J Clin Endocrinol Metab 87:4515–4521
81. Putignano P, Dubini A, Toja P et al (2001) Salivary cortisol measurement in normal-weight, obese and anorexic women: comparison with plasma cortisol. Eur J Endocrinol 145:165–171
82. Rockall AG, Babar SA, Sohaib SA et al (2004) CT and MR imaging of the adrenal glands in ACTH-independent cushing syndrome. Radiographics 24:435–452
83. Tsuiki M, Tanabe A, Takagi S, Naruse M, Takano K (2008) Cardiovascular risks and their long-term clinical outcome in patients with subclinical Cushing's syndrome. Endocr J 55:737–745
84. Tauchmanova L, Rossi R, Biondi B et al (2002) Patients with subclinical Cushing's syndrome due to adrenal adenoma have increased cardiovascular risk. J Clin Endocrinol Metab 87:4872–4878
85. Mitchell IC, Auchus RJ, Juneja K et al (2007) "Subclinical Cushing's syndrome" is not subclinical: improvement after adrenalectomy in 9 patients. Surgery 142:900–905; discussion 5 e1
86. Esposito F, Dusick JR, Cohan P et al (2006) Clinical review: early morning cortisol levels as a predictor of remission after transsphenoidal surgery for Cushing's disease. J Clin Endocrinol Metab 91:7–13
87. Ciftci AO, Senocak ME, Tanyel FC, Buyukpamukcu N (2001) Adrenocortical tumors in children. J Pediatr Surg 36:549–554

88. Sakai Y, Yanase T, Hara T, Takayanagi R, Haji M, Nawata H (1994) Mechanism of abnormal production of adrenal androgens in patients with adrenocortical adenomas and carcinomas. J Clin Endocrinol Metab 78:36–40
89. Heinbecker P, O'Neal LW, Ackerman LV (1957) Functioning and nonfunctioning adrenal cortical tumors. Surg Gynecol Obstet 105:21–33
90. D'Alva C, Abiven-Lepage G, Viallon V et al (2008) Sex steroids in androgen-secreting adrenocortical tumors: clinical and hormonal features in comparison with non tumoral causes of androgen excess. Eur J Endocrinol 159(5):641–647
91. Del Gaudio AD, Del Gaudio GA (1993) Virilizing adrenocortical tumors in adult women. Report of 10 patients, 2 of whom each had a tumor secreting only testosterone. Cancer 72:1997–2003
92. Fischler DF, Nunez C, Levin HS, McMahon JT, Sheeler LR, Adelstein DJ (1992) Adrenal carcinosarcoma presenting in a woman with clinical signs of virilization. A case report with immunohistochemical and ultrastructural findings. Am J Surg Pathol 16:626–631
93. Gabrilove JL, Sharma DC, Wotiz HH, Dorfman RI (1965) Feminizing adrenocortical tumors in the male. A review of 52 cases including a case report. medicine (Baltimore) 44:37–79
94. Burrington JD, Stephens CA (1969) Virilizing tumors of the adrenal gland in childhood: report of eight cases. J Pediatr Surg 4:291–302
95. Kenny FM, Hashida Y, Askari HA, Sieber WH, Fetterman GH (1968) Virilizing tumors of the adrenal cortex. Am J Dis Child 115:445–458
96. Loszio FA, Toth S, Kocsis J, Pavo SM (2001) Testosterone-secreting gonadotropin-responsive adrenal adenoma and its treatment with the antiandrogen flutamide. J Endocrinol Invest 24:622–627

Chapter 11
Adrenocortical Carcinoma

Patsy S.H. Soon and Stan B. Sidhu

Introduction

Adrenal tumors are common, with an estimated incidence of 7.3% from autopsy series [1]. A recent study found an overall 4.4% prevalence of incidental adrenal lesions by computed tomography (CT) [2]. The majority are benign adrenocortical adenomas. Adrenocortical carcinoma (ACC), however, is rare with an estimated prevalence of only 4–12/million population [3]. Histopathology does not always accurately predict malignancy in adrenal tumors. The prognosis for ACCs is poor with an overall 5-year survival of <40% [4, 5]. Complete en-bloc, margin-negative (R0) resection is the best treatment. Adjuvant treatment options for ACCs are fairly limited. The dismal survival rates for ACC have remained unchanged over the last 20 years. Advancement in the understanding of the pathophysiology of ACC is therefore essential for the development of more sensitive means of diagnosis and more effective treatment, resulting in better clinical outcome.

Clinical Aspects of ACC

Epidemiology

ACCs are rare cancers, accounting for only 0.02–0.2% of all cancer deaths. There is a slight female preponderance [6–9] as well as a bimodal incidence peak, with a larger peak in the 5th decade of life and a smaller one in children before the age of 5 [7, 10, 11].

S.B. Sidhu (✉)
Kolling Institute of Medical Research, University of Sydney, Sydney, NSW, Australia

Department of Endocrine and Oncology Surgery, Royal North Shore Hospital, St Leonards, NSW 2065, Australia
e-mail: stansidhu@nebsc.com.au

C. Sturgeon (ed.), *Endocrine Neoplasia*, Cancer Treatment and Research, vol 153,
DOI 10.1007/978-1-4419-0857-5_11, © Springer Science+Business Media, LLC 2010

Presentation

In the largest published series of ACC ($n = 3{,}982$), median age at diagnosis was 55 years, median tumor size was 13 cm, and distant metastases were found on presentation in 21.6% of patients [5]. About one fifth of patients with ACC present with advanced unresectable disease [6, 7]. ACCs can be functional or clinically silent. Up to 75% of patients present with symptoms of hormonal excess. Cushing's syndrome is the most common followed by either virilization or a combination of Cushing's syndrome and virilization [4, 7–9]. Approximately a third of patients present with non-specific symptoms related to the enlarging mass [7, 12]. The number of ACCs incidentally detected on imaging of the abdomen for non-related reasons is growing. Kasperlik-Zaluska et al. reported that 28.5% of their 63 patients with ACCs presented as incidentalomas [13]. The mean duration from the onset of symptoms to diagnosis of ACC varies from 6 to 16 months and appears to be independent of whether it is functional or clinically silent [14, 15].

Diagnosis

All adrenal tumors should be evaluated for hormonal activity and risk of malignancy.

Workup for functionality is described in detail in Chaps. 8, 9, and 10. To assess for the risk of malignancy, the size of the adrenal tumor is evaluated with CT or Magnetic Resonance Imaging (MRI). Size is the best preoperative indicator of malignancy, with the incidence of ACCs increasing to 25% in tumors over 6 cm [3]. Adrenal lesions that are inhomogeneous with irregular margins and irregular enhancement after intravenous contrast are suspicious for malignancy [16]. Adrenal lesions with an attenuation value of more than 10 Hounsfield units (HU) in unenhanced CT or an enhancement washout of less than 50% and a delayed attenuation of more than 35 HU are also suggestive for ACCs [17, 18].

Staging

Over 90% of reported ACC are over 6 cm in diameter [19]. Mean diameters in various series range from 11 to 15 cm [5, 6, 20, 21]. The MacFarlane classification modified by Sullivan is used to stage patients with ACC. Stages I and II of the disease are confined to the adrenal gland with a tumor size of less than or greater than 5 cm, respectively. Stage III disease is defined as invasion into adjacent organs or regional lymph nodes, while stage IV disease denotes distant metastatic disease [22, 23]. Stages I and II ACCs are potentially curable with surgery. Survival is dependent on the stage of presentation, with a reported mean of 2.1–5 years for stages I and II patients and from 4 months to 2.3 years for stage IV patients [10, 15, 24] or a 5-year actuarial survival rate of 66% for stage I, 58% for stage II and 24 and 0% for stages III and IV, respectively [6]. Older series have reported that up to 70% of patients present with disease which has spread beyond the adrenal gland [10, 12], though more recent reports describe that more patients tend to present with stage II disease [6, 9, 25], presumably due to the more frequent use of better imaging techniques.

Treatment

Surgical Resection

Surgery is the mainstay of treatment for ACC. Open adrenalectomy is recommended for excision of malignant primary adrenal lesions [4, 26, 27] as there have been some case reports that laparoscopic adrenalectomy for ACC increases the risk of peritoneal dissemination and metastases [28–30]. Completeness of surgical resection is of prime importance as it influences outcome [5, 31, 32]. Complete, en-bloc, margin-negative resection should be the surgical goal. For patients who are otherwise fit with the absence of metastasis, resection should be attempted, even for ACCs extending into the inferior vena cava (IVC) or right atrium. These tumors can be radically resected with the use of hepatic vascular exclusion with or without cardiopulmonary bypass and hypothermic circulatory arrest. A review of 65 of these cases in the literature revealed 24 patients who died after a mean survival of 13.2 ± 13.6 months (range 2–60 months) and 34 patients still alive after a mean follow up of 23.1 ± 20.4 months (range 1–80 months) [33]. Despite radical surgery with curative intent for patients with localized ACCs, however, the majority will develop metastases within 6–24 months of resection [34].

Mitotane

The adjuvant treatment of choice for ACC is mitotane (o,p'-DDD). A derivative of the insecticide dichlorodiphenyltrichloroethane (DDT), mitotane is metabolized to an active metabolite which leads to necrosis of the zona fasciculata and reticularis of the adrenal cortex and inhibition of adrenocortical hormone production [35]. Up to a third of patients have at least a partial response to mitotane [10]. The largest series of mitotane use after surgery compared to surgery alone in 177 patients with ACC from 8 centers in Italy and 47 centers in Germany was published recently. All patients had radical resection with a follow up of up to 10 years. Forty-seven of the 177 patients had mitotane after surgery, while the remainder of the patients had surgery alone. Mitotane treatment was associated with significantly longer recurrence-free survival and overall survival compared with the control groups [34]. Plasma levels of mitotane require monitoring and maintenance at 14–20 mg/L in order to obtain optimal response and lower rates of toxic side effects [36].

Chemotherapy

ACC has a 10–40% response rate to various chemotherapeutic agents. ACC tends to express the multidrug resistance gene *MDR-1* which results in the production of p-glycoprotein which is involved in the removal of the drug from the cancer cells. Because of this multidrug resistance gene, single agent chemotherapy is not favored for ACC [37]. A combination of either mitotane with etoposide, doxorubicin and cisplatin [38] or mitotane with streptozotocin [39] are the two best choices for the management of patients with advanced ACC [40]. The ongoing FIRM ACT trial is a randomized controlled trial comparing these two options in patients with locally advanced or metastatic ACC (www.firm-act.org).

A recent study assessed the use of an epidermal growth factor receptor inhibitor, erlotinib, in combination with gemcitabine after 12 weeks of treatment and found that 8 of the 10 patients had progressive disease while only one patient had a minor response, indicating that erlotinib with gemcitabine had very limited to no activity in patients with advanced ACC [41].

Radiotherapy

Radiotherapy to the tumor bed has also been used as adjuvant treatment after radical resection of ACC. Reports with small numbers of patients have described response rates of up to 42%. Fassnacht et al compared a group of 14 patients who received radiotherapy to the tumor bed with a matched control group of 14 patients. Local recurrence was significantly lower in the radiotherapy group at 14% compared to 79% in the control group. Disease-free and overall survival, however, were not significantly different between the two groups [42].

Prognosis

The prognosis for ACCs is poor with an overall 5-year survival rate of <40% [4, 7]. Prognosis is mainly dependent on tumor stage [6]. Patients with stage IV disease at the time of diagnosis have a survival rate of less than 12 months [4]. Large tumors over 12 cm have been shown to have poorer outcome in some studies. Histologic findings including high mitotic rate, atypical mitoses, high Ki-67 index, tumor necrosis and TP53 mutation have also been associated with poorer prognosis [43, 44].

In the recent report from the National Cancer Database (NCDB), the overall 5-year survival for all patients who underwent resection was 38.6% (median survival, 31.9 months) [5]. Multivariable analysis of this cohort demonstrated a higher risk of death with increasing age, poorly differentiated tumors, involved margins, and nodal or distant metastases. Survival was not affected by tumor size in this study. Overall survival for this aggressive malignancy has remained unchanged over the past several decades.

Molecular Aspects of Adrenocortical Carcinomas

To improve the dismal prognosis of this cancer, novel therapeutic targets are urgently needed, and new frontiers must therefore be explored. There has been an explosion in knowledge in molecular biology over the past decade. This has led to better understanding of the pathways of carcinogenesis, which will hopefully facilitate the discovery of newer, more superior methods of diagnosis and treatment with corresponding improvement in outcome for patients with ACCs.

Hereditary Tumor Syndromes

Adrenocortical tumors (ACTs) occur as a component of several hereditary tumor syndromes. The causative genes in these syndromes have also been found to be involved in the tumorigenesis of some sporadic ACTs. Table 11.1 summarizes these hereditary tumor syndromes and the genes/chromosomal loci involved.

Genes Associated with Sporadic Adrenocortical Tumors

TP53 Gene

The *TP53* gene is a tumor suppressor gene (TSG) which is frequently mutated in human cancers [45]. The p53 protein plays a role as a transcription factor in regulation of the cell cycle, causing cell cycle arrest or cell death in response to DNA damaging agents such as radiation and viruses [46].

TP53 mutation is thought to be a late event in the evolution of malignant transformation in ACTs. Mutations in exons 5–8 of *TP53* have been found in 20–27% of ACCs and 0–6% of ACAs [47, 48]. Patients whose ACC had *TP53* mutation had a trend towards shorter survival ($p = 0.098$) [49].

The rate of pediatric ACTs in southern Brazil is 3.4–4.2/million/year in children under 15 years old, which is 10–15 times higher than the worldwide incidence of

Table 11.1 Summary of hereditary tumor syndromes associated with ACTs

Hereditary tumor syndrome	Gene (chromosomal locus)	Manifestation of tumor syndrome
Li–Fraumeni syndrome	*TP53* (17p13) *hCHK2* (22q12.1) 1q23	Soft tissue sarcomas, osteosarcomas, breast cancer, brain tumors, leukemia, ACCs
Beckwith–Wiedemann Sydnrome	*IGF2, H19, CDKN1C, KCNQ1* (11p15)	Exomphalos, macroglossia, gigantism, ACC, nephroblastoma, hepatoblastoma, rhabdomyosarcoma
Carney Complex	*PRKAR1A* (17q22–q24) 2p16	Cardiac, endocrine, cutaneous and neural myxomatous tumors, and pigmented lesion of the skin and mucosa
Multiple Endocrine Neoplasia 1	*MEN1* (11q13)	Parathyroid, pancreatic islet cell, anterior pituitary and ACTs
Congenital Adrenal Hyperplasia	*CYP21B* (6p21.3) – most common *CYP11B* *CYP17A* *HSD3B2*	Adrenal hyperplasia, virilization, salt-wasting
Familial Adenomatous Polyposis (FAP)	*APC* (5q21–q22)	Multiple colonic polyps, gastric carcinoma, duodenal carcinoma, congenital hypertrophy of retinal pigment epithelium, ACTs

0.3–0.38/million/year [50]. This is associated with an Arg337His germline mutation of the *TP53* gene which was found in 35 of 36 pediatric ACTs in Southern Brazil [51]. Loss of heterozygosity (LOH) of the Arg337His mutation was also found in 8 of 11 (72.7%) ACTs tested which harbored the mutation [52]. The high rate of LOH of the *TP53* gene associated with mutation of that gene is consistent with Knudson's 2-hit hypothesis of loss of TSGs resulting in the disease. Interestingly, while *TP53* mutations tend to confer a poor prognosis in other cancers (multiple myeloma [53] and bladder cancer [54, 55]) and are associated with shorter survival in ACCs [49], only 1 child with the Arg337His mutation of *TP53* in Latronico's study developed metastasis, suggesting that this particular mutation may not necessarily result in a bad prognosis.

IGF2 Genes

Rearrangements, LOH and abnormal imprinting of the 11p15.5 locus, associated with elevated *IGF2* mRNA expression have all been reported in ACC [56, 57].

IGF2 overexpression has been consistently found in ACCs compared to adrenal adenomas or normal adrenal cortices [58–60]. Higher *IGF2* levels are associated with a malignant phenotype [61] and overexpression of *IGF2* is associated with an increased risk of ACC recurrence [56]. Demethylation of *IGF2* is also found more frequently in ACCs and correlates with *IGF2* mRNA expression [57]. Furthermore, LOH of the 11p15 locus has been demonstrated more frequently in ACC (67%) compared to adrenal adenomas (13%). It has been postulated that this leads to overexpression of *IGF2* because the maternal allele is lost with duplication of the paternal allele leading to a double dose of the expressed allele [57].

PEPCK (phosphoenolpyruvate carboxykinase)-IGF2 transgenic mice have 4 - 6 times the serum levels of *IGF2* as well as *IGF2* mRNA in the adrenal cortex in contrast to control mice where *IGF2* mRNA is not found. Studies with these transgenic mice have shown that the weights of the adrenal glands of these animals are significantly higher than controls, a result of hyperplasia of the zona fasciculata. Despite adrenal hyperplasia, over an 18-month period, these transgenic mice did not develop tumors in their adrenal glands, indicating that overexpression of *IGF2* alone is insufficient to cause ACT formation and that other factors are required for tumorigenesis [62].

Menin Gene

ACTs, usually adenomas, occur in up to 55% of persons with MEN1 syndrome [63–66]. As LOH of 11q13 occurs in about 20% of sporadic ACTs and adrenal lesions, mostly benign, occur in up to 40% of patients from MEN1 kindreds, *menin* was considered to be a prime candidate gene in the pathogenesis of these lesions. It was found however that although the majority of ACCs had 11q13 LOH, somatic mutations within the *menin* coding region do not occur commonly in sporadic ACTs [67] *Menin* mRNA expression by qPCR and Northern blot has also been found to be similar in ACCs, adenomas and normal adrenal cortices indicating that the *menin* gene is unlikely to play a prominent part in the pathogenesis of sporadic ACTs [68–70].

CYP21B Gene

As adrenal incidentalomas are common and there is thought to be a high frequency of mild undiagnosed congenital adrenal hyperplasia (CAH) in the population as well as an increased prevalence of ACTs in CAH patients, *CYP21B* mutations were thought to be involved in the pathogenesis of sporadic ACTs. Amongst patients with adrenal cortical adenomas, there is a 16% rate of CAH carriers and 2% rate of CAH compared to a 1–2% carrier rate in the general population [71]. There is, however, an absence of *CYP21B* mutations in the majority of patients with ACTs resulting in the conclusion that CAH is not a major predisposing factor for ACT formation [72, 73].

PRKAR1A Gene

PRKAR1A encodes the type 1α regulatory subunit of protein kinase A (PKA), the main mediator of cAMP signaling [74]. LOH of 17q22–24, the locus for *PRKAR1A* has been found in 23% of adrenal cortical adenomas and 53% of ACCs. Direct sequencing of the *PRKAR1A* gene revealed inactivating mutations in 10% of ACAs with corresponding decreased mRNA and protein levels in these tumors. These tumors were also smaller in size and exhibited paradoxical cortisol responses to dexamethasone, all features which are found in primary pigmented nodular adrenocortical disease (PPNAD). In contrast, no mutations were found in ACCs. This is consistent with PPNAD in which there has not been a case of ACC reported to date [75].

Guanine Nucleotide-Binding Protein, Alpha-Stimulating Activity Polypeptide (GNAS) Gene

Activating somatic mutations of *GNAS*, located on 20q13.2, are responsible for the McCune Albright syndrome (MAS; OMIM 174,800), a pediatric genetic disease. *GNAS* encodes the stimulatory G-protein α subunit ($G_s\alpha$) protein. In the abnormal $G_s\alpha$ protein, there is a substitution of arginine 201 by histidine or cysteine and it has decreased GTPase activity resulting in constitutive adenylate cyclase activation and consequent cAMP signalling [76–78]. MAS is a sporadic disease that predominantly affects the skeleton, skin and endocrine system. Classical manifestations include a triad of polyostotic fibrous dysplasia, large irregular café-au-lait spots and endocrine dysfunction including precocious puberty, hyperthyroidism, gigantism and Cushing's syndrome. It has been suggested that this disorder is caused by an autosomal dominant lethal gene that is compatible with viability of the fetus only when it occurs in the mosaic state, having arisen by somatic mutation during early embryogenesis [78, 79]. As the genes involved in MAS and Carney Complex (CNC) both act on the cAMP pathway, the endocrine features of both syndromes are very similar.

GNAS has been reported rarely to be mutated in sporadic adrenal adenomas. There have been no reports, however, of *GNAS* mutations in sporadic ACCs.

Evidence of the involvement of the genes above in the pathogenesis of sporadic ACTs is summarized in Table 11.2.

Signaling Pathways in Adrenocortical Tumors

Many different pathways are involved in cancer development. In ACTs, the ACTH/cAMP/PKA and Wnt pathway are thought to be important.

Table 11.2 Summary of genes and evidence of their involvement in the pathogenesis of sporadic ACTs

Gene	Evidence of involvement in sporadic ACTs
TP53	Mutation of TP53 found in 20–27% of ACCs and 0–6% of adrenal adenomas [48, 49]
IGF2	Overexpression of IGF2 mRNA in ACCs compared to adenomas [56, 58–60, 127]
MEN1	*MEN1* gene mutation in 7% of ACCs and adenomas [69, 70]
CYP21B	16% rate of CAH carriers and 2% rate of CAH in patients with adrenal adenomas compared to 1–2% carrier rate in general population [71]
PRKAR1A (17q22–q24)	Mutation of *PRKAR1A* in 10% of adrenal adenomas, not in ACCs [75]
GNAS (20q13.2)	Mutation of *GNAS* in adrenal cortical adenomas and tumors of patients with AIMAH [87, 128]

ACTH/cAMP/PKA Pathway

The binding of ACTH to its receptor, a member of the G protein-coupled receptor family, results in the dissociation of the heterotrimeric stimulatory G protein (Gs), causing the separation of the alpha-subunit (Gsα) from the β and γ subunits and stimulation of adenylate cyclase, which in turn leads to the production of cAMP from ATP. cAMP then binds to the regulatory subunits of PKA, releasing the catalytic subunits which results in phosphorylation of proteins in the cytoplasm and nucleus and subsequent signal transduction [80] (Fig. 11.1).

The ACTH/adenylate cyclase signaling pathway has been postulated to be involved in the pathogenesis of ACTs for a number of reasons. First, activating mutations of components of the adenylate cyclase pathway have been found in other human endocrine disorders, including toxic thyroid adenomas and acromegaly [81]. Second, there is a correlation between circulating ACTH levels and the size of the adrenal cortex, as seen in patients with CAH or Cushing's disease [82]. Finally, patients with CNC and MAS exhibit mutations in the *PRKAR1A* and *GNAS* genes, respectively. Both of these gene products are components of the cAMP pathway [83, 84].

In the Y1 mouse adrenocortical cells however, ACTH has been shown to have contradictory effects on the growth regulatory pathway. Its mitogenic effect activates ERK-MAPK pathway, induces transcription of *jun* and *fos* genes and weakly stimulates DNA synthesis. On the other hand, it also has an antimitogenic effect by activating the cAMP/PKA pathway, leading to degradation of c-Myc protein and Akt/PKB dephosphorylation with increased levels of the CDK inhibitor $p27^{Kip1}$[85]. Overall, however, ACTH is thought to have differentiating and growth inhibitory functions [80, 86].

Whilst no activating mutations of the *MC2R* (ACTH receptor) gene have been found in adrenal adenomas, ACCs or hyperplasias [87–89], LOH of this gene has been found in a small proportion of adrenal adenoma and ACCs [90] suggesting

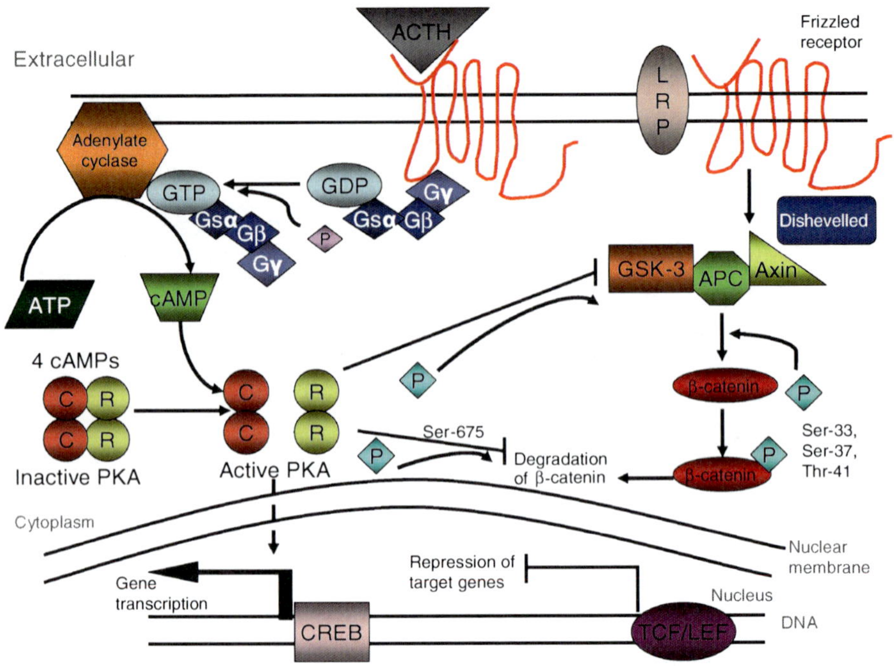

Fig. 11.1 Diagrammatic representation of ACTH/cAMP/PKA pathway (Adapted from www.biocarta.com/pathfiles/h_gsPathway.asp), Wnt pathway in the absence of Wnt ligand (Adapted from the Wnt Homepage (www.stanford.edu/~musse/wntwindow.html#diagrams)) and crosstalk between the 2 pathways. Abbreviations: *ACTH* adrenocorticotrophic hormone, *APC* Adenomatous polyposis coli, *ATP* adenosine triphosphate, *C* catalytic subunit of Protein kinase A, *cAMP* cyclic adenosine monophosphate, *CREB* cAMP response element, *GSK-3* glycogen synthase kinase 3β, *Gsα* G-protein α subunit, *Gβ* G-protein β subunit, *Gγ* G-protein γ subunit, *GDP* guanosine diphosphate, *GTP* guanosine trihosphate, *LRP* Lipoprotein receptor-related protein, *P* phosphate, *PKA* Protein kinase A, *R* regulatory subunit of Protein kinase A, *TCF/LEF* T cell-specific transcription factor/lymphoid enhancer-binding factor

that loss of the ACTH receptor resulting in loss of ACTH response may play a role in adrenocortical tumorigenesis.

Wnt Pathway

The Wnt family is comprised of a group of highly conserved growth factors with similar amino acid sequence and is responsible for developmental and homeostatic processes. The central event in the canonical Wnt signaling pathway is the accumulation of β-catenin in the cytoplasm with subsequent translocation into the nucleus. Wnt binds to its receptor complex which is composed of members of the Frizzled (Fz) family and low density lipoprotein receptor-related protein (LRP). This binding results in the inhibition of the Axin-Adenomatous polyposis coli (APC)-glycogen synthase kinase 3β (GSK-3β) complex, leading to a block in β-catenin phosphorylation by GSK-3β and accumulation of β-catenin in the cytoplasm. β-catenin then translocates into the nucleus where it interacts with the T cell-specific transcription factor/lymphoid enhancer-binding factor 1 (TCF/LEF) family of transcription factors to regulate transcription of Wnt target genes. In the absence of Wnt stimulation of its receptor, GSK-3β phosphorylates β-catenin, resulting in its ubiquitination and degradation by proteosomes [91] (Fig. 11.1).

The Wnt pathway has been noted to be involved in the pathogenesis of several cancers [92–94], in particular, in patients with Familial adenomatous polyposis (FAP) and the development of colorectal carcinomas [95]. Abnormal cytoplasmic and/or nuclear accumulation of β-catenin has been found to occur more commonly in ACCs compared to adrenal adenomas with a focal pattern in adenomas and a diffuse pattern in ACCs. Abnormal immunohistochemistry (IHC) for β-catenin was also found more frequently in non-functioning compared to functioning adrenocortical adenomas. Mutation of the β-catenin gene, however, was found with similar frequency in adrenal adenomas and ACCs. The most common mutation occurring in two thirds of the tumors tested was a point mutation in serine at the 45th position of exon 3 resulting in an amino acid substitution. As there is a higher rate of abnormal IHC for β-catenin in ACCs compared to adrenal adenomas but a similar rate of mutation of the β-catenin gene in the two groups, other components of the Wnt signaling pathway, such as *APC* or *AXIN*, may contribute to the pathogenesis of ACCs. Since β-catenin mutation occurs to a similar extent in adrenal adenomas and ACCs, it may be an early step in a common multistep pathogenesis of both lesions [96].

A recent paper by Doghman et al. highlighted the potential for novel treatment of ACTs. The study investigated the effect of the small-molecule inhibitor of the T cell factor (TCF)/β-catenin complex PKF115-584 on the H295R ACC cell-line which is known to have a mutation of the β-catenin gene. PKF115-584 inhibited β-catenin dependent transcription and proliferation of the H295R cells in a dose-dependent manner [97].

Crosstalk Between cAMP and Wnt/β-Catenin Pathways

In a study of nine adrenal PPNAD lesions and three adrenocortical adenomas with *PRKAR1A* mutations, β-catenin was found to accumulate in the cytoplasm and nucleus [98]. Mutation of the β-catenin gene has also been found in 11% of patients with germline *PRKAR1A* mutation [99]. Crosstalk between the cAMP and Wnt/β-catenin pathways are thought to play a part in the stabilization of β-catenin as PKA has been shown to phosphorylate Serine-9 of GSK-3β, inhibiting its phosphorylation of β-catenin [100]. PKA has also been shown to directly phosphorylate Serine-675 of β-catenin, leading to inhibition of its degradation, as well as facilitation of its binding to CREB-binding protein (CBP), its transcriptional coactivator [101, 102] (Fig. 11.1).

Clonal Analysis of Adrenocortical Tumors

Three clonal composition studies have shown that 60–100% of ACCs are monoclonal while 77.4–100% of adrenal hyperplasias and 12.5–43% of adenomas are polyclonal [103–105]. Interestingly, one of the studies examined both adrenal glands of a patient with ACTH-independent macronodular adrenal hyperplasia (AIMAH) and found polyclonality in two ipsilateral adrenal lesions and monoclonality in a contralateral adrenal lesion, suggestive of transition from hyperplasia to autonomous adenoma-like growth in larger nodules [104]. All three studies concur that ACCs are more often monoclonal, adrenal hyperplasia is more often polyclonal and adrenocortical adenomas can be either monoclonal or polyclonal. A polyclonal tumor would favor the idea that it developed from a group of cells under the common stimulus of a growth factor while a monoclonal tumor would suggest that it developed from a single genetically aberrant cell. The presence of monoclonal and polyclonal adenomas could be due to either different pathological mechanisms or different stages of a common multistep process. It has been suggested that progression to a monoclonal tumor could occur as a result of a first event which would initiate the growth of a polyclonal or partially monoclonal tumor with the maintenance of a normal steroid secretory pattern while a second event would confer a growth advantage in a selected clone of cells with a concomitant loss of differentiated functions and an aberrant steroid secretory pattern [103].

Comparative Genomic Hybridization Analysis

Comparative genomic hybridization (CGH) is a tool for detecting genetic aberrations in tumors and DNA copy losses identified on CGH have been shown to correlate with LOH studies on the sub-chromosomal level. These chromosomal regions of gains or losses provide a basis for the identification of protooncogenes or TSGs, respectively, within these regions. CGH analysis of adrenal adenomas and ACCs has identified clear differences between the two groups. More chromosomal changes have been identified in ACCs compared to ACAs and some studies have shown that the number of chromosomal changes increases with increasing tumor size. These findings would support the theory of an adenoma to carcinoma progression. A summary of all CGH studies performed in ACTs are listed in Table 11.3.

Loss of Heterozygosity Analysis

CGH has the limitation of not being able to detect DNA copy losses if the region affected is smaller than 10 Mb, if an allelic loss arises as a result of mitotic recombination or if one allele is lost and the other one is duplicated. LOH analysis, on the

Table 11.3 Summary of CGH results in sporadic ACTs

Study	Samples	Gains	Losses
Kjellman et al. [129]	8 ACCs	4q, 5p, 5q	2, 11q, 17p
	14 Adenomas	1q, 9q	1p
Sidhu et al. [130]	13 ACCs	5, 12	1p, 17p
	18 Adenomas	4q, 5	3q, 1p, 17p
Zhao et al. [131]	12 ACCs	20q, 5q, 9q	1p, 9p, 3p
	23 Adenomas	17q, 17p, 9p	
	6 Adrenocortical hyperplasias	17p, 17q	
Dohna et al. [132]	14 ACCs	5, 7p	9p
	8 Adenomas	5, 7p	9p
Stephan et al. [133]	25 ACCs	5, 7, 12, 16q, 20	1, 3p, 10q, 11, 14q, 15q, 17, 22q

other hand, is able to detect small deleted regions of the chromosome. It will, however, miss small deletions if the microsatellite markers used are not located in the deleted region. LOH analysis has been used to study chromosomal loci which have been linked to familial syndromes associated with ACTs (17p13, 11p15, 11q13, 17q22–24, 2p16) and found to be highly specific for ACCs. A summary of these results are shown in Table 11.4.

The numerous LOH studies have shown that LOH of 17p13 (Li–Fraumeni syndrome; LFS), 11p15 (Beckwith-Wiedemann syndrome; BWS), 11q13 (MEN1), 17q22–24 (CNC) and 2p16 (also CNC) tended to occur more frequently in sporadic ACCs compared to adrenal adenomas. Some of these studies have also shown the absence of mutations in the genes involved with the hereditary tumor syndromes at the respective loci suggesting that there are other TSGs within these loci that are involved in the pathogenesis of sporadic ACCs. One study identified a 10.4 megabase region of LOH on 17p13 in ACCs but not ACAs. From this region, the expression of two genes Acyl coenzyme-A dehydrogenase very long chain (*ACADVL)* and arachidonate 15-lipoxygenase (*ALOX15B*) were found to be significantly downregulated in ACCs compared to adrenal adenomas, suggesting that these genes may be involved in the tumorigenesis of ACCs [106].

Microarray Gene Expression Profiling Studies

Microarray gene expression analysis is a high throughput technique that allows the simultaneous analysis of the expression of thousands of genes in a tissue. By comparing gene expression profiles of two different groups, such as ACCs and adrenocortical adenomas, it is possible to identify genes which are significantly upregulated or downregulated in one group relative to the other. The assumption is that these genes are in some way involved in the pathogenesis of these tumors. Potential therapeutic targets can also be identified by this technique. A total of 6 microarray

Table 11.4 Summary of chromosomal locus and evidence of their involvement in the pathogenesis of sporadic ACTs

Chromosomal locus	Evidence of involvement in sporadic ACTs
17p13	17p13 LOH in up to 87.5% of ACCs and up to 30% of adrenal adenomas [56, 134, 135]
11p15	11p15 LOH in up to 83% of ACCs and 34% of adrenal adenomas [56, 57]
17q22–q24	LOH of 17q22–24 in 53% of ACCs and 23% of adrenal adenomas [75]
11q13	LOH of 11q13 in 100% of ACCs and 25% adrenal adenomas [69, 70, 136]
2p16	LOH of 2p16 in 92% of ACCs and no adrenal adenomas [136]

studies comparing gene expression profiles of ACCs compared to adrenal adenomas have been published. The top genes which have been found to be significantly differentially expressed in these studies are listed in Table 11.5.

As ACCs are rare tumors, most of the microarray gene expression profiling studies have been performed using small number of samples. In common across all the adrenocortical microarray gene expression studies is the overexpression of *IGF2* in ACCs compared to adrenal adenomas. No other putative pathogenic genes, however, have been identified in all the studies. This could be a result of the use of different microarray platforms, different software and algorithms used to analyze the data and different significance level cutoffs used. Contamination with normal adrenocortical, medullary or stromal tissue could also account for differences in expression profiles. Three of the 6 studies above specify a minimum amount of tumor tissue in sections used for RNA extraction (Giordano et al. >90%, Velazquez-Fernandez et al. >70% and Slater et al. >85%). Slater et al went further to verify the adrenocortical origin of the RNA by checking for mRNA expression of cytochrome P450, family 17 (*CYP17*), an enzyme involved in steroidogenesis, and only found in the cortex of the adrenal gland.

Molecular Markers in the Diagnosis of Adrenocortical Tumors

A number of studies have assessed the use of molecular markers in discriminating ACCs from adrenal adenomas.

IHC with Ki-67/MIB1 has been found to be useful in differentiating ACCs from adrenal adenomas [107–109] with a reported sensitivity of 87.5% and specificity of 95.5% in one study [108]. Combining IGF2 with Ki-67/MIB1 IHC improved sensitivity and specificity for differentiating ACCs from adrenal adenomas to 100 and 95.5%, respectively [108]. IHC with p53 has not been found to be particularly helpful because even though it is highly specific for ACCs, its sensitivity in identifying ACCs is low, ranging from 5.4–73% [107–109].

Protein expression of Matrix metalloproteinase type 2 (MMP2), also known as Gelatinase A, by IHC has been found to be high in ACCs but low in adrenal

Table 11.5 Top genes which are significantly differentially expressed in ACCs compared to adrenal adenomas in six microarray gene profiling studies

Study	Upregulated genes	Downregulated genes
Giordano et al. [58]	Insulin-like growth factor 2 (*IGF2*) Ubiquitin carrier protein E2-C (*UBCH10*) KIAA0101 gene product (*KIAA0101*) Secreted phosphoprotein 1 (*SPP1*) Chromosome 20 open reading frame 1 (*C20ORF1*)	Alcohol dehydrogenase 1 (*ADH1*) Alcohol dehydrogenase 2 (*ADH2*) Tropomodulin (*TMOD*) Stromal cell-derived factor 1 (*SDF1*) KIAA1024 protein (*KIAA1024*)
de Fraipont et al. [59]	*IGF2* Transforming growth factor, beta 2 (*TGFβ2*) Fibroblast growth factor receptor 1 (*FGFR1*) Fibroblast growth factor receptor 4 (*FGFR4*) Macrophage stimulating 1 receptor (*MST1R*) Transforming growth factor, beta receptor I (*TGFBR1*) KCNQ1 overlapping transcript 1 (*KCNQ1OT1*) Glyceraldehyde-3-phosphate dehydrogenase (*GAPD*)	Steroidogenic acute regulatory protein (StAR) Cytochrome P450, family 11, subfamily A (*CYP11A*) Hydroxy-delta-5-steroid dehydrogenase, 3 beta- and steroid delta-isomerase 1 (*HSD3B1*) Cytochrome P450, family 11, subfamily B, polypeptide 1 (*CYP11B1*) Cytochrome P450, family 21, subfamily A, polypeptide 2 (*CYP21A2*) Cytochrome P450, family 17 (*CYP17*) Protein phosphatase 1, catalytic subunit, alpha isoform (*PP1A*) S100 calcium binding protein B (*S100B*) Glypican 3 (*GPC3*) Inhibin α-chain (*INHA*) cAMP response element modulator (*CREM*) Retinoblastoma 1 (*RB1*) Nonmetastatic protein 23 (*NM23H5*) TGFβ type 3 receptor (*TGFB3*)
Velazquez et al. [137]	Ubiquitin specific peptidase 4 (*USP4*) Ubiquitin fusion degradation 1 like (*UFD1L*) Inositol polyphosphate phosphatase-like 1 (*INPPL1*) Aquaporin 3 (*AQP3*) H3 histone, family 3B (*H3F3B*)	Chemokine (CXC motif) ligand 10 (*CXCL10*) Retinoic acid receptor responder 2 (*RARRES2*) Aldehyde dehydrogenase 1 family, member A1 (*ALDH1A1*) Cytochrome b reductase 1 (*CYBRD1*) Glutathione S-transferase A4 (*GSTA4*)
Slater et al. [60]	Cathepsin H (*CTSH*) Mucolipin 3 (*MCOLN3*) Fibroblast growth factor receptor 1 (*FGFR1*) Aldo-keto reductase family 1, member C1 (*AKR1C1*) Fibronectin 1 (*FN1*)	Hypothetical protein MGC5306 (*MGC5306*) Cytoplasmic FMR1 interacting protein 2 (*CYFIP2*) Purkinje cell protein 4 (*PCP4*) Glutaminyl-peptide cyclotransferase (*QPCT*) Paralemmin (*PALM*)

(continued)

Table 11.5 (continued)

Study	Upregulated genes	Downregulated genes
Fernandez-Ranvier et al. [137]		Serpin peptidase inhibitor, clade G, member 1 *(SERPING1)* Mitochondrial ribosomal protein L48 *(MRPL48)* Transmembrane 7 superfamily member 2 *(TM7SF2)* Damage-specific DNA binding protein 1 *(DDB1)* NADH dehydrogenase Fe-S protein 8 *(NDUSF8)* Peroxiredoxin 5 *(PRDX5)*
West et al. [127]	Thyroid hormone receptor interactor *(TRIP)* Delta-like 3 *(DLL3)* Hypothetical protein FLJ22814 *(FLJ22814)* Dual oxidase 2 *(DUOX2)* Hypothetical protein FLJ10458 *(FLJ10458)*	Phenylalanine hydroxylase *(PAH)* Major histocompatibility complex, class II, DR alpha *(HLA-DRA)* Pleiomorphic adenoma gene-like 1 *(PLAGL1)* Cytochrome P450, family 11, subfamily B, polypeptide 1 *(CYP11B1)* Major histocompatibility complex, class II, DP alpha 1 *(HLA-DPA1)*

The first five studies compare expression profiles of adult ACCs and adrenal adenomas while the last study compares expression profiles of pediatric ACCs and adrenal adenomas

cortical adenomas. MMP2 protein expression in ACCs was focal in two-thirds of cases and diffuse in the remainder. It was also noted that more diffuse expression of MMP2 in ACCs was associated with shorter overall and disease-free survival [110]. Interestingly, whilst MMP2 mRNA was found more frequently in ACCs compared to adrenal adenomas, the mRNA was actually found in surrounding stromal tissue and not the neoplastic cell itself [111]. Serum levels of MMP2 have not been found to be useful in predicting either ACCs or adrenal adenomas [112].

Transcription factors have also been used as possible molecular markers which can differentiate ACCs from adrenal adenomas. A member of the nuclear receptor family of transcription factors, Steroidogenic factor 1 (SF-1) maps to 9q34. It has a key role in the development and function of the adrenal cortex [113]. A study on SF-1 knockout mice demonstrated that these mice died on postnatal day 8 with severe adrenocortical insufficiency due to an absence of the adrenal glands [114]. SF-1 heterozygous mice have also been found to develop adrenal insufficiency [115]. SF-1 protein levels have been noted to be increased in all ACTs compared to normal adrenal cortex [116]. While IHC with SF-1 has not been shown to differentiate between ACCs and adrenal adenomas [117], it is useful in distinguishing between primary ACCs and metastasis from other sites [118].

GATA-6 is from the GATA family of transcription factors, which is characterized by the binding to the DNA consensus sequence (A/T)GATA(A/G). GATA-6 plays a role in cellular maturation and differentiation [119]. GATA-6 protein expression has been found to be significantly decreased in ACCs compared to adrenal adenomas on IHC. Accordingly, ACTs with Weiss scores 4–9 had significantly lower GATA-6 level than ACTs with Weiss scores 1–3 [117].

Vascular endothelial growth factor (VEGF) plays a pivotal role in the regulation of both normal and tumor angiogenesis [120]. Angiogenesis is critical for tumor growth and metastasis [121]. VEGF has been found to be increased in the majority of cancers and is associated with a poorer outcome [122–125]. VEGF levels are significantly lower in adrenal adenomas compared to ACCs and are unrelated to tumor weight. The VEGF levels in ACCs which recurred were also higher than in those which did not recur [126]. Serum VEGF levels have not been found to be significantly different between patients with ACCs and those with adrenal adenomas [112]. VEGF, however, as a molecular marker for ACCs, has not been integrated into clinical practice.

Molecular Markers in the Prognosis of Adrenocortical Carcinomas

Several studies have noted the prognostic significance of molecular markers in ACCs [56, 59, 110]. De Fraipont's microarray study identified an 8-gene *IGF2* related cluster which could select the subgroup of patients with ACCs who were at high risk of recurrence and who would therefore benefit from adjuvant therapy [59]. Analyzing a subgroup of 40 tumors with follow up data showed that this gene cluster was not as effective as the Weiss score in terms of predicting malignancy and postoperative recurrence [59]. Another study found that LOH of the 17p13 locus in a cohort of 96 localized ACTs was a strong predictor of shorter disease free survival with a relative risk of 21.5 by multivariate analysis [56].

Many of the molecular markers described above lack specificity to achieve discrimination between ACCs and adrenal adenomas. To date, Ki-67/MIB1 and IGF2 IHC have been used in clinical practice. While IGF2 is a promising diagnostic marker, it does not predict the clinical behavior of ACCs. 17p13 LOH has been suggested as a new molecular marker which predicts tumor recurrence [56]. The search for other better molecular markers is therefore a continuing challenge.

Conclusion

Adrenocortical adenomas are common while ACCs are rare. Current methods of diagnosis do not always accurately differentiate between the two groups. ACCs are highly aggressive tumors with poor prognosis and existing treatment options are limited. Outcome for ACCs with prevailing therapies has remained unchanged for the past 2 decades. The study into the molecular biology of this cancer is therefore important to generate innovative and more sensitive means of diagnosis as well as novel and more effective therapeutic options which will translate into better patient outcome.

References

1. Abecassis M, McLoughlin MJ, Langer B, Kudlow JE (1985) Serendipitous adrenal masses: prevalence, significance, and management. Am J Surg 149:783–788
2. Bovio S, Cataldi A, Reimondo G et al (2006) Prevalence of adrenal incidentaloma in a contemporary computerized tomography series. J Endocrinol Invest 29:298–302
3. NIH (2002) NIH state-of-the-science statement on management of the clinically inapparent adrenal mass ("incidentaloma"). NIH Consens State Sci Statements 19:1–25
4. Allolio B, Fassnacht M (2006) Adrenocortical Carcinoma: Clinical Update. J Clin Endocrinol Metab 91:2027–2037
5. Bilimoria KY, Shen WT, Elaraj D et al (2008) Adrenocortical carcinoma in the United States: treatment utilization and prognostic factors. Cancer 113:3130–3136
6. Icard P, Goudet P, Charpenay C et al (2001) Adrenocortical carcinomas: surgical trends and results of a 253-patient series from the French Association of Endocrine Surgeons study group. World J Surg 25:891–897
7. Crucitti F, Bellantone R, Ferrante A, Boscherini M, Crucitti P (1996) The Italian Registry for Adrenal Cortical Carcinoma: analysis of a multiinstitutional series of 129 patients. The ACC Italian Registry Study Group. Surgery 119:161–170
8. Kasperlik-Zaluska AA, Migdalska BM, Zgliczynski S, Makowska AM (1995) Adrenocortical carcinoma. A clinical study and treatment results of 52 patients. Cancer 75:2587–2591
9. Tauchmanova L, Colao A, Marzano LA et al (2004) Andrenocortical carcinomas: twelve-year prospective experience. World J Surg 28:896–903
10. Wooten MD, King DK (1993) Adrenal cortical carcinoma Epidemiology and treatment with mitotane and a review of the literature. Cancer 72:3145–3155
11. Sidhu S, Sywak M, Robinson B, Delbridge L (2004) Adrenocortical cancer: recent clinical and molecular advances. Curr Opin Oncol 16:13–18
12. Didolkar MS, Bescher RA, Elias EG, Moore RH (1981) Natural history of adrenal cortical carcinoma: a clinicopathologic study of 42 patients. Cancer 47:2153–2161
13. Kasperlik-Zeluska AA, Roslonowska E, Slowinska-Srzednicka J et al (1997) Incidentally discovered adrenal mass (incidentaloma): investigation and management of 208 patients. Clin Endocrinol (Oxf) 46:29–37
14. Luton JP, Cerdas S, Billaud L et al (1990) Clinical features of adrenocortical carcinoma, prognostic factors, and the effect of mitotane therapy. N Engl J Med 322:1195–1201
15. Henley DJ, van Heerden JA, Grant CS, Carney JA, Carpenter PC (1983) Adrenal cortical carcinoma – a continuing challenge. Surgery 94:926–931
16. Allolio B, Hahner S, Weismann D, Fassnacht M (2004) Management of adrenocortical carcinoma. Clin Endocrinol (Oxf) 60:273–287
17. Caoili EM, Korobkin M, Francis IR, Cohan RH, Dunnick NR (2000) Delayed enhanced CT of lipid-poor adrenal adenomas. AJR Am J Roentgenol 175:1411–1415
18. Pena CS, Boland GW, Hahn PF, Lee MJ, Mueller PR (2000) Characterization of indeterminate (lipid-poor) adrenal masses: use of washout characteristics at contrast-enhanced CT. Radiology 217:798–802
19. Copeland PM (1999) The incidentally discovered adrenal mass: an update. Endocrinologist 9:415–423
20. Gomez-Rivera F, Medina-Franco H, Arch-Ferrer JE, Heslin MJ (2005) Adrenocortical carcinoma: a single institution experience. Am Surg 71:90–94

21. Kebebew E, Reiff E, Duh QY, Clark OH, McMillan A (2006) Extent of disease at presentation and outcome for adrenocortical carcinoma: have we made progress? World J Surg 30:872–878
22. Macfarlane DA (1958) Cancer of the adrenal cortex; the natural history, prognosis and treatment in a study of fifty-five cases. Ann R Coll Surg Engl 23:155–186
23. Sullivan M, Boileau M, Hodges CV (1978) Adrenal cortical carcinoma. J Urol 120:660–665
24. Cohn K, Gottesman L, Brennan M (1986) Adrenocortical carcinoma. Surgery 100:1170–1177
25. Kendrick ML, Lloyd R, Erickson L et al (2001) Adrenocortical carcinoma: surgical progress or status quo? Arch Surg 136:543–549
26. Shen WT, Sturgeon C, Duh QY (2005) From incidentaloma to adrenocortical carcinoma: the surgical management of adrenal tumors. J Surg Oncol 89:186–192
27. Kopf D, Goretzki PE, Lehnert H (2001) Clinical management of malignant adrenal tumors. J Cancer Res Clin Oncol 127:143–155
28. Iino K, Oki Y, Sasano H (2000) A case of adrenocortical carcinoma associated with recurrence after laparoscopic surgery. Clin Endocrinol (Oxf) 53:243–248
29. Ushiyama T, Suzuki K, Kageyama S, Fujita K, Oki Y, Yoshimi T (1997) A case of Cushing's syndrome due to adrenocortical carcinoma with recurrence 19 months after laparoscopic adrenalectomy. J Urol 157:2239
30. Schlamp A, Hallfeldt K, Mueller-Lisse U, Pfluger T, Reincke M (2007) Recurrent adrenocortical carcinoma after laparoscopic resection. Nat Clin Pract Endocrinol Metab 3:191–195 quiz 1 p following 5
31. Terzolo M, Berruti A (2008) Adjunctive treatment of adrenocortical carcinoma. Curr Opin Endocrinol Diabetes Obes 15:221–226
32. Dackiw AP, Lee JE, Gagel RF, Evans DB (2001) Adrenal cortical carcinoma. World J Surg 25:914–926
33. Chiche L, Dousset B, Kieffer E, Chapuis Y (2006) Adrenocortical carcinoma extending into the inferior vena cava: presentation of a 15-patient series and review of the literature. Surgery 139:15–27
34. Terzolo M, Angeli A, Fassnacht M et al (2007) Adjuvant mitotane treatment for adrenocortical carcinoma. N Engl J Med 356:2372–2380
35. van Ditzhuijsen CI, van de Weijer R, Haak HR (2007) Adrenocortical carcinoma. Neth J Med 65:55–60
36. Baudin E, Pellegriti G, Bonnay M et al (2001) Impact of monitoring plasma 1, 1-dichlorodiphenildichloroethane (o, p'DDD) levels on the treatment of patients with adrenocortical carcinoma. Cancer 92:1385–1392
37. Ahlman H, Khorram-Manesh A, Jansson S et al (2001) Cytotoxic treatment of adrenocortical carcinoma. World J Surg 25:927–933
38. Berruti A, Terzolo M, Sperone P et al (2005) Etoposide, doxorubicin and cisplatin plus mitotane in the treatment of advanced adrenocortical carcinoma: a large prospective phase II trial. Endocr Relat Cancer 12:657–666
39. Khan TS, Imam H, Juhlin C et al (2000) Streptozocin and o, p'DDD in the treatment of adrenocortical cancer patients: long-term survival in its adjuvant use. Ann Oncol 11:1281–1287
40. Schteingart DE, Doherty GM, Gauger PG et al (2005) Management of patients with adrenal cancer: recommendations of an international consensus conference. Endocr Relat Cancer 12:667–680
41. Quinkler M, Hahner S, Wortmann S et al (2008) Treatment of advanced adrenocortical carcinoma with erlotinib plus gemcitabine. J Clin Endocrinol Metab 93:2057–2062
42. Fassnacht M, Hahner S, Polat B et al (2006) Efficacy of adjuvant radiotherapy of the tumor bed on local recurrence of adrenocortical carcinoma. J Clin Endocrinol Metab 91:4501–4504
43. Stojadinovic A, Ghossein RA, Hoos A et al (2002) Adrenocortical carcinoma: clinical, morphologic, and molecular characterization. J Clin Oncol 20:941–950
44. Harrison LE, Gaudin PB, Brennan MF (1999) Pathologic features of prognostic significance for adrenocortical carcinoma after curative resection. Arch Surg 134:181–185
45. Hollstein M, Sidransky D, Vogelstein B, Harris CC (1991) p53 mutations in human cancers. Science 253:49–53

46. Levine AJ, Momand J, Finlay CA (1991) The p53 tumour suppressor gene. Nature 351:453–456
47. Ohgaki H, Kleihues P, Heitz PU (1993) p53 mutations in sporadic adrenocortical tumors. Int J Cancer 54:408–410
48. Reincke M, Karl M, Travis WH et al (1994) p53 mutations in human adrenocortical neoplasms: immunohistochemical and molecular studies. J Clin Endocrinol Metab 78:790–794
49. Sidhu S, Martin E, Gicquel C et al (2005) Mutation and methylation analysis of TP53 in adrenal carcinogenesis. Eur J Surg Oncol 31:549–554
50. Sandrini R, Ribeiro RC, DeLacerda L (1997) Childhood adrenocortical tumors. J Clin Endocrinol Metab 82:2027–2031
51. Ribeiro RC, Sandrini F, Figueiredo B et al (2001) An inherited p53 mutation that contributes in a tissue-specific manner to pediatric adrenal cortical carcinoma. Proc Natl Acad Sci USA 98:9330–9335
52. Latronico AC, Pinto EM, Domenice S et al (2001) An inherited mutation outside the highly conserved DNA-binding domain of the p53 tumor suppressor protein in children and adults with sporadic adrenocortical tumors. J Clin Endocrinol Metab 86:4970–4973
53. Chang H, Yeung J, Qi C, Xu W (2007) Aberrant nuclear p53 protein expression detected by immunohistochemistry is associated with hemizygous P53 deletion and poor survival for multiple myeloma. Br J Haematol 138:324–329
54. Sanchez-Carbayo M, Socci ND, Kirchoff T et al (2007) A polymorphism in HDM2 (SNP309) associates with early onset in superficial tumors, TP53 mutations, and poor outcome in invasive bladder cancer. Clin Cancer Res 13:3215–3220
55. Erill N, Colomer A, Verdu M et al (2004) Genetic and immunophenotype analyses of TP53 in bladder cancer: TP53 alterations are associated with tumor progression. Diagn Mol Pathol 13:217–223
56. Gicquel C, Bertagna X, Gaston V et al (2001) Molecular markers and long-term recurrences in a large cohort of patients with sporadic adrenocortical tumors. Cancer Res 61:6762–6767
57. Gicquel C, Bertagna X, Schneid H et al (1994) Rearrangements at the 11p15 locus and overexpression of insulin-like growth factor-II gene in sporadic adrenocortical tumors. J Clin Endocrinol Metab 78:1444–1453
58. Giordano TJ, Thomas DG, Kuick R et al (2003) Distinct transcriptional profiles of adrenocortical tumors uncovered by DNA microarray analysis. Am J Pathol 162:521–531
59. de Fraipont F, El Atifi M, Cherradi N et al (2005) Gene expression profiling of human adrenocortical tumors using complementary deoxyribonucleic. Acid microarrays identifies several candidate genes as markers of malignancy. J Clin Endocrinol Metab 90:1819–1829
60. Slater EP, Diehl SM, Langer P et al (2006) Analysis by cDNA microarrays of gene expression patterns of human adrenocortical tumors. Eur J Endocrinol 154:587–598
61. Boulle N, Logie A, Gicquel C, Perin L, Le Bouc Y (1998) Increased levels of insulin-like growth factor II (IGF-II) and IGF-binding protein-2 are associated with malignancy in sporadic adrenocortical tumors. J Clin Endocrinol Metab 83:1713–1720
62. Weber MM, Fottner C, Schmidt P et al (1999) Postnatal overexpression of insulin-like growth factor II in transgenic mice is associated with adrenocortical hyperplasia and enhanced steroidogenesis. Endocrinology 140:1537–1543
63. Barzon L, Pasquali C, Grigoletto C, Pedrazzoli S, Boscaro M, Fallo F (2001) Multiple endocrine neoplasia type 1 and adrenal lesions. J Urol 166:24–27
64. Skogseid B, Larsson C, Lindgren PG et al (1992) Clinical and genetic features of adrenocortical lesions in multiple endocrine neoplasia type 1. J Clin Endocrinol Metab 75:76–81
65. Burgess JR, Harle RA, Tucker P et al (1996) Adrenal lesions in a large kindred with multiple endocrine neoplasia type 1. Arch Surg 131:699–702
66. Waldmann J, Bartsch DK, Kann PH, Fendrich V, Rothmund M, Langer P (2007) Adrenal involvement in multiple endocrine neoplasia type 1: results of 7 years prospective screening. Langenbecks Arch Surg 392:437–443
67. Heppner C, Reincke M, Agarwal SK et al (1999) MEN1 gene analysis in sporadic adrenocortical neoplasms. J Clin Endocrinol Metab 84:216–219

68. Zwermann O, Beuschlein F, Mora P, Weber G, Allolio B, Reincke M (2000) Multiple endocrine neoplasia type 1 gene expression is normal in sporadic adrenocortical tumors. Eur J Endocrinol 142:689–695
69. Schulte KM, Heinze M, Mengel M et al (1999) MEN I gene mutations in sporadic adrenal adenomas. Hum Genet 105:603–610
70. Schulte KM, Mengel M, Heinze M et al (2000) Complete sequencing and messenger ribonucleic acid expression analysis of the MEN I gene in adrenal cancer. J Clin Endocrinol Metab 85:441–448
71. Baumgartner-Parzer SM, Pauschenwein S, Waldhausl W, Polzler K, Nowotny P, Vierhapper H (2002) Increased prevalence of heterozygous 21-OH germline mutations in patients with adrenal incidentalomas. Clin Endocrinol (Oxf) 56:811–816
72. Kjellman M, Holst M, Backdahl M, Larsson C, Farnebo LO, Wedell A (1999) No overrepresentation of congenital adrenal hyperplasia in patients with adrenocortical tumours. Clin Endocrinol (Oxf) 50:343–346
73. Beuschlein F, Schulze E, Mora P et al (1998) Steroid 21-hydroxylase mutations and 21-hydroxylase messenger ribonucleic acid expression in human adrenocortical tumors. J Clin Endocrinol Metab 83:2585–2588
74. Bossis I, Stratakis CA (2004) Minireview: PRKAR1A: normal and abnormal functions. Endocrinology 145:5452–5458
75. Bertherat J, Groussin L, Sandrini F et al (2003) Molecular and functional analysis of PRKAR1A and its locus (17q22–24) in sporadic adrenocortical tumors: 17q losses, somatic mutations, and protein kinase A expression and activity. Cancer Res 63:5308–5319
76. Weinstein LS, Shenker A, Gejman PV, Merino MJ, Friedman E, Spiegel AM (1991) Activating mutations of the stimulatory G protein in the McCune-Albright syndrome. N Engl J Med 325:1688–1695
77. Schwindinger WF, Francomano CA, Levine MA (1992) Identification of a mutation in the gene encoding the alpha subunit of the stimulatory G protein of adenylyl cyclase in McCune-Albright syndrome. Proc Natl Acad Sci USA 89:5152–5156
78. Lania A, Mantovani G, Spada A (2001) G protein mutations in endocrine diseases. Eur J Endocrinol 145:543–559
79. Happle R (1986) The McCune–Albright syndrome: a lethal gene surviving by mosaicism. Clin Genet 29:321–324
80. Kirschner LS (2002) Signaling pathways in adrenocortical cancer. Ann NY Acad Sci 968:222–239
81. Lyons J, Landis CA, Harsh G et al (1990) Two G protein oncogenes in human endocrine tumors. Science 249:655–659
82. Rosenberg D, Groussin L, Bertagna X, Bertherat J (2002) cAMP pathway alterations from the cell surface to the nucleus in adrenocortical tumors. Endocr Res 28:765–775
83. Lumbroso S, Paris F, Sultan C (2002) McCune–Albright syndrome: molecular genetics. J Pediatr Endocrinol Metab 15(Suppl 3):875–882
84. Kirschner LS, Carney JA, Pack SD et al (2000) Mutations of the gene encoding the protein kinase A type I-alpha regulatory subunit in patients with the Carney complex. Nat Genet 26:89–92
85. Rocha KM, Forti FL, Lepique AP, Armelin HA (2003) Deconstructing the molecular mechanisms of cell cycle control in a mouse adrenocortical cell line: roles of ACTH. Microsc Res Tech 61:268–274
86. Beuschlein F, Reincke M (2006) Adrenocortical tumorigenesis. Ann NY Acad Sci 1088:319–334
87. Fragoso MC, Domenice S, Latronico AC et al (2003) Cushing's syndrome secondary to adrenocorticotropin-independent macronodular adrenocortical hyperplasia due to activating mutations of GNAS1 gene. J Clin Endocrinol Metab 88:2147–2151
88. Latronico AC, Reincke M, Mendonca BB et al (1995) No evidence for oncogenic mutations in the adrenocorticotropin receptor gene in human adrenocortical neoplasms. J Clin Endocrinol Metab 80:875–877

89. Light K, Jenkins PJ, Weber A et al (1995) Are activating mutations of the adrenocorticotropin receptor involved in adrenal cortical neoplasia? Life Sci 56:1523–1527
90. Reincke M, Mora P, Beuschlein F, Arlt W, Chrousos GP, Allolio B (1997) Deletion of the adrenocorticotropin receptor gene in human adrenocortical tumors: implications for tumorigenesis. J Clin Endocrinol Metab 82:3054–3058
91. Gordon MD, Nusse R (2006) Wnt signaling: multiple pathways, multiple receptors, and multiple transcription factors. J Biol Chem 281:22429–22433
92. Collu GM, Brennan K (2007) Cooperation between Wnt and Notch signalling in human breast cancer. Breast Cancer Res 9:105
93. Clements WM, Wang J, Sarnaik A et al (2002) beta-Catenin mutation is a frequent cause of Wnt pathway activation in gastric cancer. Cancer Res 62:3503–3506
94. Kolligs FT, Bommer G, Goke B (2002) Wnt/beta-catenin/tcf signaling: a critical pathway in gastrointestinal tumorigenesis. Digestion 66:131–144
95. Clements WM, Lowy AM, Groden J (2003) Adenomatous polyposis coli/beta-catenin interaction and downstream targets: altered gene expression in gastrointestinal tumors. Clin Colorectal Cancer 3:113–120
96. Tissier F, Cavard C, Groussin L et al (2005) Mutations of beta-catenin in adrenocortical tumors: activation of the Wnt signaling pathway is a frequent event in both benign and malignant adrenocortical tumors. Cancer Res 65:7622–7627
97. Doghman M, Cazareth J, Lalli E (2008) The T cell factor/beta-catenin antagonist PKF115–584 inhibits proliferation of adrenocortical carcinoma cells. J Clin Endocrinol Metab 93:3222–3225
98. Gaujoux S, Tissier F, Groussin L, et al (2008) Wnt/ss-catenin and cAMP/PKA signaling pathways alterations and somatic ss-catenin gene mutations in the progression of adrenocortical tumors. J Clin Endocrinol Metab (in press)
99. Tadjine M, Lampron A, Ouadi L, Horvath A, Stratakis CA, Bourdeau I (2008) Detection of somatic beta-catenin mutations in primary pigmented nodular adrenocortical disease. Clin Endocrinol (Oxf) 69:367–373
100. Fang X, Yu SX, Lu Y, Bast RC Jr, Woodgett JR, Mills GB (2000) Phosphorylation and inactivation of glycogen synthase kinase 3 by protein kinase A. Proc Natl Acad Sci USA 97:11960–11965
101. Taurin S, Sandbo N, Qin Y, Browning D, Dulin NO (2006) Phosphorylation of beta-catenin by cyclic AMP-dependent protein kinase. J Biol Chem 281:9971–9976
102. Hino S, Tanji C, Nakayama KI, Kikuchi A (2005) Phosphorylation of beta-catenin by cyclic AMP-dependent protein kinase stabilizes beta-catenin through inhibition of its ubiquitination. Mol Cell Biol 25:9063–9072
103. Gicquel C, Leblond-Francillard M, Bertagna X et al (1994) Clonal analysis of human adrenocortical carcinomas and secreting adenomas. Clin Endocrinol (Oxf) 40:465–477
104. Beuschlein F, Reincke M, Karl M et al (1994) Clonal composition of human adrenocortical neoplasms. Cancer Res 54:4927–4932
105. Blanes A, Diaz-Cano SJ (2006) DNA and kinetic heterogeneity during the clonal evolution of adrenocortical proliferative lesions. Hum Pathol 37:1295–1303
106. Soon PS, Libe R, Benn DE et al (2008) Loss of heterozygosity of 17p13, with possible involvement of ACADVL and ALOX15B, in the pathogenesis of adrenocortical tumors. Ann Surg 247:157–164
107. Stojadinovic A, Brennan MF, Hoos A et al (2003) Adrenocortical adenoma and carcinoma: histopathological and molecular comparative analysis. Mod Pathol 16:742–751
108. Schmitt A, Saremaslani P, Schmid S et al (2006) IGFII and MIB1 immunohistochemistry is helpful for the differentiation of benign from malignant adrenocortical tumours. Histopathology 49:298–307
109. Gupta D, Shidham V, Holden J, Layfield L (2001) Value of topoisomerase II alpha, MIB-1, p53, E-cadherin, retinoblastoma gene protein product, and HER-2/neu immunohistochemical expression for the prediction of biologic behavior in adrenocortical neoplasms. Appl Immunohistochem Mol Morphol 9:215–221

110. Volante M, Sperone P, Bollito E et al (2006) Matrix metalloproteinase type 2 expression in malignant adrenocortical tumors: Diagnostic and prognostic significance in a series of 50 adrenocortical carcinomas. Mod Pathol 19:1563–1569
111. Kjellman M, Enberg U, Hoog A et al (1999) Gelatinase A and membrane-type 1 matrix metalloproteinase mRNA: expressed in adrenocortical cancers but not in adenomas. World J Surg 23:237–242
112. Kolomecki K, Stepien H, Bartos M, Kuzdak K (2001) Usefulness of VEGF, MMP-2, MMP-3 and TIMP-2 serum level evaluation in patients with adrenal tumours. Endocr Regul 35:9–16
113. Parker KL, Schimmer BP (1997) Steroidogenic factor 1: a key determinant of endocrine development and function. Endocr Rev 18:361–377
114. Luo X, Ikeda Y, Parker KL (1994) A cell-specific nuclear receptor is essential for adrenal and gonadal development and sexual differentiation. Cell 77:481–490
115. Bland ML, Jamieson CA, Akana SF et al (2000) Haploinsufficiency of steroidogenic factor-1 in mice disrupts adrenal development leading to an impaired stress response. Proc Natl Acad Sci USA 97:14488–14493
116. Pianovski MA, Cavalli LR, Figueiredo BC et al (2006) SF-1 overexpression in childhood adrenocortical tumours. Eur J Cancer 42:1040–1043
117. Kiiveri S, Liu J, Arola J et al (2005) Transcription factors GATA-6, SF-1, and cell proliferation in human adrenocortical tumors. Mol Cell Endocrinol 233:47–56
118. Sasano H, Shizawa S, Suzuki T et al (1995) Transcription factor adrenal 4 binding protein as a marker of adrenocortical malignancy. Hum Pathol 26:1154–1156
119. Parviainen H, Kiiveri S, Bielinska M et al (2007) GATA transcription factors in adrenal development and tumors. Mol Cell Endocrinol 265–266:17–22
120. Ferrara N, Davis-Smyth T (1997) The biology of vascular endothelial growth factor. Endocr Rev 18:4–25
121. Hanahan D, Folkman J (1996) Patterns and emerging mechanisms of the angiogenic switch during tumorigenesis. Cell 86:353–364
122. Brodsky SV, Mendelev N, Melamed M, Ramaswamy G (2007) Vascular density and VEGF expression in hepatic lesions. J Gastrointestin Liver Dis 16:373–377
123. Kamat AA, Merritt WM, Coffey D et al (2007) Clinical and biological significance of vascular endothelial growth factor in endometrial cancer. Clin Cancer Res 13:7487–7495
124. Herve MA, Buteau-Lozano H, Vassy R et al (2008) Overexpression of vascular endothelial growth factor 189 in breast cancer cells leads to delayed tumor uptake with dilated intratumoral vessels. Am J Pathol 172:167–178
125. Logan-Collins JM, Lowy AM, Robinson-Smith TM et al (2008) VEGF expression predicts survival in patients with peritoneal surface metastases from mucinous adenocarcinoma of the appendix and colon. Ann Surg Oncol 15:738–744
126. de Fraipont F, El Atifi M, Gicquel C, Bertagna X, Chambaz EM, Feige JJ (2000) Expression of the angiogenesis markers vascular endothelial growth factor-A, thrombospondin-1, and platelet-derived endothelial cell growth factor in human sporadic adrenocortical tumors: correlation with genotypic alterations. J Clin Endocrinol Metab 85:4734–4741
127. West AN, Neale GA, Pounds S et al (2007) Gene expression profiling of childhood adrenocortical tumors. Cancer Res 67:600–608
128. Yoshimoto K, Iwahana H, Fukuda A, Sano T, Itakura M (1993) Rare mutations of the Gs alpha subunit gene in human endocrine tumors. Mutation detection by polymerase chain reaction-primer-introduced restriction analysis. Cancer 72:1386–1393
129. Kjellman M, Kallioniemi OP, Karhu R et al (1996) Genetic aberrations in adrenocortical tumors detected using comparative genomic hybridization correlate with tumor size and malignancy. Cancer Res 56:4219–4223
130. Sidhu S, Marsh DJ, Theodosopoulos G et al (2002) Comparative genomic hybridization analysis of adrenocortical tumors. J Clin Endocrinol Metab 87:3467–3474
131. Zhao J, Speel EJ, Muletta-Feurer S et al (1999) Analysis of genomic alterations in sporadic adrenocortical lesions. Gain of chromosome 17 is an early event in adrenocortical tumorigenesis. Am J Pathol 155:1039–45

132. Dohna M, Reincke M, Mincheva A, Allolio B, Solinas-Toldo S, Lichter P (2000) Adrenocortical carcinoma is characterized by a high frequency of chromosomal gains and high-level amplifications. Genes Chromosomes Cancer 28:145–152
133. Stephan EA, Chung TH, Grant CS et al (2008) Adrenocortical carcinoma survival rates correlated to genomic copy number variants. Mol Cancer Ther 7:425–431
134. Yano T, Linehan M, Anglard P et al (1989) Genetic changes in human adrenocortical carcinomas. J Natl Cancer Inst 81:518–523
135. Soon PSH, Libe R, Benn DE et al (2008) Loss of Heterozygosity of 17p13, with possible involvement of ACADVL and ALOX15B, in the pathogenesis of adrenocortical tumors. Ann Surg 247:157–164
136. Kjellman M, Roshani L, Teh BT et al (1999) Genotyping of adrenocortical tumors: very frequent deletions of the MEN1 locus in 11q13 and of a 1-centimorgan region in 2p16. J Clin Endocrinol Metab 84:730–735
137. Velazquez-Fernandez D, Laurell C, Geli J et al (2005) Expression profiling of adrenocortical neoplasms suggests a molecular signature of malignancy. Surgery 138:1087–1094

Part IV
Pancreatic Neuroendocrine Tumors

Chapter 12
Gastrinoma

Anthony J. Chambers and Janice L. Pasieka

Introduction

Gastrinomas are uncommon tumors of the endocrine system, occurring within the pancreas and duodenum. Overproduction of the hormone gastrin by these tumors produces a sustained increase in gastric acid secretion, leading to complications of peptic ulceration known as the Zollinger–Ellison syndrome (ZES). Furthermore, gastrinomas have the potential to metastasize to regional lymph nodes, the liver and to other distant sites, and it is this malignant potential which has become increasingly important since the introduction of effective medical therapy to control gastric acid secretion. Gastrinomas can occur sporadically or in a familial pattern as a component of the multiple endocrine neoplasia type I (MEN1) syndrome. Given that the endocrinopathy associated with these tumors can be well controlled medically, the role of surgical resection in the setting of advanced disease and in patients with MEN1 syndrome is the subject of continued debate.

Historical Aspects

Islet cell tumors of the pancreas had been reported in association with peptic ulcer disease and gastric acid hypersecretion in isolated cases from as early as 1946 [1]. In 1955, Robert Zollinger and Edwin Ellison at the Ohio State University College of Medicine reported two patients with complications of severe refractory peptic ulcer disease associated with hypersecretion of gastric acid and non-insulin secreting islet cell tumors of the pancreas [2]. This triad of clinical features associated with gastrin-secreting tumors now bears the authors' names. They concluded in

J.L. Pasieka (✉)
Faculty of Medicine, Department of Surgery, University of Calgary and Tom Baker Cancer Centre, 10th Floor North Tower, Foothills Medical Center, 1403 – 29 Street NW, Calgary, AB, Canada T2N 2T9
e-mail: janice.pasieka@calgaryhealthregion.ca

C. Sturgeon (ed.), *Endocrine Neoplasia*, Cancer Treatment and Research, vol 153, DOI 10.1007/978-1-4419-0857-5_12, © Springer Science+Business Media, LLC 2010

their report that a hormonal agent produced by the islet cell tumors was responsible for the increased gastric acid secretion in these patients. The role of gastrin in the causation of ZES was first proposed by Gregory from the University of Liverpool in 1960, when he injected an extract derived from a pancreatic islet cell tumor from a patient with refractory peptic ulcer disease into an animal model and demonstrated a dramatic increase in gastric acid secretion, concluding that a "gastrin-like substance" was secreted by these tumors [3]. Gastrin was first isolated from antral mucosal cells by Gregory in 1964, and later found to be nearly identical in composition to an extracted hormone from gastrinoma [4]. The development of a radio-immunoassay for the measurement of serum gastrin concentrations by McGuigan and Trudeau in 1968 enabled the diagnosis of gastrinoma and ZES to be made on biochemical criteria [5]. Oberhelman in 1961 was the first to report the occurrence of duodenal gastrinomas in patients with ZES, prior to which the syndrome had only been associated with pancreatic islet cell tumors [6]. The first report of successful resection of gastrinoma to treat ZES was reported by Rawson in 1960, when a patient with peptic ulcer disease and hypersecretion of gastric acid underwent removal of a pancreatic islet cell tumor by Professor Stammers at the University of Birmingham [7]. The patient did not undergo gastrectomy or vagotomy, yet had a complete relief of symptoms and a marked reduction of gastric acid secretion after resection of the tumor.

Pathophysiology

Gastrin is a polypeptide hormone primarily secreted by neuroendocrine G-cells of the gastric antrum, and has a half-life in the systemic circulation of between 2 and 15 min [8]. Gastrin acts primarily by binding to cell surface receptors of the cholecystokinin family on gastric parietal and chief cells to stimulate acid and pepsin secretion [9]. It also has a trophic action in stimulating growth of gastrointestinal mucosal cells and causes relaxation of smooth muscle within the lower esophageal sphincter and sphincter of Oddi [10]. Gastrin release from antral G-cells is stimulated in response to gastric distension, to the presence of amino acids and protein within the gastric lumen and to increased vagal activity. Importantly, gastrin release is also stimulated in response to increasing levels of serum calcium, which has clinical relevance in the setting of hyperparathyroidism and MEN1 [11]. Negative feedback inhibition of gastrin release is produced in response to acid content within the lumen of the stomach. The gastrointestinal hormones somatostatin, vasoactive intestinal polypeptide, gastric inhibitory polypeptide, glucagon and calcitonin also suppress gastrin release [8, 10].

Genetic Basis

A number of genetic abnormalities are involved in the pathogenesis of gastrinoma, occurring in both the sporadic form and in tumors occurring in a familial context. Germ-line mutation of the MEN1 gene, a tumor suppressor gene located on the short arm of chromosome 11 (11q31), is responsible for the MEN1 syndrome [12]. The MEN1 gene codes for the nuclear protein *menin*, which is involved in cell growth regulation [13]. MEN1 gene mutations are inherited in an autosomal dominant pattern, and 36–42% of patients with this mutation will develop gastrinoma [14, 15]. Mutation of the MEN1 gene has also been implicated in the pathogenesis of gastrinoma occurring in the sporadic form. Somatic mutation of the MEN1 gene can be found within 17–58% of gastrinomas in patients with sporadic tumors who do not possess germ-line MEN1 mutations or a family history of MEN1-related tumors [16, 17]. The majority of mutations involve deletions, particularly in the exon 2 region of the MEN1 gene [16, 18]. Loss of heterozygosity producing a single copy of the MEN1 gene is found in up to 93% of sporadic gastrinomas [19]. It has been proposed that MEN1 gene mutation is an early event in the pathogenesis of both sporadic and familial gastrinomas, with mutations occurring equally in duodenal and pancreatic gastrinomas, and in tumors which are localized and which have metastasized [18]. The biological behavior of gastrinomas displaying the MEN1 gene mutation is similar to those where this mutation is not found, with no increased risk of metastatic disease or of recurrence after surgical resection [16, 17].

A number of other genetic mechanisms are involved in the pathogenesis of gastrinoma in addition to mutations affecting the MEN1 gene. Chromosomal deletions causing loss of heterozygosity have also been identified in gastrinomas at regions 1q (identified in 44% of gastrinomas) and 22q (identified in 96%), and have been associated with higher rates of metastatic disease [20, 21]. It has been suggested that loss of tumor suppressor genes at these locations may lead to the development of gastrinoma. Inactivation or deletion of the p16 tumor suppressor gene at chromosome 9p21, coding for the p16 protein involved in the regulation of cell growth and cell cycle inhibition, has also been demonstrated in 52% of gastrinomas [22]. A number of tyrosine kinase receptors involved in cell growth regulation have also been implicated in the pathogenesis of gastrinomas. Insulin-like growth factor-1 (IGF1) receptors are expressed by 97% of gastrinomas, and tumors with higher levels of mRNA for this receptor have increased rates of hepatic metastases and reduced disease-free survival after surgical resection [23]. Epidermal growth factor (EGF) and hepatocyte growth factor (HGF) receptors are found to be overexpressed in 14 and 18% of gastrinomas respectively, which has similarly been associated with an increased risk of metastatic disease [24]. The HER-2/neu gene, coding for an EGF-related tyrosine kinase receptor, is overexpressed in 14–100% of gastrinomas, and higher levels of expression have been found in patients with metastatic disease [25].

Clinical Features and Diagnosis

Gastrinomas are rare tumors, occurring with an incidence of less than one case per million population per year [26]. Gastrinomas occur somewhat more frequently in males, with a male to female ratio of 1.3:1 to 1.5:1 [27–30]. The tumor typically presents in late adulthood with a mean age at diagnosis of 41 to 54 years [27–31]. Patients with gastrinoma classically present with symptoms of hypersecretion of gastric acid, and 98% of patients are symptomatic at diagnosis [29] (Table 12.1). Historically, patients with gastrinoma were typically diagnosed late in the course of their disease with complications of severe refractory peptic ulcer disease. In the modern era of improved biochemical and imaging investigations, a history of peptic ulceration is absent in 29% of patients at the time of diagnosis [28].

The diagnosis of gastrinoma is based on biochemical testing, demonstrating an elevation of fasting serum gastrin (FSG) level (>150 pg/ml) in the presence of raised gastric acid secretion [32]. In patients receiving acid suppressive therapy with H2-antagonists or proton pump inhibitors (PPI), FSG is secondarily raised by these medications and, as such, these should be discontinued at least 7 days prior to testing [33]. Gastric secretory studies showing a basal acid output (BAO) of more than 15 mEq/h (more than 5 mEq/h in the presence of previous gastric resection) or a pH of less than 2 are the most commonly used criteria to determine acid hypersecretion [32]. FSG can also be elevated in other disease states that must be differentiated from ZES (Table 12.2). Most patients with gastrinoma have highly elevated

Table 12.1 Clinical presentation of gastrinoma/Zollinger–Ellison syndrome

Symptom	Percentage of patients
Abdominal pain	78–94
Peptic ulcer disease	74–96
Duodenal ulcer	60–96
Gastric ulcer	24
Proximal jejunal ulceration	29
Diarrhea	72
Gastroesophageal reflux	42
Esophageal ulceration or stricture	4–6
Gastrointestinal bleeding	27–42
Weight loss	7–18
Steatorrhea	5–10

Table 12.2 Causes of hypergastrinemia

Gastrinoma/Zollinger–Ellison syndrome
G cell hyperplasia
Helicobacter pylori infection
Retained gastric antrum
Gastric outlet obstruction
Short bowel syndrome
Associated with hypochlorhydria
Pernicious anemia
Chronic atrophic gastritis
Previous Vagotomy
Gastric acid suppressing medications
Renal impairment

gastrin levels, with 36% having levels more than ten times the normal [34]. Gastrin levels may be normal or borderline in 0.3% to 3% of patients with gastrinoma, particularly during the early stages of disease [34, 35]. When the results of FSG and acid secretory studies are borderline or nondiagnostic in patients where a clinical suspicion for gastrinoma/ZES exists, provocative testing of FSG after administration of intravenous secretin (2 mg/kg) or calcium is indicated. Following secretin injection, FSG increases from baseline levels within 2 to 3 min by more than 100 pg/ml in 94% of patients with gastrinoma, and rises by more than 50% in 84% of cases [36]. Similarly, provocative testing after calcium infusion results in a rise in gastrin of more than 50% from baseline levels in 84% of cases [36]. Combining these two investigations lead to a sensitivity of 100% for confirming the diagnosis of gastrinoma in a series of 24 patients reported by Wada and coworkers [35]. Chromogranin-A, a protein contained within the secretory granules of neuroendocrine cells, is a non-specific marker for neuroendocrine tumors and is elevated in 90% of patients with gastrinoma [37]. Chromogranin-A levels tend to correlate with those of serum gastrin, however higher levels are not associated with an increased risk of advanced or metastatic disease [37].

Site and Localization of Primary Tumors

Although ZES was first described in association with gastrin producing neuroendocrine tumors of the pancreas, the primary tumor can be located in the duodenum in an equivalent proportion of cases and may also arise uncommonly from other sites [27, 38–42]. In 90% of cases the primary tumor can be localized within the "gastrinoma triangle," a region encompassing the proximal duodenum and head of the pancreas, defined by Stabile in 1984 as located between (a) the junction of the cystic and common bile ducts (superiorly), (b) the junction of the second and third parts of the duodenum (inferiorly), and (c) the junction of the neck and body of the pancreas (medially) [43]. Duodenal gastrinomas are small tumors arising within the submucosa, and are found in the first and second parts of the duodenum in 83–92% of cases, and rarely distal to this [44] (Fig. 12.1). Mean size ranges from 0.6 to 1.3 cm in diameter and 49–80% of tumors are less than 1 cm in size, and for this reason they are rarely seen on imaging studies [27, 41, 42, 44, 45]. The pancreas is the site of gastrinoma in 17–55% of patients with sporadic ZES, and the tumor is located proximally in the head of the pancreas in 33–53% of cases [27, 29, 38–42]. Gastrinoma is the second most common functional neuroendocrine tumor of the pancreas, accounting for 36% of lesions [46]. Pancreatic gastrinomas tend to be larger than their duodenal counterparts with a mean diameter of 2.7–3.2 cm [27, 42, 45, 47]. Sporadic gastrinomas can be present in multiple sites in 11–16% of patients, and pancreatic and duodenal gastrinomas may coexist in 9–11% of cases [27, 29, 38, 42]. In contrast, greater than 75% of patients with MEN1/ZES have multiple tumors [14, 48].

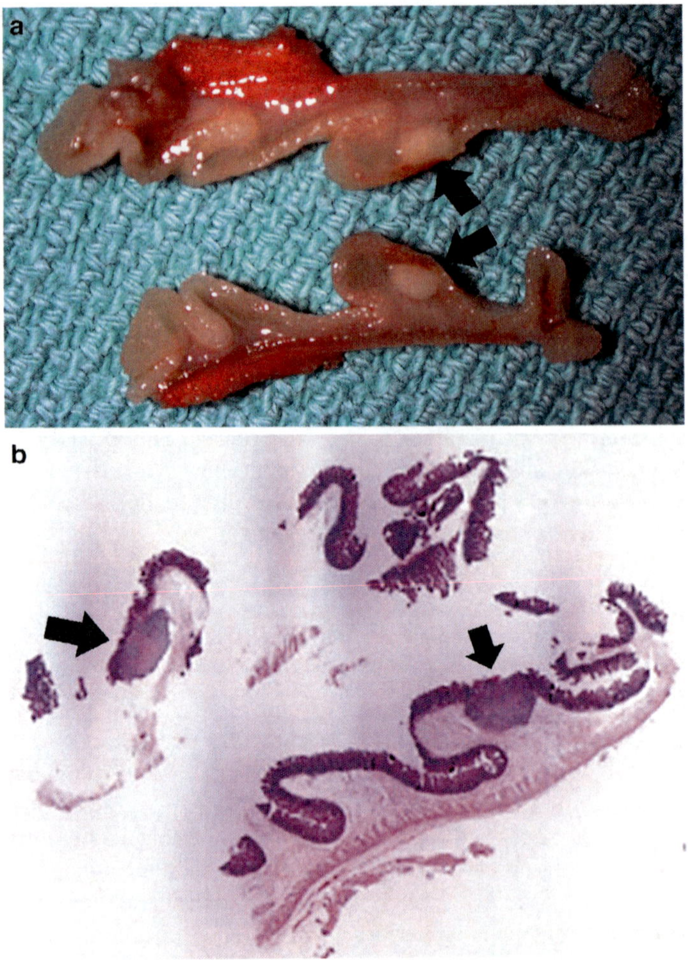

Fig. 12.1 (**a**) Operative photograph showing a 3-mm gastrinoma found within the proximal jejunum at laparotomy in a patient with Zollinger–Ellison syndrome. (**b**) Photomicrograph showing the histological appearance of the resected gastrinoma

Gastrinomas can arise in sites outside the duodenum and pancreas in rare instances, accounting for 5.6% of reported cases [49]. Primary gastrinomas have been reported in the liver, biliary tree, ovary, kidney, heart, stomach, jejunum and greater or lesser omentum [40, 49]. In 11–26% of patients with ZES undergoing laparotomy, lymph nodes involved with gastrinoma are found without identification of a primary tumor of the pancreas or duodenum, raising the possibility that gastrinoma can develop primarily in peripancreatic and periduodenal lymph nodes [40, 41, 50]. Alternatively, these nodal lesions may represent metastases from a small primary tumor that evaded detection at the time of initial operation. In a series of 176 patients with ZES undergoing laparotomy with duodenotomy and intraoperative pancreatic ultrasound, Norton and coworkers reported that involved lymph nodes were the only site of disease identified intraoperatively in 45 cases [50]. These authors concluded that lymph nodes can be the primary site of gastrinoma in 10% of patients with ZES.

Computed tomography (CT) and magnetic resonance (MR) imaging are useful as staging investigations for gastrinoma, detecting hepatic metastases with a sensitivity of 64–71% and 43–80% respectively [51]. Cross-sectional imaging with CT and MR does not usually possess the resolution to detect duodenal primary tumors due to their small size, but can detect pancreatic gastrinomas with a sensitivity of 54–71% [52]. Somatostatin receptors are expressed by 85–100% of gastrinomas, and for this reason somatostatin receptor scintigraphy (SRS) using radiolabeled octreotide can be used to detect primary gastrinomas and nodal or distant metastatic lesions [53]. SRS has a sensitivity of 11–30% for the identification of duodenal lesions, 25–77% for pancreatic lesions, 72–82% for nodal metastases and 67–100% for hepatic metastases from gastrinoma [51, 52, 54, 55]. In a study of 122 patients with ZES by Termanini and coworkers, SRS was positive for disease in 61% of patients, and was the only imaging modality that localized tumor in 12% of cases, changing the management of 47% of cases [51]. A study by Alexander and coworkers of 35 patients with gastrinoma who had preoperative SRS found that this modality was able to detect primary tumors and metastatic lesions, with a sensitivity superior to that of CT, MR and angiography combined, however was unable to identify 33% of primary tumors subsequently found at laparotomy [54].

Endoscopic ultrasound (EUS) has been shown to be useful in the detection of pancreatic neuroendocrine tumors including gastrinomas, identifying even small lesions with a sensitivity of 75–83% [52, 55, 56]. EUS can also help define the relationship of primary tumors to pancreatic ductal and vascular structures, and needle biopsy of pancreatic lesions can also be performed. EUS is less sensitive in the detection of duodenal gastrinomas due to their small size, failing to detect 60–80% of tumors in this location [52, 55].

Invasive testing involving arteriography or selective venous sampling has been utilized to assist in the localization of gastrinoma in patients where CT, MR and SRS do not localize the tumor. Selective angiography with secretin injection (SASI) involves cannulation of the right or left hepatic veins and sampling of gastrin levels from this location after intra-arterial injection of secretin, or more commonly calcium, into the gastroduodenal, hepatic, splenic, left gastric and superior mesenteric arteries [57, 58]. Secretin stimulates gastrin release from tumor present in the vascular distribution of the arterial injection, producing an increase in gastrin levels as measured in the hepatic veins. The proportion of patients with gastrinoma where the tumor can be regionalized by SASI varies from 71 to 89% [40, 41]. Selective venous sampling of gastrin levels in tributaries of the portal venous system has also been employed to assist in the localization of gastrinomas preoperatively, but is associated with a greater risk of bleeding due to the transhepatic cannulation of portal vein branches.

Whole body positron emission tomography (PET) using 11-C-5-hydroxytryptophan has been shown to be superior to CT and SRS in the detection of neuroendocrine primary tumors or their metastases [59]. PET using 68-Gallium labeled DOTA-TOC, a somatostatin analog with a greater affinity for somatostatin receptors than octreotide, has been associated with a sensitivity of 97% for the detection of neuroendocrine tumors and metastases [60].

Metastatic Disease

In one of the earliest studies involving the long-term follow-up of patients with gastrinoma, Zollinger noted that in 60% of patients the tumor behaved in a malignant fashion [61]. Metastatic disease affecting regional lymph nodes or the liver can be demonstrated in 52–69% of patients with gastrinoma on initial imaging studies or at the time of laparotomy [40, 41, 45, 46]. Involvement of regional lymph nodes, particularly peripancreatic and periduodenal nodes, can be demonstrated in 36–67% of patients with gastrinoma at the time of surgical exploration and resection [41, 45]. In a study of 185 patients, Weber and coworkers found that duodenal and pancreatic primary tumors had equivalent rates of nodal metastases, occurring in 48% of patients [45]. In contrast to distant metastatic disease, regional lymph node involvement alone has not been associated with a reduction in survival of patients with gastrinoma, with an overall 10-year survival approaching 100% [27, 30, 45]. Hepatic metastases are present in 8–22% of patients with gastrinoma at the time of initial assessment [41, 45]. Several authors have found that pancreatic gastrinomas are more frequently associated with hepatic metastases than were duodenal gastrinomas (52% vs. 5%) [27, 45]. The size of the primary tumor was associated with an increased risk of hepatic metastases, with tumors smaller than 1 cm having a 4% risk of hepatic metastases, tumors 1–3 cm in size having metastases in 28% of cases, and tumors greater than 3 cm in size having hepatic metastases in 61% of cases [45]. The development of hepatic metastases significantly worsens survival and is associated with a 10-year survival rate of 26–30% [30, 45]. Peritoneal or omental metastases occur in 6%, bone metastases in 3–7% and lung metastases in 2% of cases [29, 62].

Management and Operative Strategy

With the introduction of effective medical therapy for the control of gastric acid hypersecretion in patients with ZES, the role of surgery in the management of patients with gastrinoma has shifted from the control of gastric acid secretion to the requirement for oncological resection of the primary tumor to prevent disease progression and metastatic spread [63]. Complete surgical resection of the primary tumor and involved regional lymph nodes may be curative in patients with gastrinoma that have not metastasized to distant sites. Inspection and palpation of the duodenum and pancreas is performed after complete mobilization of these structures and can successfully detect 61–71% of primary gastrinomas [44, 47, 64]. Intraoperative ultrasound (IOS) can improve the ability to localize primary tumors of the pancreas and identify metastatic disease within the liver, but is not more sensitive than palpation in the detection of duodenal primaries [44, 64]. Small primary tumors within the duodenum are best identified by inspection and palpation of the mucosal surface via a longitudinal duodenotomy of the second portion of the duodenum. This maneuver was first recommended by Thompson and coworkers in 1989 [65, 66]. After introducing routine duodenotomy to the operative exploration of patients with ZES, Norton and coworkers showed a significant improvement in the ability to localize the primary tumors from 76 to 98% of cases, due to an increase in the rate of detection of small duodenal gastrinomas [67]. Patients in this study undergoing routine duodenotomy had significantly higher rates of long-term biochemical cure post-operatively (occurring in 52% of patients undergoing duodenotomy vs. 26% of patients who did not) [67]. In a subsequent report by these authors of their experience with 160 consecutive patients undergoing laparotomy for ZES, overall the primary tumor could be identified and resected in 94% of cases, and in 100% of those who underwent duodenotomy [40].

Options for resection of the primary gastrinoma are dependent on the location and size of the tumor. The majority of duodenal lesions are small and can be resected locally, either using a submucosal resection via duodenotomy for lesions less than 4–5 mm, or with an elliptical resection of the full-thickness of the duodenal wall for larger lesions [52, 65, 68] (Fig. 12.2). Lesions of the pancreas can be enucleated or formally resected depending on their size and location within the gland. Lesions within the head of the pancreas smaller than 3 cm can be enucleated in most cases [27, 41, 69]. Care should be taken to avoid injury to the pancreatic duct at the time of enucleation, and IOS may aid in the identification and preservation of ductal structures [70]. Pancreaticoduodenectomy may be required for large tumors (>5 cm) of the head of the pancreas, those in close proximity to the pancreatic duct with a high probability of ductal injury and those with grossly involved

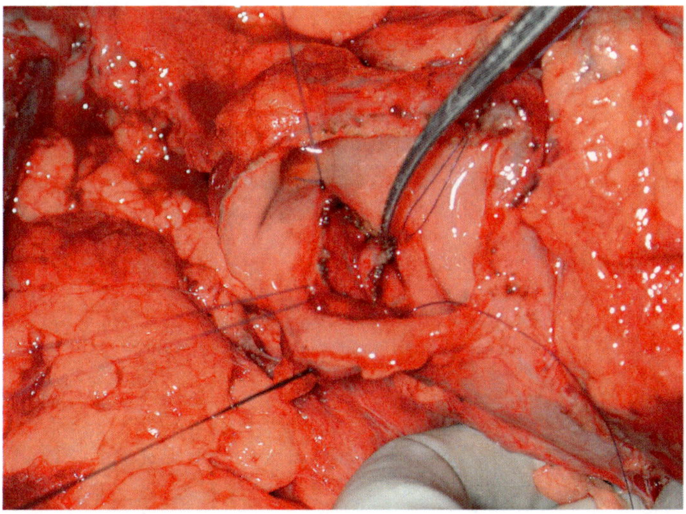

Fig. 12.2 Operative photograph showing the local resection of a duodenal gastrinoma identified by inspection of the mucosal surface after duodenotomy

regional lymph nodes [71]. Distal pancreatectomy is the procedure of choice for the rare gastrinoma located in the body or tail of the pancreas [27, 41]. Preservation of the spleen can be performed in this setting; however, splenectomy may facilitate the removal of lymph nodes in the region of the splenic hilum and is preferred on oncological grounds [68]. Spread to regional lymph nodes can be demonstrated in 36–67% of patients with gastrinoma and can serve as a source of persistent gastrin secretion, and therefore resection of regional lymph node groups should occur at the time of resection of the primary tumor [40, 41, 44]. A summary of the surgical strategies for the management of ZES is shown in Table 12.3.

Outcomes after surgery for resection of gastrinoma can be measured in terms of normalization of biochemical tests, control of symptoms, rates of disease recurrence and overall survival. In a study of 160 patients undergoing operative exploration for ZES where the primary tumor could be identified in 94% of cases, Norton and coworkers were able to achieve a disease free state with normal secretin-stimulated gastrin levels and no evidence of disease on imaging in 51% of patients [40].

Table 12.3 Surgical strategies for Zollinger–Ellison syndrome

Clinical scenario	Strategy	References
1. *Sporadic pancreatic gastrinoma*		
size <3 cm	Enucleation (open or laparoscopic)	[27, 41]
Size >3 cm	En-bloc resection	[27, 41]
2. *Sporadic duodenal gastrinoma*		
Solitary/small	Local resection	[65, 68]
Multiple/large/ local invasion	Pancreaticoduodenectomy	[71]
3. *Metastatic gastrinoma*	– Assess resectability and symptom control on PPIs	
	– Consider surgical cytoreduction of hepatic metastases if >70-90% of tumor volume removable followed by	[74, 75]
	– Multimodaility medical therapy: PPI, octreotide, radionuclide therapies, hepatic artery embolization, mTOR inhibitors	[82–85]
4. *MEN1/ZES*		
Biochemical or image detected <2 cm	Duodenotomy, 80% distal pancreatectomy and enucleation of NETs – head of pancreas	[68, 89]
	– Assess lymph nodes at laparotomy and resect if positive (or)	[95]
	Duodenotomy, local resection of pancreatic NETs	
	– Assess lymph nodes at laparotomy and resect if positive (or) Treat medically with PPIs	[89]
Image detected >2 cm	Duodenotomy and en-bloc pancreatic resection with regional lymph nodes	[45, 73, 97, 98]

MEN1, multiple endocrine neoplasia type 1; mTOR, mammalian target of rapamycin; NET, neuroendocrine tumor; PPI, proton pump inhibitors; Zes, Zollinger Ellison syndrome

Table 12.4 Outcomes after surgery for gastrinoma

Author	Year	*N*	MEN1	Localized and resected	Initial biochemical cure	Long-term cure	References
Norton	2006	160	21%	94%	51%	41%	[40]
Ellison	2006	106	25%	–	42% sporadic	26% sporadic 4% MEN1	[27]
Jordan	1999	51	14%	87%	–	31% sporadic 3% MEN1	[38]
Kaplan	1990	30	10%	74%	43%	–	[39]
Stabile	1984	45	–	80%	–	9%	[43]

Patients in this study were followed for a mean period of 12 years and during this time 41% remained disease-free. Other institutions have reported long-term biochemical cure of 31–48% of patients after surgical resection of gastrinoma [38, 39]. A summary of the biochemical cure rates associated with surgery for gastrinoma is shown in Table 12.4. Following the successful surgical resection of gastrinoma, gastric BAO is reduced by 75–80% at 3 to 6 months post-operatively [31, 72]. Gastric acid secretion remains elevated in as many as 40–67% of patients after successful resection of gastrinoma even where serum gastrin levels fall to within the normal range, and for this reason acid-suppressing medical therapy may be a long-term requirement [31, 72]. Discontinuation of acid-suppressing medications is possible in 41–57% of patients following successful resection of gastrinoma, with a reduction in dosage achievable in 82% [31, 72].

Surgical resection is the only modality capable of achieving cure in patients with ZES and, given the malignant potential of the primary tumor, this has an important role in preventing the progression to metastatic disease. In their study comparing the long-term follow-up of 160 patients undergoing surgical resection of gastrinoma with 35 patients managed non-operatively, Norton and coworkers found that significantly fewer patients undergoing surgical resection developed hepatic metastases during long-term follow-up (5% vs. 29%) [40]. Survival was significantly higher for patients who underwent surgery in this study, with 15-year disease-specific survival 98% for surgically resected patients and 74% for those managed non-operatively. In those patients who did not undergo surgery, 90% of deaths were secondary to progressive metastatic disease. In a study of 106 patients with gastrinoma managed at a single institution over a 50-year period, Ellison and coworkers found that patients undergoing macroscopically-complete resection of disease had a significantly greater long-term survival than those who had incomplete resection of disease or who did not undergo surgery (10-year survival 85% vs. 30%) [27].

Management of Advanced and Metastatic Disease

Gastrinomas may present as locally advanced tumors with invasion into surrounding structures, or with hepatic and other distant metastases (Fig. 12.3). The management of patients with locally advanced or disseminated disease requires a

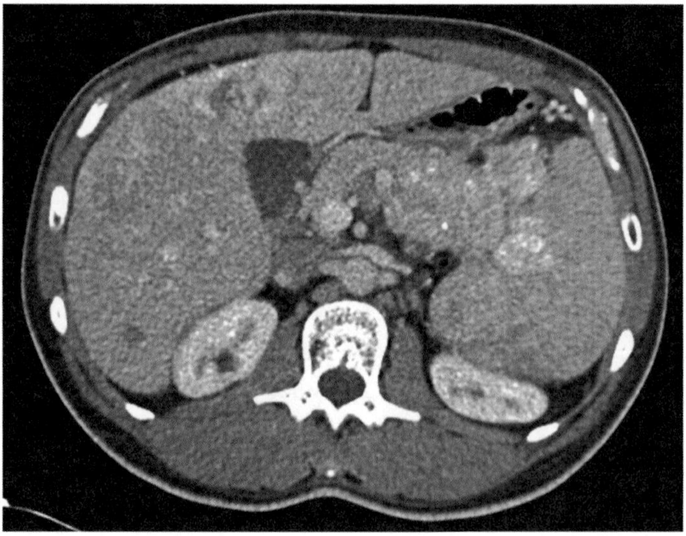

Fig. 12.3 Computed tomography showing a large pancreatic gastrinoma with local invasion that was assessed as being unresectable

multimodality approach to treatment. Medical therapy with PPI is highly effective in the control of gastric hypersecretion and for this reason the role of surgical palliative debulking for the control of endocrinopathy is limited. In the modern era of PPI, patients with metastatic gastrinoma may survive for prolonged periods, and to date the evidence for aggressive surgical resection in the presence of distant metastases is limited to small case series only [73]. Most authors agree, however, that surgical debulking of functional pancreatic neuroendocrine tumor metastases does appear to provide a palliative benefit in patients with endocrinopathy (Fig. 12.4).

In a series of 213 patients with gastrinoma, hepatic metastases occurred in 32% of cases, and diffuse involvement of the liver or extrahepatic distant metastases were present in 75% of these cases [74]. The remaining 19 patients had disease confined to the liver that was considered completely resectable. Patients undergoing resection of hepatic metastases had a 5-year survival rate of 85% which was superior to those patients with hepatic disease who were not resectable. In addition, 29% of patients remained free of hepatic disease on imaging at 5 years. Although selection bias likely played a significant role in these results, others have also demonstrated a survival benefit associated with the aggressive surgical debulking of neuroendocrine tumor metastases [75, 76]. Radiofrequency ablation (RFA) and cryotherapy ablation can be used to treat hepatic metastases that are not amenable to surgical resection. In a series of 25 patients undergoing RFA for hepatic neuroendocrine tumor metastases, Gillams and coworkers reported that control of progression of hepatic disease was achieved in 76% of cases with a median survival of 53 months, and that this treatment was associated with minimal morbidity (12%) [77].

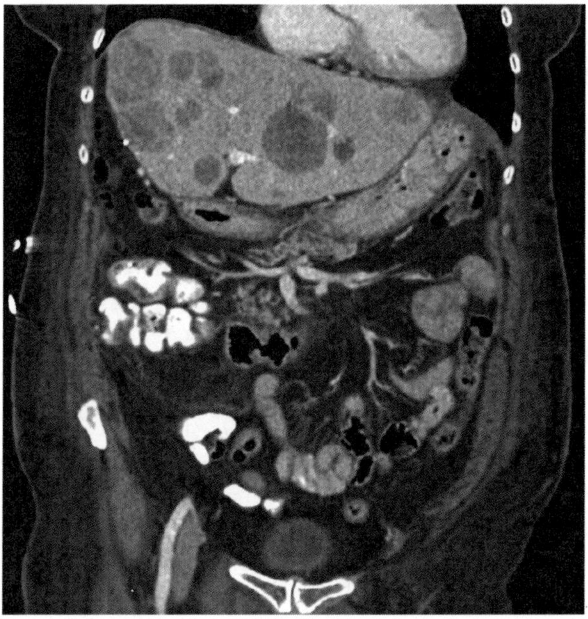

Fig. 12.4 Computed tomography of a patient with metastatic gastrinoma who underwent right hemihepatectomy for cytoreduction of hepatic metastases. Progression of disease subsequently led to the development of multiple metastases within the hepatic remnant

Hepatic artery chemoembolization has also been employed in the management of multiple hepatic neuroendocrine tumor metastases. In a phase-II trial of hepatic artery chemoembolization using doxorubicin followed by gelatin-impregnated foam embolization in 24 patients with metastatic neuroendocrine tumors, Ruszniewski and coworkers found a complete response in 8%, 33% had a reduction in size of metastases, and stabilization of disease occurred in 80% [78]. Radioembolization of the hepatic artery using 90-Yttrium-bound resin or glass microspheres has also been used in the treatment of hepatic neuroendocrine tumor metastases including those from gastrinoma, and has been associated with partial response on imaging criteria in 60.5% of patients [79].

Systemic therapy with cytotoxic chemotherapy or interferon-alpha (IFN-A) has a limited role in the management of disseminated metastatic gastrinoma, and the results associated with these treatments have proven disappointing. Grama and coworkers treated 18 patients with metastatic gastrinoma with a combination of 5-fluorouracil, streptozocin, doxorubicin and IFN-A, yet could only document a radiological response to therapy in 17% of cases [80]. A study of 84 patients with locally advanced or metastatic pancreatic neuroendocrine tumors treated with combination 5-fluorouracil, doxorubicin and streptozocin by Kouvaraki reported a partial or complete radiological response in 39% of patients; however, none of the 11 patients with metastatic gastrinoma displayed a response to therapy [81].

Radionuclide therapy with 111-Indium labeled octreotide has been associated with a clinical response in 53% of patients with metastatic neuroendocrine tumors including gastrinomas, with stabilization of disease in 35% of cases [82]. The somatostatin analog DOTA-TOC radiolabelled with 90-Yttrium or 177-Lutetium has recently been found to have a partial response in 25% of patients and stabilization of disease in 55% [83].

In addition to PPI to control gastric acid hypersecretion, somatostatin analogs including octreotide and lantreotide are also employed in the management of patients with metastatic gastrinoma to reduce both tumor gastrin production and also for a possible effect on tumor growth. In a small series of 15 patients with metastatic gastrinoma treated with subcutaneous octreotide, 53% of cases demonstrated a radiological response, with stabilization of progressive disease in 47% and partial tumor regression in 6% [84]. The mean duration of clinical response was 25 months.

Several medical agents targeting growth factor receptors and related signaling pathways have recently been studied for the management of metastatic neuroendocrine tumors. Sirolimus and everolimus are inhibitors of the mammalian target of rapamycin (mTOR), a serine-threonine kinase involved in cell-cycle and growth regulation and apoptosis via the PI3K/AKT/mTOR signaling pathway. In a phase II study, everolimus combined with long acting octreotide therapy was associated with a partial response in 14.8% and disease stabilization in 70% of patients with metastatic neuroendocrine tumors [85].

Management of Gastrinoma in Patients with MEN1

Gastrinoma occurs in the context of the MEN1 syndrome in 19–26% of cases, and management of the gastrinomas occurring as part of this syndrome is controversial [27, 41, 48]. The role of surgery in the management of MEN1/ZES is less clearly defined than for sporadic tumors due to the excellent long-term survival associated with this condition, the low rates of long-term cure of ZES after surgical resection in these patients, and the effectiveness of medical control of ZES with medical therapy.

ZES occurring in the context of MEN1 displays important differences in biological behavior compared with sporadic tumors. The mean age of onset of ZES in patients with MEN1 is 34–42 years which is younger than for sporadic gastrinomas, and is rare before the age of 24 years [15, 86–88]. In patients from verified MEN1 kindreds, most cases are detected on screening biochemical testing or pancreatic imaging, with only 28% of patients having symptoms of ZES at the time of diagnosis [88]. The duodenum is the most common site of gastrinoma in patients with MEN1, occurring in 88% of cases, with synchronous tumors of the duodenum and the pancreas occurring in 24% [87, 89]. ZES is the most common functional endocrinopathy in patients with MEN1 (42–60%), with insulinoma (19%), vasoactive intestinal polypeptide producing tumors (4%) and non-functional tumors (35%) also occurring [86, 90].

The long-term survival of patients with MEN1/ZES is excellent, and there is evidence that gastrinomas occurring in the context of MEN1 have a lower malignant potential than sporadic tumors. Hepatic metastases are present in only 3–4% of MEN1 patients with gastrinoma at the time of diagnosis, which is significantly lower than for patients with sporadic tumors (21%) [87, 89]. Hepatic metastases will develop in long-term follow-up in 14–23% of MEN1 patients [15, 87, 91]. Fourteen percent of MEN1/ZES patients exhibit an aggressive form of the disease with the development of hepatic metastases and yet still have a 5-year survival rate of 88% [91]. A number of studies have found that the long-term survival of patients with MEN1 and gastrinoma is superior to that seen in patients with sporadic gastrinoma [87]. In a study of 231 patients with gastrinoma, of which 45 had MEN1, patients with MEN1 had a 10-year survival of 93% compared with 74% for patients with sporadic tumors [87]. In contrast to these reports, Ellison and coworkers found that long-term survival for sporadic and MEN1 patients with gastrinoma were equivalent [27]. Death from metastatic disease is rare in patients with MEN1/ZES. The overall 15-year survival is 94% [88, 89, 92].

Since gastrinomas occurring as part of MEN1 are indolent tumors, the role of surgical resection in reducing the risk of developing metastatic disease has been questioned. PPI use is effective in normalizing gastric acid secretion and in controlling symptoms of ZES in MEN1 [93]. Since the introduction of effective medical therapy for the control of gastric acid hypersecretion, patients with MEN1/ZES no longer die from complications of severe peptic ulcer disease, and long-term survival can be expected [92]. The surgical treatment of hyperparathyroidism in patients with MEN1/ZES is important prior to considering intervention for gastrinoma, as hypercalcemia is a potent stimulus for gastrin release from these tumors. Normalization of FSG occurs in 40–83% of patients following successful surgical treatment of hyperparathyroidism in MEN1/ZES [15, 88].

The rate of biochemical cure of MEN1/ZES is much lower than for sporadic tumors [41]. Patients with MEN1 display a field defect with hyperplasia and multiple microtumors of gastrin-staining cells in the duodenum [94]. For this reason, long-term biochemical cure after surgery for MEN1/ZES patients is rare, achieved in as little as 0–6% of cases [27, 41, 95]. Postoperative normalization of FSG occurs in 68% of MEN1 patients without hepatic metastases undergoing surgical resection for gastrinoma, but this rate falls to 33% with provocative testing with intravenous secretin, implying that most patients harbor microscopic foci of residual disease [89, 95]. Given the low probability of long-term biochemical cure of ZES and the effectiveness of medical therapy, the role of surgical resection in the management of MEN1/ZES has been questioned.

Surgical resection has been advocated by some authors for all MEN1 patients with biochemical or radiological evidence of ZES, with the aim of reducing the risk of developing metastatic disease [68, 89, 96]. Others have reserved surgical resection for tumors of more than 2–3 cm in size, citing the low risk of hepatic metastases with smaller tumors [45, 73, 97, 98]. In a study of 55 patients with MEN1 and pancreatic neuroendocrine tumors, Kouvaraki and coworkers found that patients who underwent surgical resection had significantly higher overall 10-year survival compared with those who did not (81% vs. 34%) [99]. As there is an absence of good prospective or randomized data examining the role of surgery, the indications for surgical resection for patients with MEN1/ZES remain institution specific.

The extent of the surgical resection for MEN1/ZES is also a recent subject of controversy. As duodenal tumors are present in 88% of cases, routine duodenotomy is required the time of laparotomy in all patients with MEN1 where gastrin levels are elevated preoperatively, even when a pancreatic tumor is identified [87, 89]. Distal subtotal pancreatectomy, removing 80% of the pancreas with enucleation of lesions from the head of the gland, has been recommended by Thompson for all MEN1 patients due to the high incidence of concomitant neuroendocrine tumors of the body and tail of the gland, and the risk of developing recurrent tumors in this location [89]. Recently a focused approach to resection of pancreatic neuroendocrine tumors, leaving a larger pancreatic remnant and enucleating lesions in the body of the gland, has been adopted by the University of Michigan due to the high incidence of recurrent disease on long-term follow-up, which was seen in 77% of patients [95]. Pancreaticoduodenectomy has been performed for resection of gastrinomas in the head of the pancreas, although the effects of such an approach on long-term survival are not known [14]. Critics of this approach cite the higher morbidity of the procedure and the difficulty of reoperation for neuroendocrine tumors developing in the pancreatic remnant [73]. Pancreaticoduodenectomy may be indicated in MEN1 patients with large tumors (<5 cm), tumors located close to the pancreatic duct, patients with multiple duodenal tumors or patients with extensive nodal involvement [73]. Total pancreatectomy has also been performed for neuroendocrine tumors occurring in MEN1 at some institutions [52]. Although this eliminates the risk of pancreatic tumor recurrence, it is associated with high rates of perioperative morbidity and mortality, and results in pancreatic exocrine and endocrine insufficiency.

Regional lymph nodes are involved in as many as 66% of patients with MEN1/ZES, and may appear normal in size at the time of operative exploration [89]. Dissection of peripancreatic nodes, nodes along the common hepatic artery and within the porta hepatis has been recommended for patients with MEN1 with duodenal gastrinomas or pancreatic tumors <3 cm in size [89]. An aggressive approach to nodal dissection is controversial in patients with MEN1 as the presence of nodal metastases has not been associated with a reduced survival in these patients, yet can be the source of persistent or recurrent disease [27, 30, 45].

Summary

The management of gastrinoma has evolved due to advances in medical therapies, diagnostic and imaging investigations and improvements in surgical technique. Complete surgical resection with curative intent is the procedure of choice for sporadic gastrinomas. Surgery has an important role in the ongoing management of selected patients with MEN1/ZES syndrome. The management of advanced and disseminated disease in patients with gastrinoma involves a multimodality approach to treatment, with surgical resection or ablation of metastatic lesions, medical and systemic therapies providing treatment options for both the control of tumor growth and control of the endocrinopathy.

References

1. Seiler S, Zinninger MM (1946) Massive islet cell tumor of the pancreas without hypoglycemia. Surg Gynecol Obstet 82:301
2. Zollinger RM, Ellison EH (1955) Primary peptic ulcerations of the jejunum associated with islet cell tumors of the pancreas. Ann Surg 142:709–723 discussion, 24–28
3. Gregory RA, Tracy HJ, French JM, Sircus W (1960) Extraction of a gastrin-like substance from a pancreatic tumour in a case of Zollinger–Ellison syndrome. Lancet 1:1045–1048
4. Gregory RA, Grossman MI, Tracy HJ, Bentley PH (1967) Nature of the gastric secretagogue in Zollinger–Ellison tumours. Lancet 2:543–544
5. McGuigan JE, Trudeau WL (1968) Immunochemical measurement of elevated levels of gastrin in the serum of patients with pancreatic tumors of the Zollinger–Ellison variety. N Engl J Med 278:1308–1313
6. Oberhelman HA Jr, Nelsen TS, Johnson AN Jr, Dragstedt LR 2nd (1961) Ulcerogenic tumors of the duodenum. Ann Surg 153:214–227
7. Rawson AB, England MT, Gillam GG, French JM, Stammers FA (1960) Zollinger–Ellison syndrome with diarrhoea and malabsorption. Observations on a patient before and after pancreatic islet-cell tumour removal with-out resort. Lancet 2:131–134
8. Dockray GJ, Varro A, Dimaline R, Wang T (2001) The gastrins: their production and biological activities. Annu Rev Physiol 63:119–139
9. Noble F, Wank SA, Crawley JN et al (1999) International Union of Pharmacology. XXI. Structure, distribution, and functions of cholecystokinin receptors. Pharmacol Rev 51:745–781
10. Orlando LA, Lenard L, Orlando RC (2007) Chronic hypergastrinemia: causes and consequences. Dig Dis Sci 52:2482–2489
11. Trudeau WL, McGuigan JE (1969) Effects of calcium on serum gastrin levels in the Zollinger–Ellison syndrome. N Engl J Med 281:862–866
12. Bartsch D, Kopp I, Bergenfelz A et al (1998) MEN1 gene mutations in 12 MEN1 families and their associated tumors. Eur J Endocrinol 139:416–420
13. Cavallari I, D'Agostino DM, Ferro T et al (2003) In situ analysis of human menin in normal and neoplastic pancreatic tissues: evidence for differential expression in exocrine and endocrine cells. J Clin Endocrinol Metab 88:3893–3901
14. Bartsch DK, Fendrich V, Langer P, Celik I, Kann PH, Rothmund M (2005) Outcome of duodenopancreatic resections in patients with multiple endocrine neoplasia type 1. Ann Surg 242:757–764 discussion 64–66
15. Burgess JR, Greenaway TM, Parameswaran V, Challis DR, David R, Shepherd JJ (1998) Enteropancreatic malignancy associated with multiple endocrine neoplasia type 1: risk factors and pathogenesis. Cancer 83:428–434
16. Goebel SU, Heppner C, Burns AL et al (2000) Genotype/phenotype correlation of multiple endocrine neoplasia type 1 gene mutations in sporadic gastrinomas. J Clin Endocrinol Metab 85:116–123
17. Kawamura J, Shimada Y, Komoto I et al (2005) Multiple endocrine neoplasia type 1 gene mutations in sporadic gastrinomas in Japan. Oncol Rep 14:47–52
18. Wang EH, Ebrahimi SA, Wu AY, Kashefi C, Passaro E Jr, Sawicki MP (1998) Mutation of the MENIN gene in sporadic pancreatic endocrine tumors. Cancer Res 58:4417–4420

19. Zhuang Z, Vortmeyer AO, Pack S et al (1997) Somatic mutations of the MEN1 tumor suppressor gene in sporadic gastrinomas and insulinomas. Cancer Res 57:4682–4686
20. Chen YJ, Vortmeyer A, Zhuang Z, Huang S, Jensen RT (2003) Loss of heterozygosity of chromosome 1q in gastrinomas: occurrence and prognostic significance. Cancer Res 63:817–823
21. Wild A, Langer P, Celik I, Chaloupka B, Bartsch DK (2002) Chromosome 22q in pancreatic endocrine tumors: identification of a homozygous deletion and potential prognostic associations of allelic deletions. Eur J Endocrinol 147:507–513
22. Serrano J, Goebel SU, Peghini PL, Lubensky IA, Gibril F, Jensen RT (2000) Alterations in the p16INK4a/CDKN2A tumor suppressor gene in gastrinomas. J Clin Endocrinol Metab 85:4146–4156
23. Furukawa M, Raffeld M, Mateo C et al (2005) Increased expression of insulin-like growth factor I and/or its receptor in gastrinomas is associated with low curability, increased growth, and development of metastases. Clin Cancer Res 11:3233–3242
24. Peghini PL, Iwamoto M, Raffeld M et al (2002) Overexpression of epidermal growth factor and hepatocyte growth factor receptors in a proportion of gastrinomas correlates with aggressive growth and lower curability. Clin Cancer Res 8:2273–2285
25. Goebel SU, Iwamoto M, Raffeld M et al (2002) Her-2/neu expression and gene amplification in gastrinomas: correlations with tumor biology, growth, and aggressiveness. Cancer Res 62:3702–3710
26. Yao JC, Eisner MP, Leary C et al (2007) Population-based study of islet cell carcinoma. Ann Surg Oncol 14:3492–3500
27. Ellison EC, Sparks J, Verducci JS et al (2006) 50-year appraisal of gastrinoma: recommendations for staging and treatment. J Am Coll Surg 202:897–905
28. Roy PK, Venzon DJ, Shojamanesh H et al (2000) Zollinger–Ellison syndrome. Clinical presentation in 261 patients. Medicine (Baltimore) 79:379–411
29. Soga J, Yakuwa Y (1998) The gastrinoma/Zollinger–Ellison syndrome: statistical evaluation of a Japanese series of 359 cases. J Hepatobiliary Pancreat Surg 5:77–85
30. Yu F, Venzon DJ, Serrano J et al (1999) Prospective study of the clinical course, prognostic factors, causes of death, and survival in patients with long-standing Zollinger–Ellison syndrome. J Clin Oncol 17:615–630
31. Fraker DL, Norton JA, Saeed ZA, Maton PN, Gardner JD, Jensen RT (1988) A prospective study of perioperative and postoperative control of acid hypersecretion in patients with Zollinger–Ellison syndrome undergoing gastrinoma resection. Surgery 104:1054–1063
32. Roy PK, Venzon DJ, Feigenbaum KM et al (2001) Gastric secretion in Zollinger–Ellison syndrome. Correlation with clinical expression, tumor extent and role in diagnosis – a prospective NIH study of 235 patients and a review of 984 cases in the literature. Medicine (Baltimore) 80:189–222
33. Dhillo WS, Jayasena CN, Lewis CJ et al (2006) Plasma gastrin measurement cannot be used to diagnose a gastrinoma in patients on either proton pump inhibitors or histamine type-2 receptor antagonists. Ann Clin Biochem 43:153–155
34. Berna MJ, Hoffmann KM, Serrano J, Gibril F, Jensen RT (2006) Serum gastrin in Zollinger–Ellison syndrome: I. Prospective study of fasting serum gastrin in 309 patients from the National Institutes of Health and comparison with 2229 cases from the literature. Medicine (Baltimore) 85:295–330
35. Wada M, Komoto I, Doi R, Imamura M (2002) Intravenous calcium injection test is a novel complementary procedure in differential diagnosis for gastrinoma. World J Surg 26:1291–1296
36. Berna MJ, Hoffmann KM, Long SH, Serrano J, Gibril F, Jensen RT (2006) Serum gastrin in Zollinger–Ellison syndrome: II. Prospective study of gastrin provocative testing in 293 patients from the National Institutes of Health and comparison with 537 cases from the literature. evaluation of diagnostic criteria, proposal of new criteria, and correlations with clinical and tumoral features. Medicine (Baltimore) 85:331–364
37. Tomassetti P, Migliori M, Simoni P et al (2001) Diagnostic value of plasma chromogranin A in neuroendocrine tumours. Eur J Gastroenterol Hepatol 13:55–58

38. Jordan PH Jr (1999) A personal experience with pancreatic and duodenal neuroendocrine tumors. J Am Coll Surg 189:470–482
39. Kaplan EL, Horvath K, Udekwu A et al (1990) Gastrinomas: a 42-year experience. World J Surg 14:365–375 discussion 75–76
40. Norton JA, Fraker DL, Alexander HR et al (2006) Surgery increases survival in patients with gastrinoma. Ann Surg 244:410–419
41. Norton JA, Fraker DL, Alexander HR et al (1999) Surgery to cure the Zollinger–Ellison syndrome. N Engl J Med 341:635–644
42. Pipeleers-Marichal M, Donow C, Heitz PU, Kloppel G (1993) Pathologic aspects of gastrinomas in patients with Zollinger–Ellison syndrome with and without multiple endocrine neoplasia type I. World J Surg 17:481–488
43. Stabile BE, Morrow DJ, Passaro E Jr (1984) The gastrinoma triangle: operative implications. Am J Surg 147:25–31
44. Zogakis TG, Gibril F, Libutti SK et al (2003) Management and outcome of patients with sporadic gastrinoma arising in the duodenum. Ann Surg 238:42–48
45. Weber HC, Venzon DJ, Lin JT et al (1995) Determinants of metastatic rate and survival in patients with Zollinger–Ellison syndrome: a prospective long-term study. Gastroenterology 108:1637–1649
46. Phan GQ, Yeo CJ, Hruban RH, Lillemoe KD, Pitt HA, Cameron JL (1998) Surgical experience with pancreatic and peripancreatic neuroendocrine tumors: review of 125 patients. J Gastrointest Surg 2:472–482
47. Sugg SL, Norton JA, Fraker DL et al (1993) A prospective study of intraoperative methods to diagnose and resect duodenal gastrinomas. Ann Surg 218:138–144
48. Ruszniewski P, Podevin P, Cadiot G et al (1993) Clinical, anatomical, and evolutive features of patients with the Zollinger–Ellison syndrome combined with type I multiple endocrine neoplasia. Pancreas 8:295–304
49. Wu PC, Alexander HR, Bartlett DL et al (1997) A prospective analysis of the frequency, location, and curability of ectopic (nonpancreaticoduodenal, nonnodal) gastrinoma. Surgery 122:1176–1182
50. Norton JA, Alexander HR, Fraker DL, Venzon DJ, Gibril F, Jensen RT (2003) Possible primary lymph node gastrinoma: occurrence, natural history, and predictive factors: a prospective study. Ann Surg 237:650–657 discussion 7–9
51. Termanini B, Gibril F, Reynolds JC et al (1997) Value of somatostatin receptor scintigraphy: a prospective study in gastrinoma of its effect on clinical management. Gastroenterology 112:335–347
52. Tonelli F, Fratini G, Nesi G et al (2006) Pancreatectomy in multiple endocrine neoplasia type 1-related gastrinomas and pancreatic endocrine neoplasias. Ann Surg 244:61–70
53. Hofland LJ, Liu Q, Van Koetsveld PM et al (1999) Immunohistochemical detection of somatostatin receptor subtypes sst1 and sst2A in human somatostatin receptor positive tumors. J Clin Endocrinol Metab 84:775–780
54. Alexander HR, Fraker DL, Norton JA et al (1998) Prospective study of somatostatin receptor scintigraphy and its effect on operative outcome in patients with Zollinger–Ellison syndrome. Ann Surg 228:228–238
55. Proye C, Malvaux P, Pattou F et al (1998) Noninvasive imaging of insulinomas and gastrinomas with endoscopic ultrasonography and somatostatin receptor scintigraphy. Surgery 124:1134–1143 discussion 43–44
56. Bansal R, Tierney W, Carpenter S, Thompson N, Scheiman JM (1999) Cost effectiveness of EUS for preoperative localization of pancreatic endocrine tumors. Gastrointest Endosc 49:19–25
57. Imamura M, Takahashi K, Adachi H et al (1987) Usefulness of selective arterial secretin injection test for localization of gastrinoma in the Zollinger–Ellison syndrome. Ann Surg 205:230–239
58. Dhillo WS, Jayasena CN, Jackson JE et al (2005) Localization of gastrinomas by selective intra-arterial calcium injection in patients on proton pump inhibitor or H2 receptor antagonist therapy. Eur J Gastroenterol Hepatol 17:429–433

59. Orlefors H, Sundin A, Garske U et al (2005) Whole-body (11)C-5-hydroxytryptophan positron emission tomography as a universal imaging technique for neuroendocrine tumors: comparison with somatostatin receptor scintigraphy and computed tomography. J Clin Endocrinol Metab 90:3392–3400
60. Gabriel M, Decristoforo C, Kendler D et al (2007) 68Ga-DOTA-Tyr3-octreotide PET in neuroendocrine tumors: comparison with somatostatin receptor scintigraphy and CT. J Nucl Med 48:508–518
61. Zollinger RM, Martin EW Jr, Carey LC, Sparks J, Minton JP (1976) Observations on the postoperative tumor growth behavior of certain islet cell tumors. Ann Surg 184:525–530
62. Gibril F, Doppman JL, Reynolds JC et al (1998) Bone metastases in patients with gastrinomas: a prospective study of bone scanning, somatostatin receptor scanning, and magnetic resonance image in their detection, frequency, location, and effect of their detection on management. J Clin Oncol 16:1040–1053
63. Ellison EC, Sparks J (2003) Zollinger–Ellison syndrome in the era of effective acid suppression: are we unknowingly growing tumors? Am J Surg 186:245–248
64. Norton JA (1999) Intraoperative methods to stage and localize pancreatic and duodenal tumors. Ann Oncol 10(Suppl 4):182–184
65. Thompson NW, Pasieka J, Fukuuchi A (1993) Duodenal gastrinomas, duodenotomy, and duodenal exploration in the surgical management of Zollinger–Ellison syndrome. World J Surg 17:455–462
66. Thompson NW, Vinik AI, Eckhauser FE (1989) Microgastrinomas of the duodenum. A cause of failed operations for the Zollinger–Ellison syndrome. Ann Surg 209:396–404
67. Norton JA, Alexander HR, Fraker DL, Venzon DJ, Gibril F, Jensen RT (2004) Does the use of routine duodenotomy (DUODX) affect rate of cure, development of liver metastases, or survival in patients with Zollinger–Ellison syndrome? Ann Surg 239:617–625 discussion 26
68. Akerstrom G, Hessman O, Hellman P, Skogseid B (2005) Pancreatic tumours as part of the MEN-1 syndrome. Best Pract Res Clin Gastroenterol 19:819–830
69. NCCN practice guidelines in oncology: neuroendocrine tumors V.1.2008. National comprehensive cancer network, 2008. http://www.nccn.org/professionals/physician_gls/PDF/neuroendocrine.pdf. Accessed July 20 2008
70. Zeiger MA, Shawker TH, Norton JA (1993) Use of intraoperative ultrasonography to localize islet cell tumors. World J Surg 17:448–454
71. Sarmiento JM, Farnell MB, Que FG, Nagorney DM (2002) Pancreaticoduodenectomy for islet cell tumors of the head of the pancreas: long-term survival analysis. World J Surg 26:1267–1271
72. Metz DC, Benya RV, Fishbeyn VA et al (1993) Prospective study of the need for long-term antisecretory therapy in patients with Zollinger–Ellison syndrome following successful curative gastrinoma resection. Aliment Pharmacol Ther 7:247–257
73. Norton JA, Jensen RT (2004) Resolved and unresolved controversies in the surgical management of patients with Zollinger–Ellison syndrome. Ann Surg 240:757–773
74. Norton JA, Doherty GM, Fraker DL et al (1998) Surgical treatment of localized gastrinoma within the liver: a prospective study. Surgery 124:1145–1152
75. Sarmiento JM, Heywood G, Rubin J, Ilstrup DM, Nagorney DM, Que FG (2003) Surgical treatment of neuroendocrine metastases to the liver: a plea for resection to increase survival. J Am Coll Surg 197:29–37
76. Touzios JG, Kiely JM, Pitt SC et al (2005) Neuroendocrine hepatic metastases: does aggressive management improve survival? Ann Surg 241:776–783 discussion 83–85
77. Gillams A, Cassoni A, Conway G, Lees W (2005) Radiofrequency ablation of neuroendocrine liver metastases: the Middlesex experience. Abdom Imaging 30:435–441
78. Ruszniewski P, Rougier P, Roche A et al (1993) Hepatic arterial chemoembolization in patients with liver metastases of endocrine tumors. A prospective phase II study in 24 patients. Cancer 71:2624–2630
79. Kennedy AS, Dezarn WA, McNeillie P et al (2008) Radioembolization for unresectable neuroendocrine hepatic metastases using resin 90Y-microspheres: early results in 148 patients. Am J Clin Oncol 31:271–279

80. Grama D, Eriksson B, Martensson H et al (1992) Clinical characteristics, treatment and survival in patients with pancreatic tumors causing hormonal syndromes. World J Surg 16:632–639
81. Kouvaraki MA, Ajani JA, Hoff P et al (2004) Fluorouracil, doxorubicin, and streptozocin in the treatment of patients with locally advanced and metastatic pancreatic endocrine carcinomas. J Clin Oncol 22:4762–4771
82. De Jong M, Valkema R, Jamar F et al (2002) Somatostatin receptor-targeted radionuclide therapy of tumors: preclinical and clinical findings. Semin Nucl Med 32:133–140
83. Frilling A, Weber F, Saner F et al (2006) Treatment with (90)Y- and (177)Lu-DOTATOC in patients with metastatic neuroendocrine tumors. Surgery 140:968–976 discussion 76–77
84. Shojamanesh H, Gibril F, Louie A et al (2002) Prospective study of the antitumor efficacy of long-term octreotide treatment in patients with progressive metastatic gastrinoma. Cancer 94:331–343
85. Yao JC, Phan AT, Chang DZ et al (2006) Phase II study of RAD001 (everolimus) and depot octreotide (Sandostatin LAR) in patients with advanced low grade neuroendocrine carcinoma (LGEP NET). J Clin Oncol 24:4042
86. Gibril F, Schumann M, Pace A, Jensen RT (2004) Multiple endocrine neoplasia type 1 and Zollinger–Ellison syndrome: a prospective study of 107 cases and comparison with 1009 cases from the literature. Medicine (Baltimore) 83:43–83
87. Jensen RT (1998) Management of the Zollinger–Ellison syndrome in patients with multiple endocrine neoplasia type 1. J Intern Med 243:477–488
88. Shepherd JJ, Challis DR, Davies PF, McArdle JP, Teh BT, Wilkinson S (1993) Multiple endocrine neoplasm, type 1. Gastrinomas, pancreatic neoplasms, microcarcinoids, the Zollinger–Ellison syndrome, lymph nodes, and hepatic metastases. Arch Surg 128:1133–1142
89. Thompson NW (1998) Current concepts in the surgical management of multiple endocrine neoplasia type 1 pancreatic-duodenal disease. Results in the treatment of 40 patients with Zollinger–Ellison syndrome, hypoglycaemia or both. J Intern Med 243:495–500
90. Dean PG, van Heerden JA, Farley DR et al (2000) Are patients with multiple endocrine neoplasia type I prone to premature death? World J Surg 24:1437–1441
91. Gibril F, Venzon DJ, Ojeaburu JV, Bashir S, Jensen RT (2001) Prospective study of the natural history of gastrinoma in patients with MEN1: definition of an aggressive and a nonaggressive form. J Clin Endocrinol Metab 86:5282–5293
92. Wilson SD, Krzywda EA, Zhu Y et al (2008) The influence of surgery in MEN1 syndrome: observations over 150 years. Surgery 144:695–702
93. Metz DC, Soffer E, Forsmark CE et al (2003) Maintenance oral pantoprazole therapy is effective for patients with Zollinger–Ellison syndrome and idiopathic hypersecretion. Am J Gastroenterol 98:301–307
94. Anlauf M, Perren A, Meyer CL et al (2005) Precursor lesions in patients with multiple endocrine neoplasia type 1-associated duodenal gastrinomas. Gastroenterology 128:1187–1198
95. Hausman MS Jr, Thompson NW, Gauger PG, Doherty GM (2004) The surgical management of MEN-1 pancreatoduodenal neuroendocrine disease. Surgery 136:1205–1211
96. Skogseid B, Oberg K, Eriksson B et al (1996) Surgery for asymptomatic pancreatic lesion in multiple endocrine neoplasia type I. World J Surg 20:872–876 discussion 7
97. Norton JA, Fang TD, Jensen RT (2006) Surgery for gastrinoma and insulinoma in multiple endocrine neoplasia type 1. J Natl Compr Canc Netw 4:148–153
98. Triponez F, Goudet P, Dosseh D et al (2006) Is surgery beneficial for MEN1 patients with small (< or = 2 cm), nonfunctioning pancreaticoduodenal endocrine tumor? An analysis of 65 patients from the GTE. World J Surg 30:654–662 discussion 63–64
99. Kouvaraki MA, Shapiro SE, Cote GJ et al (2006) Management of pancreatic endocrine tumors in multiple endocrine neoplasia type 1. World J Surg 30:643–653

Chapter 13
Insulinoma

Kimberly Vanderveen and Clive Grant

Insulinoma remains a very rare tumor, and the first challenge to making the diagnosis is to consider it. Although these tumors are typically benign, they can cause severe and often bizarre symptoms. The diagnosis is established with biochemical confirmation of hypoglycemia and endogenous hyperinsulinemia after fasting, and is distinguished from the postprandial hyperinsulinemic hypoglycemia of Noninsulinoma Pancreatogenous Hyperinsulinemia Syndrome (NIPHS). Operative removal of the tumor is the mainstay of treatment, but is predicated on precise preoperative localization. Multiple imaging options are available, including: transabdominal ultrasound, computed tomography, endoscopic ultrasound (EUS), angiography with intraarterial calcium stimulation testing, and intraoperative ultrasound (IOUS). Patients with MEN-1 syndrome virtually always have multiple pancreatic neuroendocrine tumors, and evaluation and treatment of these patients is different than for sporadic disease. Surgical excision of the disease is the only cure; in the rare case of malignant disease, an aggressive surgical and multimodal approach is recommended, even for palliation of hypoglycemia.

> I think someone picked him for a "nut" ... about a year ago he noticed that he would develop a tremor, sweating, and nervousness after going without food or after severe exertion. He discovered taking sugar would prevent the recurrence of these attacks. ... About three weeks ago I saw him in one of his typical attacks caused by his going without breakfast and not having enough candy. He resembled an acute alcoholic, great motor activity, dancing and talking, squinting and frowning, apparently having hallucination of sight and hearing, negativistic and difficult to control. I had great difficulty in getting him to take a coca cola full of syrup, but after taking it, he recovered in about five minutes. ... Several times he has become comatose. ... This man is not a nut but has become rather soured on his professional confreres because he has not got to first base on a diagnosis. [He] is an exceptional case and I can find nothing about hypoglycemia. Try and get someone interested in him and don't let him die because he sure will if he goes too long without carbohydrate. {Referral letter to Dr. Davis at The Mayo Clinic, 1926[1]}

C. Grant (✉)
Mayo Clinic, Department of Surgery, 200 First Street SW, Mayo W12,
Rochester, MN 55905, USA
e-mail: cgrant@mayo.edu

C. Sturgeon (ed.), *Endocrine Neoplasia*, Cancer Treatment and Research, vol 153,
DOI 10.1007/978-1-4419-0857-5_13, © Springer Science+Business Media, LLC 2010

The above referral letter describes the presenting symptoms of the first patient ever diagnosed and subsequently operated for insulinoma. This description is illustrative of the nature of insulinomas in many respects. The patient displayed both neuroglycopenic and adrenergic response symptoms typical of hypoglycemia, and his symptoms were indeed prevented and treated with ingestion of sugar. Furthermore, the bizarre nature of his symptoms resulted in a prolonged delay (over 4 years) in his diagnosis and treatment, which is still unfortunately true of patients today. The patient, an orthopedic surgeon, was ultimately taken to the operating room by Dr. Will Mayo in 1926, at which point he was found to have unresectable malignant insulinoma. He subsequently died 1 month later due to uncontrollable hypoglycemia [1, 2].

History

Paul Langerhans, who was a medical student working under Virchow, first identified pancreatic islet cells in 1869 [3]. Over the next 40 years, work with pancreatic extracts ultimately resulted in the 1922 discovery of insulin by Banting and Best, which subsequently won them the Nobel Prize [4]. In 1926, Dr. Will Mayo first attempted surgical resection of an insulinoma in the patient described above, but was unable to cure the patient due to bulky metastatic disease [1, 2]. In 1929, the first successful surgical resection (enucleation) of a benign insulinoma was performed by Roscoe Graham of Toronto [5]. However, it wasn't until 1935 that basic diagnostic criteria were established by Franz and Whipple [6]. "Whipple's triad" of (1) hypoglycemia (plasma glucose less than 50 mg/dl), (2) symptoms of hypoglycemia, and (3) symptom resolution after glucose administration still serves as the basis for initial diagnostic evaluation today.

Physiology

The pancreatic islets contain several different cell types with different secretory profiles. The beta cell secretes insulin, which is manufactured as an inactive precursor, proinsulin. Proinsulin consists of two peptide chains and an inactive "connecting" peptide (C-peptide). Proinsulin is cleaved prior to secretion, and equimolar amounts of C-peptide and active insulin are released [7]. Insulin has a shorter half-life than C-peptide (4–6 min vs. 11–14 min), which is important for diagnostic testing as elevated insulin levels, if indeed from an endogenous source, should also be accompanied by elevated C-peptide levels [8]. Manufactured insulin compounds do not contain C-peptide, and therefore low or undetectable C-peptide levels in the setting of hyperinsulinemia should raise the suspicion of surreptitious insulin administration or a medication error.

Epidemiology

Endogenous hyperinsulinemia may result from two distinct pancreatic pathologies: insulinoma and non-insulinoma pancreatogenous hyperinsulinemia syndrome (NIPHS – discussed below). Insulinoma is an islet cell neoplasm, characterized by the excessive unregulated secretion of insulin which results in the clinical symptoms of hypoglycemia. Insulinomas remain rare tumors, with an approximated incidence of 4 per 1 million person years [9]. Sporadic tumors are most often single and benign, whereas islet cell neoplasms in patients with MEN-1 syndrome are typically multiple and have a higher risk of malignancy [10]. Multiple Endocrine Neoplasia – Type I (MEN-1) syndrome is the only documented risk factor for insulinoma. MEN-1 syndrome results from a mutation in the *menin* gene on the long arm of chromosome 11, which predisposes patients to pituitary, parathyroid, and upper gastrointestinal neuroendocrine tumors (predominantly in the pancreas and duodenum) [11]. Pancreatic and duodenal neuroendocrine tumors are the second most common manifestation of the disease, and affect more than 50% of patients, and are the leading cause of mortality [10, 12]. This most commonly manifests as gastrinomas (resulting in Zollinger–Ellison syndrome), insulinomas, and/or non-functional pancreatic tumors; however, rarely manifests with glucagonomas, VIP-omas, carcinoids, or PP-omas. Because of the persistent risk of malignancy and the multicentric nature of the disease, long-term management of MEN 1 patients requires close lifelong surveillance, and thoughtfully timed surgical interventions.

Clinical Presentation

Even today, to make the diagnosis, the first step is to consider it. The diagnosis of patients with hyperinsulinemia is therefore often delayed (sometimes years), as the presenting symptoms can be vague and sometimes bizarre, and it is such a rare tumor as to be hardly considered at all. It is not uncommon for patients to be initially diagnosed with a psychiatric disorder. Mild hypoglycemia stimulates autonomic and adrenergic activation, resulting in sweating, tachycardia, tremor, anxiety, hunger, and weakness. Severe hypoglycemia (<50 mg/dl), results in neurologic dysfunction and symptoms of neuroglycopenia: confusion, visual disturbances, loss of consciousness, seizures, or rarely focal neurologic deficits resembling stroke. Neuroglycopenic symptomatology is the "red flag" that should prompt suspicion and evaluation for hyperinsulinemia. Symptoms are usually induced by fasting and can be precipitated by exercise; while variable between patients, the specific set of symptoms are generally typical and reproducible for each patient but may progressively worsen over time. Documentation of fasting hypoglycemia at the time of symptoms is essential. In contrast, *postprandial* hypoglycemia symptoms suggest NIPHS rather than insulinoma. Prior to diagnosis and treatment, many insulinoma patients gain weight due to increased oral intake as their frequency and severity of symptoms progress, and as they learn to abort/prevent symptoms with food intake.

Family history (of endocrine disease) and social history (access to injectable insulin or oral hypoglycemic medication) should be sought.

At the Mayo clinic, 339 patients with either insulinoma or NIPHS have been surgically treated in the last 25 years. Table 13.1 lists the demographics of this

Table 13.1 Mayo Clinic Series, Operations for Endogenous Hyperinsulinemia, July 1982–December 2007 (339 operations in 258 patients)

Characteristics	Number (range)	Percent
Demographics		
Male/Female (ratio)	134:201 (1:1.5)	40:60
Mean age (years)	50.2 year (12–86)	–
Sporadic/NIPHS/MEN	254:68:17	65:20:5
Primary/reoperations	308:31	91:9
Presentation		
Duration of symptoms (months)	41.6 m (0–360)	–
Mean fasting glucose nadir (mg/dL)	38.6 (14–63)	–
Patients with glucose nadir >40 mg/dl	131	39
Mean C-peptide with glucose nadir (pmol/L)	2,393 (1.2–14,000)	–
Tumor location[a]		
Uncinate	35	13
Head	70	26
Neck	20	8
Body	64	24
Tail	78	29
Tumor size[a]		
Mean	1.6 cm (0.1–7)	
<1 cm	56	21
1–1.5 cm	98	37
1.6–2 cm	59	22
>2 cm	54	20
Palpable at operation	244	91
Single/multiple tumor(s)	247:20	93:7
Operative procedures		
Enucleation	173	51
Distal pancreatectomy (+/– splenectomy)	144	43
Distal pancreatectomy plus enucleation	1	0.3
Partial pancreatectomy	1	0.3
Subtotal pancreatectomy	1	0.3
Pancreaticoduodenectomy	8	2.4
Laparoscopic resection	5	1.5
Open/close	3	0.9
Complications		
Pancreatic (leak, hemorrhage, etc.)	62	18
Non-pancreatic (wounds, DVT, pneumonia)	45	13
Cure rate	326	97

MEN Multiple endocrine neoplasia

[a]Insulinomas only ($n=267$ tumors, 3 open/close, 1 failed resection)

cohort. The average age of presentation was 50 years (range 12–86 years), with a slight predominance of women vs. men (1.5:1). Slightly less than six percent of insulinoma cases were associated with MEN-1 syndrome.

Diagnostic Evaluation

Biochemical Testing

While Whipple's triad still serves as the basis for initial diagnostic evaluation, the diagnostic criteria have been scientifically sharpened to four concomitant criteria that are reliable in establishing a diagnosis of endogenous hyperinsulinemia:

- Plasma glucose less than 45–50 mg/dl
- Elevated insulin level (>6 μU/ml by IRMA or >3 μU/ml by ICMA)
- C-peptide levels (≥200 pmol/L)
- Negative screening for sulfonylureas.

While a classic inpatient 72-h fast was performed for diagnosis in the past and remains a solid "gold standard"; much shorter supervised fasts can safely be performed in the outpatient setting. Based on a patient's usual timing for the onset of hypoglycemic symptoms, a patient can begin the fast at home the evening prior to testing with a carefully supervised office visit scheduled to coincide with the usual time of symptoms. On arrival to the clinic, an IV is started and initial serum glucose level drawn. Serial measurements of glucose by reflectance-meter are then performed until neuroglycopenic symptoms arise (and glucose levels are documented below 50 mg/dl), at which point serum levels of glucose, insulin, C-peptide, and beta-hydroxybutyrate are drawn. Glucagon (1 mg IV) is then administered and glucose is monitored every 10 min for an additional 30 min to allow for measurement of beta-hydroxybutyrate and glucose response. These additional tests provide additional sensitivity, as insulin levels may be unreliable in a couple of scenarios (hemolyzed blood samples, insulin levels at the lower limit of detection). As insulin's activity is antiketogenic and glycogenic, β-hydroxybutyrate level ≤2.7 mmol/L at the time of documented hypoglycemia (glucose ≤50 mg/dl), or an increase in the plasma glucose of >25 mg/dl within 30 min of a 1 mg IV glucagon bolus are "surrogate" markers of hyperinsulinemia [13]. If the patient's glucose does not drop during the outpatient supervision, he/she can be admitted to the hospital to continue the fast for the remaining 72 h as necessary. Low (suppressed) C-peptide levels in the setting of hyperinsulinemic hypoglycemia suggest exogenous insulin administration.

Insulin-to-glucose ratios have long been promoted by some groups as a confirmatory test [14, 15]. However, in our experience, all such ratios have been inaccurate. The key to making the diagnosis is to recognize that any measurable insulin (according to the detection level in each laboratory) in the setting of severe hypoglycemia (<45–50 mg/dl) is pathologic.

Noninsulinoma Pancreatogenous Hyperinsulinemia Syndrome

NIPHS is a condition of endogenous hyperinsulinism not caused by a functional tumor. These patients, in contrast to patients with an insulinoma, have diffuse islet cell hyperplasia and/or nesidioblastosis which results in an exaggerated insulin response to glucose ingestion [16]. Therefore, these patients do not experience fasting hypoglycemia; rather, they develop symptomatic *postprandial* hypoglycemia (typically 1–3 h after meals). NIPHS is most often encountered in the setting of prior gastric surgery – most-commonly Roux en Y gastric bypass for obesity, but also occasionally seen with anti-reflux or ulcer surgery. While the timing of symptoms and the pathology responsible for NIPHS is different than that of insulinoma, the biochemical profile of these patients is identical. Sometimes glucose measurements fall well below 30 mg/dl with concomitantly elevated insulin and C-peptide levels; and their symptomatology (adrenergic and neuroglycopenic) can be equally as bizarre and debilitating as in patients with insulinoma. As with insulinoma, the symptoms and biochemical confirmation of neuroglycopenia are the keys to the diagnosis, as many patients who have had gastric surgery may also have postprandial symptoms of diaphoresis, weakness, dizziness, or flushing with rapid gastric emptying ("dumping syndrome"). The key to differentiating NIPHS and insulinoma reflects the difference in pathophysiology – insulinoma causes unregulated, persistent, excessive insulin secretion (resulting in fasting hypoglycemia); whereas NIPHS results from diffuse islet cell hypertrophy with associated hyperresponsiveness.

NIPHS is diagnosed with a mixed meal test – the patient performs supervised ingestion of a premixed meal replacement (or ingestion of the inciting food type), with serial serum measurements of glucose, insulin, and C-peptide at baseline every 30 min. A positive test confirms hyperinsulinism with concomitant hypoglycemia and elevated C-peptide. Additional confirmation can be documented by a negative 72-h fast, negative imaging studies, and selective arterial calcium stimulation (SACS) testing with elevated response in more than one arterial distribution (oftentimes all three distributions). In cases of severe, debilitating symptoms that have failed medical management, distal pancreatectomy has been performed for an effective reduction in islet cell mass.

Localization

Insulinomas are routinely small (1–2 cm) and can be difficult to localize; however, preoperative localization is essential to operative success. The availability and success rates of imaging and localization techniques vary by institution. Our algorithm at the Mayo Clinic is presented in Fig. 13.1. The sensitivities and specificities of the different techniques at our institution are presented in Table 13.2. Each technique and its strengths and shortcomings is discussed below.

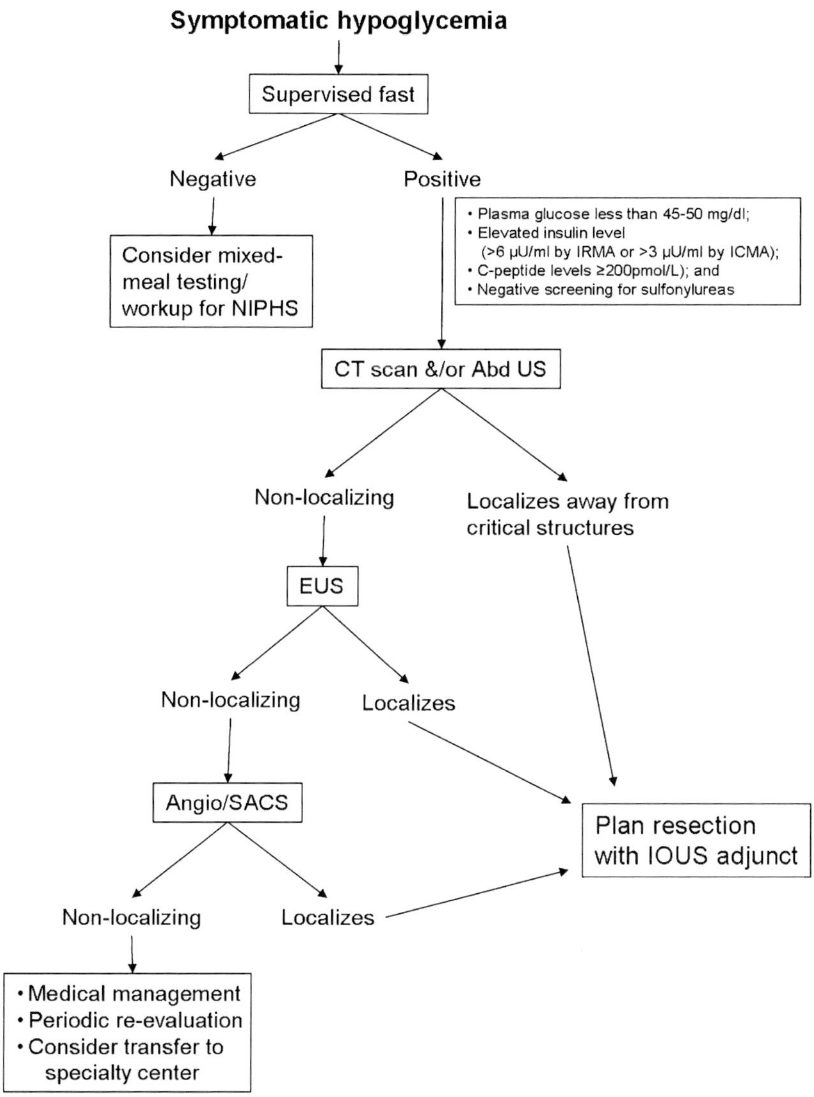

Fig. 13.1 Diagnostic algorithm for patients with suspected hyperinsulinemic hypoglycemia. *Abd US* Transabdominal Ultrasonography; *EUS* Endoscopic Ultrasonography; *Angio/SACS* Angiography with Selective Arterial Calcium Stimulation; *IOUS* Intraoperative Ultrasonography

Computed Tomography (CT scan)

Helical CT scan is typically one of the first imaging tests ordered after positive biochemical studies. CT is non-invasive, and is particularly useful in preoperative planning as it can identify the precise anatomic location, size, and relationship of

Table 13.2 Mayo Clinic Series, July 1982–February 2007

Statistic	Trans-abd US	CT scan	EUS	SACS	IOUS
Total studies (n)	299	209	42	97	242
True Pos (n)	137	85	25	90	204
Sensitivity (%)	60.9	60.3	83.3	100	97.6
False Pos (n)	13	10	3	6	5
Specificity (%)	80.6	84.8	62.5	14.3	86.1
PPV (%)	91	89	89	94	98
False neg (n)	88	56	5	0	5

Localization studies for endogenous hyperinsulinemia. *Trans-abd US* Transabdominal ultrasound; *EUS* endoscopic ultrasound; *SACS* Angiography with selective arterial calcium stimulation; *IOUS* intraoperative ultrasound

the tumor to other important structures. CT scan can also identify lymphadenopathy, invasion of surrounding structures, and metastatic lesions suggestive of malignant disease. Furthermore, these images are typically easily interpreted by the operating surgeon. With the recent advances in CT imaging (increased speed, resolution, and image-reconstruction software), CT sensitivity has improved. Despite these improvements, CT scan still may fail to localize over 30% of tumors. Figure 13.2 shows a CT scan and surgical specimen of a patient with malignant insulinoma invading the spleen.

Transabdominal Ultrasound

Prior to the recent advances in CT imaging, we relied heavily on transabdominal ultrasonography as our primary imaging modality. We still routinely order ultrasound on almost all patients, with similar sensitivity to CT scan. Abdominal ultrasound, like CT scan, can accurately identify the size, location, and relationship of the tumor to surrounding structures, and like CT scan, it is non-invasive. Its usefulness can be limited by patients with abdominal obesity, and occasionally by bowel gas interference. Ingestion of 12 oz. of water prior to scanning can improve imaging and reduce gas interference. The most important limitation of ultrasound is its dependence on the experience of the radiologist. In addition the images are not as easily interpreted by surgeons.

Endoscopic Ultrasound (EUS)

EUS can also provide useful information about tumor size and proximity to surrounding structures, but requires operator expertise in both advanced endoscopy and ultrasound. The images obtained are typically less helpful to the operating surgeon.

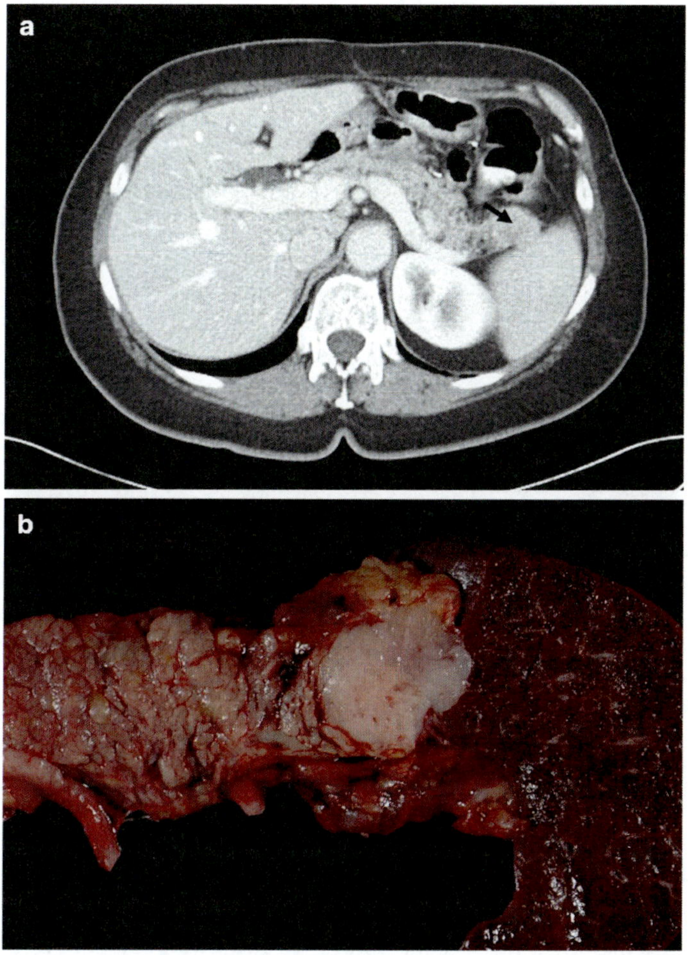

Fig. 13.2 *Panel a*: CT scan demonstrating a tumor in the tail of the pancreas (*arrow*) with concern for invasion of the splenic hilum. *Panel b*: Surgical specimen (same patient as Panel a) demonstrating a malignant insulinoma with direct invasion of the spleen

Complications are rare (e.g., pancreatitis, perforation). Because of these drawbacks, we reserve EUS for patients with non-localizing CT scans or abdominal ultrasounds, and for assistance with operative planning in patients with pancreatic head tumors in close proximity to the common bile duct or main pancreatic duct. However, EUS is potentially more sensitive than either CT scan or abdominal ultrasound in identifying small tumors (identifying 83% of otherwise non-localizing tumors at our institution) and its role in insulinoma localization will likely become even more prominent in the future.

Arteriography with Selective Arterial Calcium Stimulation (SACS)

A small percentage of patients will have a negative or indeterminate CT scan, trans-abdominal ultrasound, and EUS. We therefore turn to angiography with SACS testing. Since 1996, when we implemented this additional combined technique, we have been able to localize or regionalize 100% of tumors. SACS involves sequential, selective catheterization of the gastroduodenal, splenic, and superior mesenteric arteries with simultaneous separate venous catheterization of the right hepatic vein for blood sampling. Arteriograms of each respective artery are first performed, and may identify a tumor, which is seen as a hypervascular "blush." For the calcium stimulation phase of the test, calcium gluconate (0.025 mEq/kg) is sequentially injected into the superior mesenteric, splenic, and gastroduodenal arteries and blood samples are taken from the hepatic vein at 0, 20, 40, and 60 sec after each injection (Fig. 13.3). A greater than two-fold increase in hepatic vein insulin levels is considered a positive result. This "regionalizes" the site of insulin secretion within the pancreas by its arterial supply, but does not truly "localize" the tumor itself. Furthermore, recognition of aberrant arterial anatomy at the time of angiography must be accounted for as this may affect the accuracy of the "regionalization." Success and risk of this complex procedure is very dependent on the experience and skill of the interventional radiologist performing the procedure. In patients with NIPHS, typically more than one distribution (and often all three) is positive, although there may be a "gradient" of stimulation response [16].

Intraoperative Ultrasound (IOUS)

IOUS is extremely helpful in confirming tumor location, anatomic relationships (e.g., to the pancreatic and biliary ducts and vasculature – Fig. 13.4), and detecting (or excluding) the presence of multiple tumors. We have used IOUS since 1982 on almost all patients operated on for insulinoma, and almost all tumors (>97%) were visualized by IOUS. Although this may slightly increase the operative time, the information obtained can be invaluable in planning the approach to enucleation and help prevent surgical complications.

Nuclear Imaging

OctreoScan, although useful in other neuroendocrine tumors, is rarely used for insulinomas, as the majority of tumors lack somatostatin receptors with high affinity for octreotide [17].

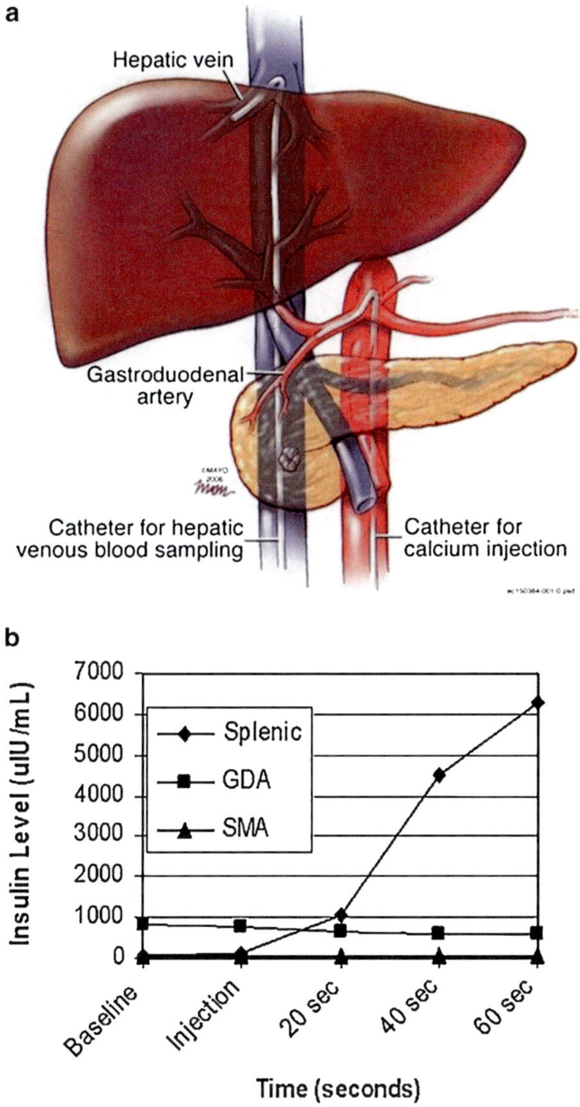

Fig. 13.3 *Panel a*: Catheter placement for Selective Arterial Calcium Stimulation (SACS). *Panel b*: SACS in a patient with MEN-1 and negative imaging studies regionalizes the insulinoma to the tail of the pancreas

Magnetic Resonance Imaging (MRI)

We have had very limited experience with magnetic resonance imaging (MRI) for insulinoma. It is more expensive than CT scan and its images are less easily interpreted by the operating surgeon. Given our success with the combination of CT

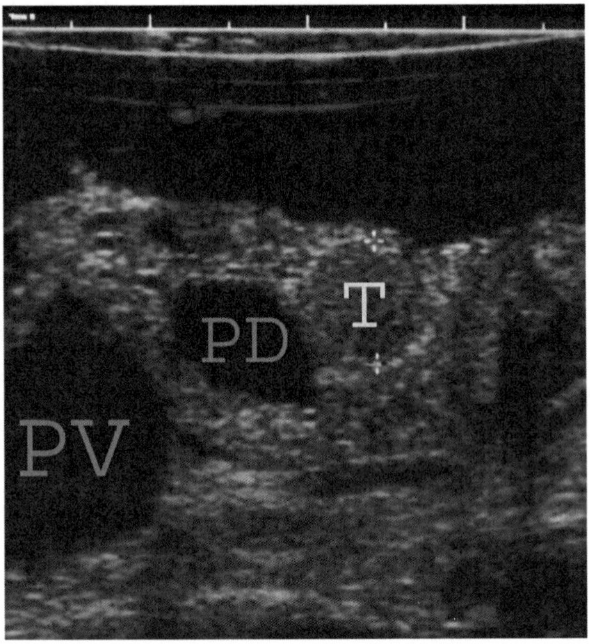

Fig. 13.4 Intraoperative ultrasound in a patient who had undergone a pancreaticoduodenectomy for a benign insulinoma incorrectly localized to the pancreatic head, with persistent hypoglycemia postoperatively. At reoperation, IOUS was performed demonstrating the tumor in the body of the pancreas (T). The relationship of the tumor to the main pancreatic duct (PD) and the portal vein (PV) is seen

scan, transabdominal ultrasound, and EUS, we have rarely needed to add MRI, but have done so in select patients (e.g., previously operated patients with otherwise non-localizing studies).

Management

Perioperative care

Patients with insulinomas are typically admitted the night prior to operation for intravenous dextrose administration (to prevent fasting hypoglycemia). The choice of the surgical approach depends on several important factors that are assessed preoperatively: (1) tumor location within the pancreas (e.g., head, body, tail); (2) location in relation to the pancreatic duct; (3) sporadic vs. MEN-1 associated disease; and (4) suspected malignancy. Intraoperatively, dextrose-free fluids are administered, the blood glucose is monitored every 15–20 min, and bolus doses of dextrose given only if the glucose level falls below 40 mg/dl. After tumor excision, continued glucose monitoring typically demonstrates a prompt rise in glucose levels, typically to levels of 150–200 mg/dl depending on whether the tumor is enucleated or pancreatic resection was necessary.

Surgical Treatment

Open Approach

The abdomen is usually accessed through a bilateral subcostal incision, and an extended Kocher maneuver is performed to allow access to the head and uncinate process. In addition, medial mobilization of the spleen and distal pancreas is performed as indicated if the tumor location is suspected in that portion of the gland. Complete mobilization of the pancreas in this manner facilitates optimal bimanual palpation of the gland and visualization by IOUS. Bimanual exam should identify the majority of tumors (>90% in our experience), but does not eliminate the need for IOUS. IOUS is an extremely useful adjunct to help confirm tumor location and proximity to the pancreatic duct, specifically to aid the surgeon in the safest approach to excise the tumor. Moreover, it can assist in identifying additional occult tumors. Enucleation is the procedure of choice for benign insulinomas, and can safely be performed even when tumors are directly adjacent to the common bile duct or major pancreatic ducts, as they typically displace but do not invade or constrict the duct. Dilation of the pancreatic duct is a sign of tumor invasion and malignancy. Benign insulinomas are typically firm, well circumscribed, and reasonably easy to differentiate from the surrounding normal pancreatic parenchyma – there is often a distinct plane between the tumor and normal pancreatic parenchyma. The enucleation bed is observed for a leak and the site can either be oversewn or left open. Closed-suction drainage is often used.

When enucleation is not possible (either due to size, tumor location, or concerns of malignancy) distal pancreatectomy with or without splenectomy (for body and tail lesions), or rarely pancreaticoduodenectomy (for head and uncinate lesions) may be required. These are performed in the standard manner. In cases of suspected or proven malignancy, peripancreatic lymphadenectomy should also be performed for staging and locoregional control. If splenectomy is performed, the patient should be vaccinated against encapsulated organisms (Haemophilus, Pneumococcus, and Meningococcus), which is ideally performed either 2 weeks before or 2 weeks after operation.

"Blind distal pancreatectomy" – where progressive pancreatic resection starting from the tail and moving toward the head until hypoglycemia resolves – is of historical significance, but is no longer advised as it carries a high rate of surgical failure, with obvious surgical risks. In the rare case of a patient with non-localizing preoperative studies who is taken for exploration and has no identifiable tumor by palpation or IOUS, we would advise abdominal closure and referral to a tertiary referral center. Similarly, patients who have previously been operated (either with prior enucleation, resection, or MEN 1 disease) should be evaluated and treated at a tertiary referral center as preoperative localization and surgical planning is critical.

Laparoscopic Approach

Laparoscopic resection of islet cell tumors was first reported in 1996 by Gagner et al, and has since been reported by multiple centers with good results in selected patients [18, 19, 30, 31, 32]. Principles of laparoscopic resection are similar to open surgery, with enucleation (when feasible) being the procedure of choice. This requires both advanced laparoscopic skill and experience with laparoscopic IOUS. Tumor location should be confirmed preoperatively by imaging. Laparoscopic enucleation can be performed either with electrocautery (e.g., Endoshears, hook cautery) or other sealing device (e.g., Harmonic® scalpel). When distal pancreatectomy is performed for pancreatic tail tumors, the pancreas (and splenic vessels if splenectomy if performed) is often transected with an endoscopic stapling device. Scenarios that should prompt conversion to open procedure are: (1) uncontrolled hemorrhage; (2) poor visualization; (3) technical difficulty/anatomy precluding safe resection; or (4) findings suggestive of malignancy. Laparoscopic resections should not be attempted in patients with MEN-1, questionable localization, or if tumor location or anatomy (proximity to ducts or vasculature) impair laparoscopic visualization/safety.

Special Consideration: MEN 1

The surgical goals in patients with MEN 1 are: (1) cure the hyperinsulinism (and, if present, gastrinomas as well); (2) safely excise and/or debulk associated non-functioning islet cell tumors so as to minimize the future risk of malignancy; and (3) minimize long-term complications (e.g., diabetes). Surgical treatment in patients with MEN 1 must be individualized to each patient's pattern of disease, and has resulted in two main approaches. For patients whose disease is most prominent in the body or tail of the pancreas, distal pancreatectomy and enucleation of all accessible pancreatic head tumors is the option of choice (Fig. 13.5). For patients with dominant disease in the pancreatic head, pancreaticoduodenectomy with enucleation of additional tumors in the tail may be required. Other manifestations of the disease (e.g., hypercalcemia from hyperparathyroidism, Zollinger–Ellison syndrome) should be considered when discussing operative strategy and timing of interventions. Duodenotomy with palpation of the duodenal wall and excision of any palpable submucosal carcinoids should be part of the operative approach in patients with hypergastrinemia. Because of the importance of thorough palpation

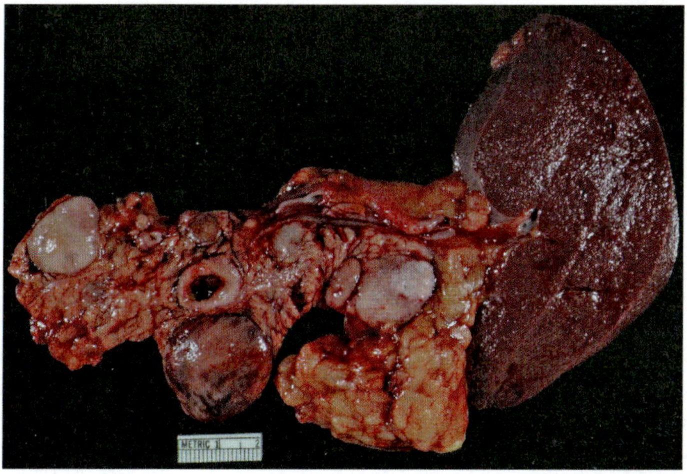

Fig. 13.5 Distal pancreatectomy specimen in a patient with MEN-1 and insulinoma, demonstrating multiple islet cell tumors

and examination of both the pancreas and duodenum in these patients, a laparoscopic approach is not advised.

Postoperative care

Transient hyperglycemia (usually around 200 mg/dl) is typically observed for the first few postoperative days, and this is a reassuring sign of surgical success. Close monitoring of blood glucose (initially every 30 min in the recovery room, and ultimately spaced out to every 12–24 h) is required, as many patients transiently require exogenous insulin for glycemic control. Therefore, we typically avoid dextrose in the patient's IV fluids for the first 24 h, and administer insulin as needed for patients with glucose levels over 200 mg/dl. Most patients will have normalization of their glucose levels within 2–3 weeks of surgery, and are nearly euglycemic by the time of hospital discharge. Drainage tubes are typically removed after the patient resumes a normal diet provided there is no sign of pancreatic leak.

Complications

Complications may occur in up to 40–50% of patients [19–22], many of whom are minor and few who require reoperation. Pancreatic complications (hemorrhage, abscess, pancreatitis, or pancreatic fistula) account for approximately half to two-thirds of perioperative morbidity. Pancreatic fistulas typically close spontaneously without operative re-intervention within a few weeks as long as adequate drainage is maintained. Non-pancreatic complications (such as DVT, pneumonia, and wound infections) also occur, but death is rare. At our institution, there have been no postoperative deaths since 1941 (over 330 patients). Complication rates with laparoscopic resections appear to be similar to open surgery, but with enhanced laparoscopic skills and careful patient selection, this represents a very plausible surgical approach.

Follow-up

Except for patients with MEN-1 syndrome, follow-up in patients with benign insulinomas is basically unnecessary. Prognosis is excellent, with greater than 97% of patients achieving a long-term cure. Return of hypoglycemic signs and symptoms should prompt reevaluation and suspicion of recurrence in the previous enucleation site, and may be an indicator of previously undiagnosed MEN-1 syndrome, or may suggest malignant disease.

Malignant Disease

The prognosis for patients with malignant insulinoma is better than for patients with exocrine pancreatic adenocarcinoma, and therefore an aggressive approach is recommended for these patients as their tumors are typically slow-growing, and highly symptomatic. Primary tumor resection in combination with debulking of metastatic disease through surgical resection, tumor ablation (radiofrequency ablation, cryoablation, or ethanol ablation), chemoembolization, or hepatic arterial chemoperfusion can provide good palliation with minimal morbidity [23–26]. In the last 15 years, chemotherapeutic options (such as streptozocin monotherapy or in combination with 5-FU, doxorubicin, or chlorozotocin) have yielded reasonable response rates – both in tumor regression and symptom palliation [26, 27]. A multi-disciplinary approach has resulted in some long-term (20–30 year) survivors [23]. For patients with disease not amenable to resection (e.g., high surgical risk, anatomic considerations, unresectable metastatic disease), medical management (e.g., diazoxide or somatostatin analogs) can help alleviate symptoms by reducing insulin secretion [27, 28]. As only limited treatment data are available due to the rarity of this disease, creative strategies for palliation should be customized for the individual patient, pattern of disease, and severity of symptoms. We have used a continuous glucose-infusion pump in one patient with inoperable disease with severe uncontrolled hyperinsulinism. Novel therapies based on molecular targets in insulinoma (GLP-1 receptor-based therapies) remain in the preclinical stages of development, but may have future value [29].

References

1. van Heerden JA, Churchward MM (1999) Dr. Dickinson Ober Wheelock – a case of sporadic insulinoma or multiple endocrine neoplasia type 1? Mayo Clinic Proc 74:735–738
2. Wilder RM, Allan FN, Power MH et al (1927) Carcinoma of the islets of the pancreas: hyperinsulinism and hypoglycemia. JAMA 89:348
3. Morrison H (1937) Contributions to the microscopic anatomy of the pancreas by Paul Langerhans [Berlin, 1869]. [Translated from German]. Bull Hist Med 5:259–267
4. Banting FG (1937) Early work on insulin. Science 85:594–596
5. Howland G, Campbell CW, Maltby EJ et al (1929) Dysinsulinism: convulsions and coma due to islet cell tumor of the pancreas with operation and cure. JAMA 93:674
6. Whipple AO, Frantz VK (1935) Adenoma of Islet cells with Hyperinsulinism: a review. Ann Surg 101:1299–1335
7. Starr JI, Rubenstein AH (1974) Metabolism of endogenous proinsulin and insulin in man. J Clin Endocrinol Metab 38:305–308
8. Service FJ (1995) Hypoglycemic disorders. N Engl J Med 332:1144–1152
9. Service FJ, McMahon MM, O'Brien PC, Ballard DJ (1991) Functioning insulinoma–incidence, recurrence, and long-term survival of patients: a 60-year study. Mayo Clin Proc 66:711–719
10. Doherty GM (2005) Multiple endocrine neoplasia type 1. J Surg Oncol 89:143–150
11. Larsson C, Skogseid B, Oberg K et al (1988) Multiple endocrine neoplasia type 1 gene maps to chromosome 11 and is lost in insulinoma. Nature 332:85–87
12. Doherty GM, Thompson NW (2003) Multiple endocrine neoplasia type 1: duodenopancreatic tumours. J Inst Med 253:590–598
13. O'Brien T, O'Brien PC, Service FJ (1993) Insulin surrogates in insulinoma. J Clin Endocrinol Metab 77:448–451
14. Pasieka JL, McLeod MK, Thompson NW, Burney RE (1992) Surgical approach to insulinomas. Assessing the need for preoperative localization. Arch Surg 127:442–447
15. Finlayson E, Clark OH (2004) Surgical treatment of insulinomas. Surg Clin North Am 84:775–785
16. Service GJ, Thompson GB, Service FJ et al (2005) Hyperinsulinemic hypoglycemia with nesidioblastosis after gastric-bypass surgery. N Engl J Med 353:249–254
17. Slooter GD, Mearadji A, Breeman WA et al (2001) Somatostatin receptor imaging, therapy and new strategies in patients with neuroendocrine tumours. Br J Surg 88:31–40
18. Assalia A, Gagner M (2004) Laparoscopic pancreatic surgery for islet cell tumors of the pancreas. World J Surg 28:1239–1247
19. Pierce RA, Spitler JA, Hawkins WG et al (2007) Outcomes analysis of laparoscopic resection of pancreatic neoplasms. Surg Endosc 21:579–586
20. Menegaux F, Schmitt G, Mercadier M, Chigot JP (1993) Pancreatic insulinomas. Am J Surg 165:243–248
21. Doherty GM, Doppman JL, Shawker TH et al (1991) Results of a prospective strategy to diagnose, localize, and resect insulinomas. Surgery 110:989–996
22. Phan GQ, Yeo CJ, Hruban RH et al (1998) Surgical experience with pancreatic and peripancreatic neuroendocrine tumors: review of 125 patients. J Gastrointest Surg 2:472–482
23. Hirshberg B, Cochran C, Skarulis MC et al (2005) Malignant insulinoma: spectrum of unusual clinical features. Cancer 104:264–272
24. Sarmiento JM, Que FG, Grand CS et al (2002) Concurrent resections of pancreatic islet cell cancers with synchronous hepatic metastases: outcomes of an aggressive approach. Surgery 132:976–982
25. Siperstein AE, Berber E (2001) Cryoablation, percutaneous alcohol injection, and radiofrequency ablation for treatment of neuroendocrine liver metastases. World J Surg 25:693–696

26. Starke A, Saddig C, Mansfeld L et al (2005) Malignant metastatic insulinoma-postoperative treatment and follow-up. World J Surg 29:789–793
27. Moertel CG, Lefkopoulo M, Lipsitz S et al (1992) Streptozocin-doxorubicin, streptozocin-fluorouracil or chlorozotocin in the treatment of advanced islet-cell carcinoma. N Engl J Med 326:519–523
28. Goode PN, Farndon JR, Anderson J et al (1986) Diazoxide in the management of patients with insulinoma. World J Surg 10:586–592
29. Wicki A, Wild D, Storch D et al (2007) [Lys40(Ahx-DTPA-111In)NH2]-Exendin-4 is a highly efficient radiotherapeutic for glucagon-like peptide-1 receptor-targeted therapy for insulinoma. Clin Cancer Res 13:3696–3705
30. Gagner M, Pomp A, Herrera MF (1996) Early experience with laparoscopic resections of islet cell tumors. Surgery 120:1051–1054
31. Mabrut JY, Fernandez-Cruz L, Azagra JS et al (2005) Laparoscopic pancreatic resection: results of a multicenter European study of 127 patients. Surgery 137:597–605
32. Kaczirek K, Asari R, Scheuba C, Niederle B (2005) Organic hyperinsulinism and endoscopic surgery. Wien Klin Wochenschrt 117:19–25

Chapter 14
Rare Neuroendocrine Tumors of the Pancreas

Shih-Ping Cheng and Gerard M. Doherty

Neuroendocrine tumors of the pancreas are rare tumors. The annual incidence of pancreatic neuroendocrine tumors is approximately 4–12 cases per million population, which is much lower than that reported from autopsy series (about 1%) [1, 2]. Neuroendocrine tumors comprise only a minor number of all pancreatic tumors. By incidence, neuroendocrine carcinomas account for 1.3% of all pancreatic cancers. However, in prevalence analyses they represent about 10% of all pancreatic cancers because of the better outcome than exocrine carcinomas [3]. With the development of more sensitive imaging techniques, the number of patients with pancreatic neuroendocrine tumors has increased [4, 5]. This, however, probably does not reflect an actual increase in incidence but rather an improvement in the diagnostic methods.

The endocrine pancreas is composed of the islets of Langerhans, with four main cell types: the glucagon, insulin, somatostatin, and pancreatic polypeptide (PP) cells. These cells have many histological similarities to neural cells, such as the secretory granules and the expression of the so-called neuronal markers. It was believed that pancreatic endocrine cells arise from a neuroectodermal origin [6]. This hypothesis was challenged by convincing evidence that the endocrine and exocrine lineages develop from common progenitors in the foregut endoderm [7]. There is still a debate on whether neuroendocrine tumors of the pancreas originate from the islets of Langerhans [8]. These tumors are frequently called "islet cell tumors," even though it is now believed that they arise from multipotent stem cells in the ductal epithelium that differentiate toward the neuroendocrine phenotype [9, 10]. These tumors may produce hormones that are normally not found in the adult pancreas, such as gastrin and vasoactive intestinal polypeptide (VIP).

Pancreatic neuroendocrine tumors are a heterogeneous group of benign and malignant neoplasms. Malignancy cannot be reliably predicted based on tumor histopathology. The only well-accepted proofs of malignancy are evidence of invasion of adjacent organs, spread to regional lymph nodes or distant metastases. The

G.M. Doherty (✉)
University of Michigan, 2920 Taubman Center, 1500 East Medical Center Drive, Ann Arbor, MI 48109, USA
e-mail: gerardd@umich.edu

C. Sturgeon (ed.), *Endocrine Neoplasia*, Cancer Treatment and Research, vol 153,
DOI 10.1007/978-1-4419-0857-5_14, © Springer Science+Business Media, LLC 2010

Table 14.1 Classification of neuroendocrine tumors of the pancreas (WHO classification 2004)

1. Well-differentiated neuroendocrine tumor
Benign: confined to pancreas, <2 cm in size, non-angioinvasive, ≤2 mitoses/HPF and ≤2% Ki-67-positive cells
Functioning: insulinoma
Non-functioning
Benign or low-grade malignant (uncertain malignant potential): confined to pancreas, ≥2 cm in size, >2 mitoses/HPF, >2% Ki-67-positive cells, or angioinvasive
Functioning: gastrinoma, insulinoma, VIPoma, glucagonoma, somatostatinoma, or ectopic hormonal syndrome
Non-functioning
2. Well-differentiated neuroendocrine carcinoma (Low-grade malignant): invasion of adjacent organs and/or metastases
Functioning: gastrinoma, insulinoma, VIPoma, glucagonoma, somatostatinoma, or ectopic hormonal syndrome
Non-functioning
3. Poorly-differentiated neuroendocrine carcinoma (High-grade malignant)

HPF high power fields; *VIP* vasoactive intestinal polypeptide

World Health Organization (WHO) classification scheme is based on both histopathological and functional parameters [11]. According to the WHO classification, the vast majority of pancreatic neuroendocrine tumors are well-differentiated tumors or carcinomas (Table 14.1).

Presentation

Pancreatic neuroendocrine tumors can be divided into functioning and nonfunctioning tumors. The terms "functional/functioning" are used to denote the clinical manifestations of certain syndromes related to tumors that secrete hormones and peptides at supraphysiological levels [12]. Depending on the predominant hormone secreted, these tumors are referred to as VIPomas, glucagonomas, and somatostatinomas (Table 14.2). Control of the hormonal syndrome should be achieved preoperatively to stabilize the patient for the operation (Table 14.3). Sometimes resection may be an important part of the control of the hormonal syndrome.

Nonfunctioning tumors may also secrete a number of amines and peptides, with blood levels above the normal range. These amines and peptides do not produce recognizable clinical syndromes because the secreted amount may be too small or they are functionally inert precursor hormones. Some secreted peptides, such as PP and chromogranin A, are not associated with specific clinical symptoms and signs. These tumors are considered nonfunctioning. The tumors that stain positively for various markers should still be considered nonfunctioning in the absence of elevated serum levels of specific hormones.

The frequency of presentation with typical symptoms has decreased in recent years [13]. The widespread use of cross-sectional imaging has led to more frequent

Table 14.2 Characteristics of rare neuroendocrine tumors of the pancreas

Tumor	Syndrome	Location		Malignancy (%)	MEN-1 (%)
		Pancreas (%)	Duodenum (%)		
VIPoma	Watery diarrhea Hypokalemia Achlorhydria	85	15	40–50	1
Glucagonoma	Necrolytic migratory erythema Diabetes mellitus Cachexia Panhypoaminoacidemia Thromboembolism	100	–	70–90	3
Somatostatinoma	Steatorrhea/diarrhea Diabetes mellitus Gallstones	50 (syndrome common)	50 (syndrome rare)	80	1[a]
PPoma or non-functioning	Symptoms from pancreatic mass and/or liver metastases	100	–	80	50

[a]Up to 50% of patients with duodenal somatostatinomas have von Recklinghausen disease.
MEN-1 multiple endocrine neoplasia type 1; *VIP* vasoactive intestinal polypeptide; *PP* pancreatic polypeptide

Table 14.3 Management of hormone syndromes in rare pancreatic neuroendocrine tumors

Tumor	Syndrome	Management
VIPoma	Watery diarrhea	Rehydration with intravenous fluids
	Hypokalemia	Correction of electrolyte imbalance (K^+, Mg^{++}, $HCO3^-$)
	Achlorhydria	Somatostatin analogue
		Cholecystectomy[a]
Glucagonoma	Necrolytic migratory erythema	Total parenteral nutrition ± zinc
	Diabetes mellitus	Diabetes control
	Cachexia	Anticoagulation for deep venous thrombosis
	Panhypoaminoacidemia	Somatostatin analogue
	Thromboembolism	Cholecystectomy[a]
		Vena cava filter[a]
Somatostatinoma	Steatorrhea/diarrhea	Pancreatic enzyme supplementation
	Diabetes mellitus	Diabetes control
	Gallstones	Cholecystectomy[a]

[a]Specific operative measures to improve long-term symptomatic management
VIP vasoactive intestinal polypeptide

identification of small incidental tumors, with a trend toward lesser likelihood of malignancy [14]. Currently, approximately 50% of pancreatic neuroendocrine tumors are reported to be nonfunctioning, about 25% are insulinomas, and about 15% are gastrinomas [15, 16]. VIPoma and other functioning tumors are a small fraction among neuroendocrine tumors. Because nonfunctioning tumors are not heralded by the symptoms of hormone excess, it was thought that nonfunctioning tumors tend to be larger and more advanced at the time of diagnosis [17]. Nonetheless, functioning and nonfunctioning neuroendocrine tumors usually follow a similar clinical course [18]. Extensive screening for secreted hormones in asymptomatic patients is not recommended [19, 20].

Most pancreatic neuroendocrine tumors are sporadic; however, they may develop in a familial context of multiple endocrine neoplasia type 1 (MEN-1), von Hippel–Lindau disease, von Recklinghausen disease, or tuberous sclerosis [21]. The most frequent condition associated with pancreatic neuroendocrine tumors is MEN-1 (15–30%) [15]. The possibility of the presence of MEN-1 should always be considered before applying any kind of therapy because there is a great difference in the management of these tumors.

VIPoma

VIP is a peptide hormone with close structural homology to secretin [22]. The syndrome that is associated with VIP-producing neuroendocrine tumors has been referred to as the Verner–Morrison syndrome, WDHA (Watery Diarrhea, Hypokalemia, Achlorhydria) syndrome, or pancreatic cholera. Nearly 100% of patients present with severe watery secretory diarrhea, which persists even when fasting. During the initial stages of the disease, diarrhea may be intermittent but becomes profuse and continuous with progression of the tumor. If inadequately treated, the resulting dehydration and electrolyte disturbances may cause renal failure and ultimately cardiac arrest [23]. Weight loss is often remarkable due to substantial fluid loss. Hypokalemia, paradoxically associated with low bicarbonate levels, is present in nearly every patient. Achlorhydria or hypochlorhydria is present in over two thirds of the patients. Flushing of the face and trunk, characterized by a patchy erythema and urticaria, is seen in approximately 20% of the patients.

The mean age of patients at diagnosis is approximately 50 years, with a slightly higher incidence in women [22]. The diagnosis of VIPoma requires the presence of the triad – secretory diarrhea, elevated fasting VIP levels, and a pancreatic neuroendocrine tumor. The stool volume is usually more than 3 L per day. Volumes less than 700 mL/day without treatment essentially exclude the diagnosis. A definitive diagnosis is aided by the determination of plasma VIP concentrations, which are typically 2–10 multiples of the upper limit of the normal range.

VIPomas usually occur in the pancreas, mostly from the pancreatic tail (Fig. 14.1). The mean size at the time of diagnosis is 5.2 cm [22]. Approximately 50% of pancreatic VIPomas are malignant, of which three quarters have either

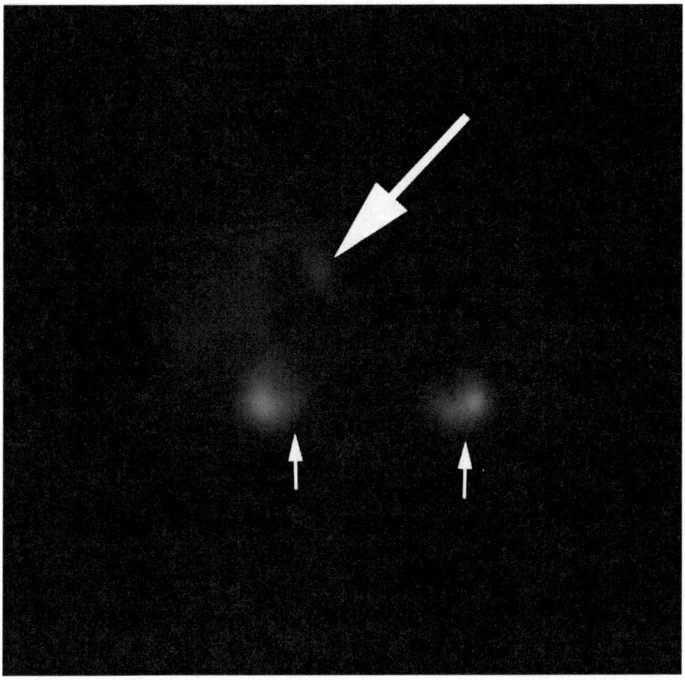

Fig. 14.1 Somatostatin receptor scintigraphy from patient with VIPoma. This image shows a large nodal metastasis rather than the primary tumor (*large arrow*) at the level of the upper poles of the kidneys (*smaller arrows*)

hepatic, distant, or lymph node metastases at presentation. Compared with pancreatic VIPomas, extrapancreatic lesions have a lower rate of malignancy and metastases [24].

Once the syndrome is diagnosed, the first step in the management of these patients is the correction of potentially life-threatening dehydration and electrolyte abnormalities. Usually, this requires hospital admission with intensive intravenous therapy. Somatostatin analog treatment can stop the diarrhea and allow for rehydration and correction of electrolyte derangements in the majority of these patients, and may even reduce tumor size [25].

Glucagonoma

Glucagon is a 29-amino acid single chain peptide hormone produced by the alpha cells of the pancreatic islets, which counteracts the effects of insulin on glucose metabolism [26]. The glucagonoma syndrome is characterized by the four D's: dermatitis, diabetes, deep venous thrombosis, and depression [27]. The hallmark clinical finding is necrolytic migratory erythema, which occurs in nearly all glucagonoma patients at some time during their clinical illness. This pathognomic rash often starts in the groin and perineum, and subsequently spreads centrifugally to the distal extremities and face [28]. The lesions have a cyclic nature, with progression from erythema to vesiculation, to crusting, to resolution over one to two weeks. Most patients complain of pain and intense pruritus at the site of the rash.

Generalized hypoaminoacidemia is a universal finding in glucagonoma syndrome patients [27]. Pathological levels of glucagon promote protein degradation, resulting in decreased blood amino acid concentration [29]. Weight loss and cachexia are common, probably resulting from the catabolic effects of glucagon. In 80% of patients with hyperglucagonemia, mild diabetes mellitus develops at the expense of tissue glycogen stores [28]. Angular stomatitis, cheilitis, and glossitis are also common manifestations. Deep venous thrombosis and/or pulmonary embolism have been reported to occur in up to 30% of patients with glucagonoma syndrome. Thromboembolic events account for over 50% of all deaths related to the glucagonoma syndrome [30].

Patients typically present in the 5th or 6th decade of life with an even gender distribution. Diagnostic criteria of glucagonoma syndrome include raised fasting plasma glucagon concentration, together with demonstrable tumor and characteristic clinical features [30]. Serum glucagon levels greater than 1,000 pg/mL are diagnostic of the syndrome, while levels between 150 and 1,000 pg/mL are suggestive. Tumors arise almost exclusively in the pancreas, usually in the tail (Fig. 14.2).

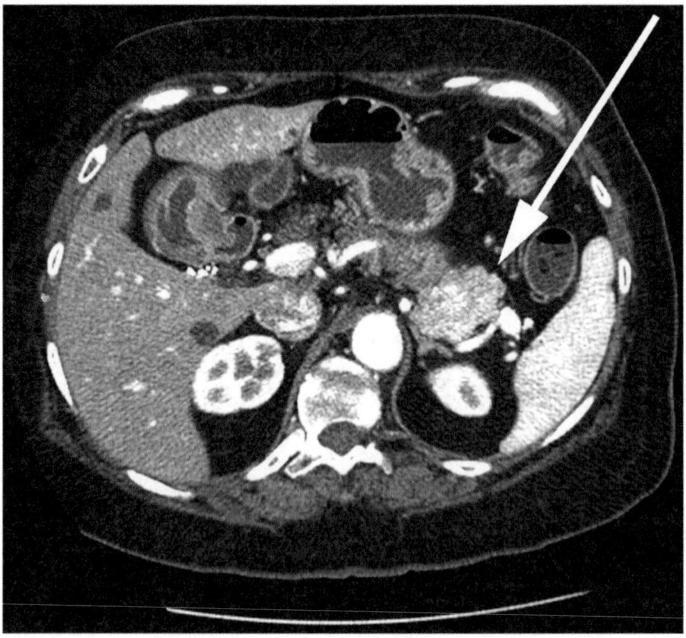

Fig. 14.2 CT scan of a VIPoma in the distal pancreas. The typical hypervascular tumor is indicated by the *white arrow*

The average size of glucagonomas is 5.8 cm, and 60–80% of them exhibit metastasis at diagnosis [28, 31, 32].

The patients often experience marked palliation by aggressive nutritional supplementation, which tends to heal the skin lesions [33]. Somatostatin analog treatment usually, and sometimes dramatically, improves most of the manifestations [28, 34]. In addition, these patients should be considered for prophylactic anticoagulation and/or vena cava filter placement.

Somatostatinoma

Somatostatin is a 14-amino acid polypeptide, with a biologic half life of 2–4 min [12]. Oversecretion by somatostatin-producing tumors results in multisecretory insufficiency and gastrointestinal symptoms, collectively termed the "somatostatinoma syndrome" or "inhibitory syndrome" [35]. The classic triad of the syndrome is hyperglycemia (suppression of insulin release), cholelithiasis (suppression of cholecystokinin release and of gallbladder contractility), and malabsorption (diarrhea or steatorrhea due to suppression of pancreatic exocrine function). Diabetes tends to be mild and can be controlled usually with oral hypoglycemic agents. Gallbladder stones are generally asymptomatic [36]. Additional features include hypochlorhydria, dyspepsia, abdominal pain, weight loss, and anemia. Many patients have only a partial expression of the syndrome, probably due to the short half-life of somatostatin, making it difficult to affect the target tissues via circulation [37, 38].

There are two distinct clinicopathological forms of somatostatinoma: pancreatic and duodenal. Most pancreatic somatostatinomas are located in the head region. The majority of extrapancreatic somatostatinomas are found in the duodenum but they can also occur in the jejunum or biliary tract [38]. Most duodenal tumors are located near the ampulla of Vater and present with obstruction of the bile duct, pancreatitis, or gastrointestinal bleeding (Fig. 14.3). Compared with the pancreatic counterpart, duodenal somatostatinomas are seldom associated with somatostatinoma syndrome [39]. There is a strong association between duodenal somatostatinomas and von Recklinghausen disease. Psammoma bodies (psammomatous calcification) are characteristic histological features of somatostatinomas and are most frequently associated with duodenal tumors [40].

The mean age at diagnosis is 53 years with a slight female preponderance [38]. The diagnosis is established by demonstrating elevated fasting plasma somatostatin levels in patients with a relevant history and the presence of a pancreatic tumor. The majority of somatostatinomas are discovered incidentally during cholecystectomy or in the course of various imaging studies. The average size at the time of diagnosis is 5–6 cm in pancreatic tumors and 2–5 cm in duodenal tumors [39, 41]. In earlier series, nearly 30% of duodenal and 70% of pancreatic somatostatinomas were associated with metastases at presentation [42]. Nonetheless, it has been shown that there is no statistically significant difference in the rate of metastases

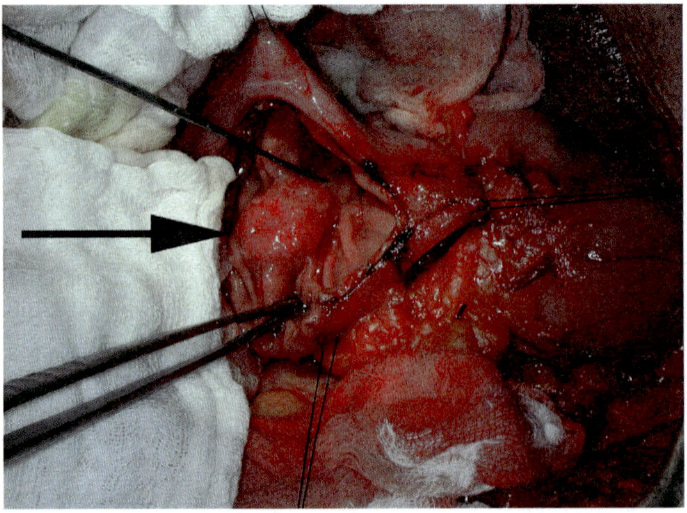

Fig. 14.3 An intraoperative photograph of a typical duodenal somatostatinoma. This tumor is in the second portion of the duodenum adjacent to the ampulla of Vater

and malignancy between the two groups, although sporadic tumors are more frequently malignant than those linked to familial syndromes [40].

PPoma and Non-functioning Neuroendocrine Tumor

PP is a 36-amino acid polypeptide secreted by PP cells. Plasma PP levels are increased in about three quarters of patients with pancreatic neuroendocrine tumors. In general, PP does not appear to cause distinct symptoms, although some patients with PPoma may present with watery diarrhea [43]. There is no evidence suggesting that PPomas and other tumors without elevation of PP levels differ in biological behavior. However, elevated PP levels may be helpful as a monitoring tool.

Nonfunctioning tumors, by definition, are not associated with a hormone-related clinical syndrome. They may be found incidentally or manifest due to symptoms related to local expansion. Significant back pain and cachexia are infrequent. Some patients may complain of vague abdominal pain (35–78%), dyspepsia, anorexia/nausea (45%), or weight loss (20–35%), while others may be totally asymptomatic [20]. In one study, 35% of nonfunctioning tumors were discovered incidentally [44]. Intra-abdominal hemorrhage can occasionally be seen (4–20%). Tumors arising in the pancreatic head or uncinate process may cause obstruction of the common bile duct (17–50%). At an advanced stage these tumors tend to grow into surrounding structures, and may lead to gastrointestinal obstruction or bleeding [43]. Vascular involvement may result in portal hypertension or intestinal ischemia (Fig. 14.4).

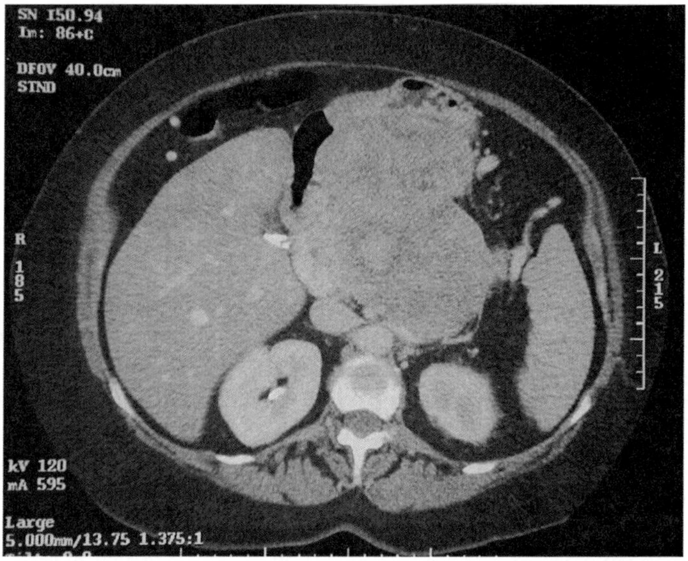

Fig. 14.4 A large non-functional tumor of the pancreas. These tumors can become quite large prior to causing symptoms

The peak incidence of nonfunctioning tumors is during the fifth decade, with an equal gender distribution [20]. Sporadic nonfunctioning tumors are typically solitary. They are commonly located in the pancreatic head (45–60%), but can also be found anywhere within the pancreas. Some authors report that nonfunctioning tumors are larger at detection than functioning tumors, whereas others fail to find a difference in size between the two groups [17, 45, 46]. Most patients (59–80%) present with synchronous liver metastases at diagnosis.

In patients with MEN-1 syndrome, nonfunctioning tumors are currently the most common tumors of the pancreaticoduodenal region [47]. MEN-1-related tumors occur at an earlier age and demonstrate a more benign course than do sporadic tumors. Most frequently, these tumors become symptomatic in the fourth or fifth decade, whereas the biochemical abnormalities often develop in the third decade. Neuroendocrine tumors associated with MEN-1 will be further discussed in Chapter 16.

Diagnosis

Diagnosis is suspected based on the patient's clinical manifestations, laboratory tests, and imaging studies. The biochemical diagnosis is based on peptide hormones and amines released from the neuroendocrine tumors. An accurate analysis of specific markers related to the hormonal syndrome, such as VIP from a VIPoma and glucagon from glucagonoma, is critical to determine the appropriate perioperative management [48]. There are also general tumor markers, including chromogranin A, PP, and neuron-specific enolase. Chromogranin A is considered the best serum marker currently available with the highest specificity (80–100%) [49]. Serial evaluation of chromogranin A is very helpful in the follow-up of neuroendocrine tumors [50].

A multimodality imaging approach is usually exploited to characterize the primary tumor and to determine the extent of the metastatic disease. Determination of functionality is not possible with any of the available imaging methods [51]. Computed tomographic (CT) scan is usually the radiological imaging modality of choice. The characteristic appearance of neuroendocrine tumors is hyperattenuation during early arterial phase of imaging. With magnetic resonance imaging (MRI), neuroendocrine tumors have low signal intensity on T1-weighted fat-suppressed images and high signal intensity on T2-weighted images [52, 53]. T2-weighted images are particularly useful for identifying nodal metastasis because lymph nodes appear bright against the dark background.

In experienced hands, Endoscopic ultrasound (EUS) is probably the most sensitive technique for detecting small pancreatic tumors and regional lymphadenopathy [5, 54]. An additional advantage of EUS is the ability to perform EUS-guided fine needle aspiration (FNA) biopsy. However, it is generally agreed that pancreatic tumors should not be biopsied prior to attempted resection [55]. For patients in whom surgery is not an option and the results of FNA will change the management of the patient, FNA may be undertaken.

High-affinity somatostatin receptors have been identified in most neuroendocrine tumors [51, 56]. Somatostatin receptor scintigraphy (SRS) has emerged as the functional imaging technique of choice with high sensitivity and specificity (90 and 80%, respectively), as well as for the evaluation of receptor status before treatment with somatostatin analogs [51]. The combined use of CT scan (or MRI) and SRS is always recommended because the detection of an unsuspected lesion often alters the management of the patient.

Operative Management

Surgery remains the treatment of choice and must always be considered because complete resection of the tumor is the only chance of cure for neuroendocrine tumors. The goals of operative exploration are: (1) accurate staging, (2) complete resection, and (3) preparation for nonoperative management if complete resection is not feasible [48]. Sometimes demonstration of nodal or liver metastases at operation is the only indication that the bland-appearing resected tumor is malignant. The exploration must be very thorough and meticulous, and must investigate all sites of potential metastasis, in particular locoregional lymph node basins. Intraoperative ultrasound is extremely useful for anatomic staging of the tumor. When an abdominal operation is undertaken, a cholecystectomy should be performed in anticipation of somatostatin analog or embolization therapy.

Neuroendocrine tumors should be removed according to oncological principles. There is a general consensus that curative surgery should also be aimed at metastatic disease, including disease localized to the liver [15]. This may necessitate major resections of the pancreas and adjacent structures, liver resection, or pulmonary metastasectomy in some patients. The 5-year survival of patients treated with hepatic resection, ranging from 47 to 76%, is better than 30–40% in untreated patients [20]. Some authors have advocated organ-preserving surgery for appropriate low-grade carcinomas [14, 57]. The options include enucleation and segmental resections with regional lymphadenectomy. The role of lymphadenectomy is supported by the fact that recurrence-free survival is possible in patients with positive lymph nodes who undergo complete resection [14].

When complete resection is not feasible, palliative resection (debulking) may provide relief from hormonal or local tumor-related symptoms, and theoretically, improve the efficacy of other treatment by decreasing the overall tumor burden. Cytoreductive surgery, following multidisciplinary discussions, should remove at least 90% of the involved tissue to achieve effective symptom control [2]. It may be difficult to justify palliative resection in an asymptomatic patient with metastatic disease. However, in selected, good-risk patients with debilitating symptoms (e.g., pain) or complications (e.g., bleeding or biliary/gastric outlet obstruction), palliative resection may be helpful [58, 59]. The decision to perform debulking surgery should be highly individualized.

Liver-Directed Therapies

The most common cause of death from these tumors is hepatic failure. Virtually all patients with distant metastases have liver metastases. Overall, liver metastasis is the rate-limiting step for survival in patients with neuroendocrine tumors [60]. Locoregional ablative procedures are alternative options in patients who are not candidates for hepatectomy. These interventions have been used mainly in the functioning metastatic tumors to improve symptoms of hypersecretion. There is insufficient evidence to define the role of ablative strategies in nonfunctioning tumors. Radiofrequency ablation (RFA) is usually limited to patients with no more than 8–10 lesions, and a diameter of the lesions below 4 cm. No data exist as to whether RFA has any effect on survival [20].

The metastatic lesions in the liver are typically hypervascular and derive their blood supply mainly from the hepatic artery. Selective embolization alone or in combination with intra-arterial chemotherapy (chemoembolization) is an established procedure for reducing hormonal symptoms as well as liver metastases [61]. In a retrospective study, chemoembolization seemed to be more effective than embolization alone in patients with pancreatic tumors, whereas the addition of intra-arterial chemotherapy did not benefit patients with carcinoid tumors [62].

The procedure is accompanied by a symptomatic response of 50–100%, biochemical response of 22–92%, and tumor volume response of 25–86% [20]. To prevent hormonal crises, preparation with somatostatin analogs is necessary.

Liver transplantation can be an option in patients with metastases confined to the liver. Meta-analysis of 103 patients who underwent liver transplantation for neuroendocrine tumor revealed that the overall 2- and 5-year survival rates are 60 and 47%, respectively, but recurrence-free 5-year survival does not exceed 24% [63]. The small benefit achieved by liver transplantation must be weighed against medical treatment options and the favorable biology of these tumors. It should be regarded as a low-yield intervention [19].

Nonoperative Management

Following complete surgical resection, additional (adjuvant) treatment in the absence of radiographically demonstrable residual disease is not recommended, even if general tumor marks remain elevated. On the other hand, when surgical options are exhausted, medical treatment options may be helpful in patients with unresectable tumors. Treatment is directed at both controlling symptoms of hormone excess and managing tumor growth.

Biotherapy, particularly somatostatin analog therapy, has become increasingly important in the management of neuroendocrine tumors. Many investigators have reported that somatostatin analogs are an effective treatment in the control of symptoms in functioning tumors, especially in patients with VIPomas and glucagonomas [2, 64]. Apart from their potent antisecretory action, there is debate as to whether somatostatin analogs also reduce the tumor size [18, 65, 66]. Clinical observations indicate that they are tumorostatic rather than tumoricidal agents. After months or even years of therapy, most tumors develop resistance. Dose escalation usually becomes ineffective with time. Interferon-α is given for the same indications as somatostatin analogs but has more pronounced side effects. A recent study has shown that the response rate of interferon therapy is comparable to that of somatostatin analogs [18]. The combination of somatostatin analogs and interferon-α does not increase the therapeutic efficacy.

Contrary to biotherapy, several studies suggest that pancreatic neuroendocrine tumors are more responsive to chemotherapy than are carcinoid tumors [67]. Chemotherapy is indicated in progressive tumors after biotherapy has failed. Streptozocin-based combinations remain the standard therapy for well-differentiated tumors [68, 69]. Given the fact that no chemotherapy regimen is curative, the physician must weigh the expected side effects and the patient's life quality against a realistic expectation of efficacy. For poorly-differentiated carcinomas, the cisplatin/etoposide combination has a definite role with a short-lasting response of 40–60% [67]. External irradiation has occasionally been attempted for locally advanced tumors, but most neuroendocrine tumors are relatively radioresistant [19].

Prognosis

The behavior of neuroendocrine tumors is rather heterogeneous, with many exhibiting long periods of slow growth, spontaneous standstill, or even tumor regression, while others show explosive growth and disseminated metastases. The WHO classification using histopathological criteria places these tumors in three risk groups [11]. It can be used reliably to predict the survival of patients with pancreatic neuroendocrine tumors [57, 70, 71]. On the basis of the WHO classification, a tumor node metastasis (TNM) classification and grading systems have been proposed by the European Neuroendocrine Tumor Society (ENETS) [72].

In addition to tumor differentiation, the most important determinant of long-term survival remains the stage of the disease at the time of diagnosis and resectability. Aggressive treatment in selected patients may dramatically improve outcome [57, 73]. Tumor size is often considered an important prognostic factor [4, 20, 74]. Some studies revealed a better outcome in functioning tumors [14, 17], while others found no difference in survival for functioning vs. nonfunctioning tumors [45, 75, 76]. Because of the improved control of hormone excess, the cause of death in patients with functioning tumors is mainly malignant disease. In general, functionality does not affect tumor biology in pancreatic neuroendocrine tumors.

It is unclear whether nodal metastasis has a similar prognostic impact on distant metastasis. Some studies have found that nodal metastases do not influence survival [57, 77], while others found that nodal metastases are a poor prognostic factor [71]. It is believed that lymph node metastases may not negatively affect overall survival, but they may decrease the cure rate [60]. More sophisticated markers, including mitotic rate and proliferative index evaluated by Ki-67, are also important determinants of prognosis and have been incorporated into the WHO classification and ENETS grading systems. Overall, a 5-year survival is reported to be 30–65% [2, 20, 78]. Using the Surveillance Epidemiology and End Results (SEER) data, Fesinmeyer and colleagues found that patients with neuroendocrine cancer have a median survival of 27 months vs. 4 months in patients with exocrine cancer of the pancreas [79].

Summary

Neuroendocrine tumors of the pancreas are uncommon but fascinating tumors. Functioning tumors may be suspected based on the presence of characteristic symptoms and/or syndromes. Incidentally discovered, nonfunctioning tumors are drawing attention with increasing frequency. In contrast to ductal adenocarcinoma, most of the pancreatic neuroendocrine tumors are slow-growing but exhibit varying degrees of malignancy. Long-term survival can be expected in some patients even in the presence of metastases. They are best managed with a customized multimodality approach, addressing both hormonal production and the extent of disease. The only curative treatment is complete resection, but long-term palliation can often be achieved by other means including cytoreductive surgery, locoregional ablation of liver metastases, biotherapy particularly with somatostatin analogs, and chemotherapy. Because of the frequently indolent natural history of these tumors, the expected efficacy of treatment must be weighed against possible adverse effects.

References

1. Barakat MT, Meeran K, Bloom SR (2004) Neuroendocrine tumours. Endocr Relat Cancer 11:1–18
2. O'Toole D, Salazar R, Falconi M, Kaltsas G, Couvelard A, de Herder WW, Hyrdel R, Nikou G, Krenning E, Vullierme MP, Caplin M, Jensen R, Eriksson B (2006) Rare functioning pancreatic endocrine tumors. Neuroendocrinology 84:189–195
3. Yao JC, Eisner MP, Leary C, Dagohoy C, Phan A, Rashid A, Hassan M, Evans DB (2007) Population-based study of islet cell carcinoma. Ann Surg Oncol 14:3492–3500
4. Warner RR (2005) Enteroendocrine tumors other than carcinoid: a review of clinically significant advances. Gastroenterology 128:1668–1684
5. Jani N, Khalid A, Kaushik N, Brody D, Bauer K, Schoedel K, Ohori NP, Moser AJ, Lee K, McGrath K (2008) EUS-guided FNA diagnosis of pancreatic endocrine tumors: new trends identified. Gastrointest Endosc 67:44–50
6. Pearse AG (1969) The cytochemistry and ultrastructure of polypeptide hormone-producing cells of the APUD series and the embryologic, physiologic and pathologic implications of the concept. J Histochem Cytochem 17:303–313
7. Edlund H (2002) Pancreatic organogenesis–developmental mechanisms and implications for therapy. Nat Rev Genet 3:524–532
8. Regitnig P, Spuller E, Denk H (2001) Insulinoma of the pancreas with insular-ductular differentiation in its liver metastasis–indication of a common stem-cell origin of the exocrine and endocrine components. Virchows Arch 438:624–628
9. Heitz PU, Kasper M, Polak JM, Kloppel G (1982) Pancreatic endocrine tumors. Hum Pathol 13:263–271
10. Mansour JC, Chen H (2004) Pancreatic endocrine tumors. J Surg Res 120:139–161
11. Heitz PU, Komminoth P, Perren A et al (2004) Tumors of the endocrine pancreas. In: DeLellis RA, Lloyd RV, Heitz PU, Eng C (eds) World Health Organization Classification of tumors. Pathology and genetics of tumors of endocrine organs. IARC Press, Lyon, pp 175–208
12. Oberg K, Kvols L, Caplin M, Delle Fave G, de Herder W, Rindi G, Ruszniewski P, Woltering EA, Wiedenmann B (2004) Consensus report on the use of somatostatin analogs for the management of neuroendocrine tumors of the gastroenteropancreatic system. Ann Oncol 15:966–973
13. Thompson GB, van Heerden JA, Grant CS, Carney JA, Ilstrup DM (1988) Islet cell carcinomas of the pancreas: a twenty-year experience. Surgery 104:1011–1017
14. Vagefi PA, Razo O, Deshpande V, McGrath DJ, Lauwers GY, Thayer SP, Warshaw AL, Fernandez-Del Castillo C (2007) Evolving patterns in the detection and outcomes of pancreatic neuroendocrine neoplasms: the Massachusetts General Hospital experience from 1977 to 2005. Arch Surg 142:347–354
15. Plockinger U, Rindi G, Arnold R, Eriksson B, Krenning EP, de Herder WW, Goede A, Caplin M, Oberg K, Reubi JC, Nilsson O, Delle Fave G, Ruszniewski P, Ahlman H, Wiedenmann B (2004) Guidelines for the diagnosis and treatment of neuroendocrine gastrointestinal tumours. A consensus statement on behalf of the European Neuroendocrine Tumour Society (ENETS). Neuroendocrinology 80:394–424

16. Ito T, Tanaka M, Sasano H, Osamura YR, Sasaki I, Kimura W, Takano K, Obara T, Ishibashi M, Nakao K, Doi R, Shimatsu A, Nishida T, Komoto I, Hirata Y, Imamura M, Kawabe K, Nakamura K (2007) Preliminary results of a Japanese nationwide survey of neuroendocrine gastrointestinal tumors. J Gastroenterol 42:497–500
17. Phan GQ, Yeo CJ, Hruban RH, Littemoe KD, Pitt HA, Cameron JL (1998) Surgical experience with pancreatic and peripancreatic neuroendocrine tumors: Review of 125 patients. J Gastrointest Surg 2:473–482
18. Faiss S, Pape UF, Bohmig M, Dorffel Y, Mansmann U, Golder W, Riecken EO, Wiedenmann B (2003) Prospective, randomized, multicenter trial on the antiproliferative effect of lanreotide, interferon alfa, and their combination for therapy of metastatic neuroendocrine gastroenteropancreatic tumors – the International Lanreotide and Interferon Alfa Study Group. J Clin Oncol 21:2689–2696
19. Wiedenmann B, Jensen RT, Mignon M, Modlin CI, Skogseid B, Doherty GM, Oberg K (1998) Preoperative diagnosis and surgical management of neuroendocrine gastroenteropancreatic tumors: general recommendations by a consensus workshop. World J Surg 22:309–318
20. Falconi M, Plockinger U, Kwekkeboom DJ, Manfredi R, Korner M, Kvols L, Pape UF, Ricke J, Goretzki PE, Wildi S, Steinmuller T, Oberg K, Scoazec JY (2006) Well-differentiated pancreatic nonfunctioning tumors/carcinoma. Neuroendocrinology 84:196–211
21. Anlauf M, Garbrecht N, Bauersfeld J, Schmitt A, Henopp T, Komminoth P, Heitz PU, Perren A, Kloppel G (2007) Hereditary neuroendocrine tumors of the gastroenteropancreatic system. Virchows Arch 451(Suppl. 1):S29–S38
22. Ghaferi AA, Chojnacki KA, Long WD, Cameron JL, Yeo CJ (2008) Pancreatic VIPomas: subject review and one institutional experience. J Gastrointest Surg 12:382–393
23. Verner JV, Morrison AB (1958) Islet cell tumor and a syndrome of refractory watery diarrhea and hypokalemia. Am J Med 25:374–380
24. Soga J, Yakuwa Y (1998) Vipoma/diarrheogenic syndrome: a statistical evaluation of 241 reported cases. J Exp Clin Cancer Res 17:389–400
25. Kraenzlin ME, Ch'ng JL, Wood SM, Carr DH, Bloom SR (1985) Long-term treatment of a VIPoma with somatostatin analogue resulting in remission of symptoms and possible shrinkage of metastases. Gastroenterology 88:185–187
26. Fanelli CG, Porcellati F, Rossetti P, Bolli GB (2006) Glucagon: the effects of its excess and deficiency on insulin action. Nutr Metab Cardiovasc Dis 16(Suppl. 1):S28–S34
27. Mallinson CN, Bloom SR, Warin AP, Salmon PR, Cox B (1974) A glucagonoma syndrome. Lancet 2:1–5
28. Chastain MA (2001) The glucagonoma syndrome: a review of its features and discussion of new perspectives. Am J Med Sci 321:306–320
29. Almdal TP, Heindorff H, Bardram L, Vilstrup H (1990) Increased amino acid clearance and urea synthesis in a patient with glucagonoma. Gut 31:946–948
30. Stacpoole PW (1981) The glucagonoma syndrome: clinical features, diagnosis, and treatment. Endocr Rev 2:347–361
31. Haga Y, Yanagi H, Urata J, Inada M, Shimada S, Nitahata N, Tanimura M (1995) Early detection of pancreatic glucagonoma. Am J Gastroenterol 90:2216–2223
32. Wermers RA, Fatourechi V, Wynne AG, Kvols LK, Lloyd RV (1996) The glucagonoma syndrome. Clinical and pathologic features in 21 patients. Medicine (Baltimore) 75:53–63
33. Alexander EK, Robinson M, Staniec M, Dluhy RG (2002) Peripheral amino acid and fatty acid infusion for the treatment of necrolytic migratory erythema in the glucagonoma syndrome. Clin Endocrinol (Oxf) 57:827–831
34. Kindmark H, Sundin A, Granberg D, Dunder K, Skogseid B, Janson ET, Welin S, Oberg K, Eriksson B (2007) Endocrine pancreatic tumors with glucagon hypersecretion: a retrospective study of 23 cases during 20 years. Med Oncol 24:330–337
35. Krejs GJ, Orci L, Conlon JM, Ravazzola M, Davis GR, Raskin P, Collins SM, McCarthy DM, Baetens D, Rubenstein A, Aldor TA, Unger RH (1979) Somatostatinoma syndrome. Biochemical, morphologic and clinical features. N Engl J Med 301:285–292

36. Mittendorf EA, Shifrin AL, Inabnet WB, Libutti SK, McHenry CR, Demeure MJ (2006) Islet cell tumors. Curr Probl Surg 43:685–765
37. House MG, Yeo CJ, Schulick RD (2002) Periampullary pancreatic somatostatinoma. Ann Surg Oncol 9:869–874
38. Garbrecht N, Anlauf M, Schmitt A, Henopp T, Sipos B, Raffel A, Eisenberger CF, Knoefel WT, Pavel M, Fottner C, Musholt TJ, Rinke A, Arnold R, Berndt U, Plockinger U, Wiedenmann B, Moch H, Heitz PU, Komminoth P, Perren A, Kloppel G (2008) Somatostatin-producing neuroendocrine tumors of the duodenum and pancreas: incidence, types, biological behavior, association with inherited syndromes, and functional activity. Endocr Relat Cancer 15:229–241
39. Tanaka S, Yamasaki S, Matsushita H, Ozawa Y, Kurosaki A, Takeuchi K, Hoshihara Y, Doi T, Watanabe G, Kawaminami K (2000) Duodenal somatostatinoma: a case report and review of 31 cases with special reference to the relationship between tumor size and metastasis. Pathol Int 50:146–152
40. Soga J, Yakuwa Y (1999) Somatostatinoma/inhibitory syndrome: a statistical evaluation of 173 reported cases as compared to other pancreatic endocrinomas. J Exp Clin Cancer Res 18:13–22
41. Larsson LI, Hirsch MA, Holst JJ, Ingemansson S, Kuhl C, Jensen SL, Lundqvist G, Rehfeld JF, Schwartz TW (1977) Pancreatic somatostatinoma. Clinical features and physiological implications. Lancet 1:666–668
42. Mao C, Shah A, Hanson DJ, Howard JM (1995) Von Recklinghausen's disease associated with duodenal somatostatinoma: contrast of duodenal versus pancreatic somatostatinomas. J Surg Oncol 59:67–73
43. Kouvaraki MA, Solorzano CC, Shapiro SE, Yao JC, Perrier ND, Lee JE, Evans DB (2005) Surgical treatment of non-functioning pancreatic islet cell tumors. J Surg Oncol 89:170–185
44. Gullo L, Migliori M, Falconi M, Pederzoli P, Bettini R, Casadei R, Delle Fave G, Corleto VD, Ceccarelli C, Santini D, Tomassetti P (2003) Nonfunctioning pancreatic endocrine tumors: a multicenter clinical study. Am J Gastroenterol 98:2435–2439
45. White TJ, Edney JA, Thompson JS, Karrer FW, Moor BJ (1994) Is there a prognostic difference between functional and nonfunctional islet cell tumors? Am J Surg 168:627–630
46. Tomassetti P, Campana D, Piscitelli L, Casadei R, Santini D, Nori F, Morselli-Labate AM, Pezzilli R, Corinaldesi R (2005) Endocrine pancreatic tumors: factors correlated with survival. Ann Oncol 16:1806–1810
47. Doherty GM (2003) Multiple endocrine neoplasia type 1: duodenopancreatic tumors. Surg Oncol 12:135–143
48. Doherty GM (2005) Rare endocrine tumours of the GI tract. Best Pract Res Clin Gastroenterol 19:807–817
49. de Herder WW (2007) Biochemistry of neuroendocrine tumours. Best Pract Res Clin Endocrinol Metab 21:33–41
50. Nehar D, Lombard-Bohas C, Olivieri S, Claustrat B, Chayvialle JA, Penes MC, Sassolas G, Borson-Chazot F (2004) Interest of Chromogranin A for diagnosis and follow-up of endocrine tumours. Clin Endocrinol (Oxf) 60:644–652
51. Ricke J, Klose KJ, Mignon M, Oberg K, Wiedenmann B (2001) Standardisation of imaging in neuroendocrine tumours: results of a European delphi process. Eur J Radiol 37:8–17
52. Rha SE, Jung SE, Lee KH, Ku YM, Byun JY, Lee JM (2007) CT and MR imaging findings of endocrine tumor of the pancreas according to WHO classification. Eur J Radiol 62:371–377
53. Rockall AG, Reznek RH (2007) Imaging of neuroendocrine tumours (CT/MR/US). Best Pract Res Clin Endocrinol Metab 21:43–68
54. Rosch T, Lightdale CJ, Botet JF, Boyce GA, Sivak MV Jr, Yasuda K, Heyder N, Palazzo L, Dancygier H, Schusdziarra V et al (1992) Localization of pancreatic endocrine tumors by endoscopic ultrasonography. N Engl J Med 326:1721–1726
55. Goldin SB, Bradner MW, Zervos EE, Rosemurgy AS 2nd (2007) Assessment of pancreatic neoplasms: review of biopsy techniques. J Gastrointest Surg 11:783–790

56. Intenzo CM, Jabbour S, Lin HC, Miller JL, Kim SM, Capuzzi DM, Mitchell EP (2007) Scintigraphic imaging of body neuroendocrine tumors. Radiographics 27:1355–1369
57. Schurr PG, Strate T, Rese K, Kaifi JT, Reichelt U, Petri S, Kleinhans H, Yekebas EF, Izbicki JR (2007) Aggressive surgery improves long-term survival in neuroendocrine pancreatic tumors: an institutional experience. Ann Surg 245:273–281
58. Solorzano CC, Lee JE, Pisters PW, Vauthey JN, Ayers GD, Jean ME, Gagel RF, Ajani JA, Wolff RA, Evans DB (2001) Nonfunctioning islet cell carcinoma of the pancreas: survival results in a contemporary series of 163 patients. Surgery 130:1078–1085
59. McEntee GP, Nagorney DM, Kvols LK, Moertel CG, Grant CS (1990) Cytoreductive hepatic surgery for neuroendocrine tumors. Surgery 108:1091–1096
60. Norton JA (2006) Surgery for primary pancreatic neuroendocrine tumors. J Gastrointest Surg 10:327–331
61. Chamberlain RS, Canes D, Brown KT, Saltz L, Jarnagin W, Fong Y, Blumgart LH (2000) Hepatic neuroendocrine metastases: does intervention alter outcomes? J Am Coll Surg 190:432–445
62. Gupta S, Johnson MM, Murthy R, Ahrar K, Wallace MJ, Madoff DC, McRae SE, Hicks ME, Rao S, Vauthey JN, Ajani JA, Yao JC (2005) Hepatic arterial embolization and chemoembolization for the treatment of patients with metastatic neuroendocrine tumors: variables affecting response rates and survival. Cancer 104:1590–1602
63. Lehnert T (1998) Liver transplantation for metastatic neuroendocrine carcinoma: an analysis of 103 patients. Transplantation 66:1307–1312
64. Maton PN, Gardner JD, Jensen RT (1989) Use of long-acting somatostatin analog SMS 201–995 in patients with pancreatic islet cell tumors. Dig Dis Sci 34:28S–39S
65. Florio T (2008) Molecular mechanisms of the antiproliferative activity of somatostatin receptors (SSTRs) in neuroendocrine tumors. Front Biosci 13:822–840
66. Hejna M, Schmidinger M, Raderer M (2002) The clinical role of somatostatin analogues as antineoplastic agents: much ado about nothing? Ann Oncol 13:653–668
67. Toumpanakis C, Meyer T, Caplin ME (2007) Cytotoxic treatment including embolization/chemoembolization for neuroendocrine tumours. Best Pract Res Clin Endocrinol Metab 21:131–144
68. Kouvaraki MA, Ajani JA, Hoff P, Wolff R, Evans DB, Lozano R, Yao JC (2004) Fluorouracil, doxorubicin, and streptozocin in the treatment of patients with locally advanced and metastatic pancreatic endocrine carcinomas. J Clin Oncol 22:4762–4771
69. Moertel CG, Lefkopoulo M, Lipsitz S, Hahn RG, Klaassen D (1992) Streptozocin-doxorubicin, streptozocin-fluorouracil or chlorozotocin in the treatment of advanced islet-cell carcinoma. N Engl J Med 326:519–523
70. Fischer L, Kleeff J, Esposito I, Hinz U, Zimmermann A, Friess H, Buchler MW (2008) Clinical outcome and long-term survival in 118 consecutive patients with neuroendocrine tumours of the pancreas. Br J Surg 95:627–635
71. Bettini R, Boninsegna L, Mantovani W, Capelli P, Bassi C, Pederzoli P, Delle Fave GF, Panzuto F, Scarpa A, Falconi M (2008) Prognostic factors at diagnosis and value of WHO classification in a mono-institutional series of 180 non-functioning pancreatic endocrine tumours. Ann Oncol 19:903–908
72. Rindi G, Kloppel G, Alhman H, Caplin M, Couvelard A, de Herder WW, Erikssson B, Falchetti A, Falconi M, Komminoth P, Korner M, Lopes JM, McNicol AM, Nilsson O, Perren A, Scarpa A, Scoazec JY, Wiedenmann B (2006) TNM staging of foregut (neuro)endocrine tumors: a consensus proposal including a grading system. Virchows Arch 449:395–401
73. Touzios JG, Kiely JM, Pitt SC, Rilling WS, Quebbeman EJ, Wilson SD, Pitt HA (2005) Neuroendocrine hepatic metastases: does aggressive management improve survival? Ann Surg 241:776–785
74. Ohike N, Morohoshi T (2005) Pathological assessment of pancreatic endocrine tumors for metastatic potential and clinical prognosis. Endocr Pathol 16:33–40
75. Lo CY, van Heerden JA, Thompson GB, Grant CS, Soreide JA, Harmsen WS (1996) Islet cell carcinoma of the pancreas. World J Surg 20:878–884

76. Hochwald SN, Zee S, Conlon KC, Colleoni R, Louie O, Brennan MF, Klimstra DS (2002) Prognostic factors in pancreatic endocrine neoplasms: an analysis of 136 cases with a proposal for low-grade and intermediate-grade groups. J Clin Oncol 20:2633–2642
77. Kazanjian KK, Reber HA, Hines OJ (2006) Resection of pancreatic neuroendocrine tumors: results of 70 cases. Arch Surg 141:765–770
78. Lepage C, Rachet B, Coleman MP (2007) Survival from malignant digestive endocrine tumors in England and Wales: a population-based study. Gastroenterology 132:899–904
79. Fesinmeyer MD, Austin MA, Li CI, De Roos AJ, Bowen DJ (2005) Differences in survival by histologic type of pancreatic cancer. Cancer Epidemiol Biomarkers Prev 14:1766–1773

Part V
Multiple Endocrine Neoplasia

Chapter 15
The Menin Gene

Hsin-Chieh Jennifer Shen and Steven K. Libutti

Introduction

Multiple endocrine neoplasia type 1 (MEN-1; OMIM# 131100) is inherited as a dominant syndrome caused by mutations in the *MEN-1* tumor suppressor gene [1, 2]. MEN-1 patients are predisposed to develop multiple endocrine tumors, primarily affecting parathyroid, anterior pituitary, endocrine pancreas, and adrenal cortex. Some patients might also develop nonhormonal manifestations, such as carcinoid tumors, facial angiofibromas, meningiomas, smooth muscle tumors, collagenomas, and lipomas. More than 95% of MEN-1 patients develop clinical symptoms of the disorder by the fifth decade [3, 4]; however, the earliest occurrence has been reported at as early as 5 years of age [5]. Most MEN-1-associated tumors are non-metastatic but clinical manifestations are generally related to overproduction of hormones, such as parathyroid hormone, insulin, glucagon, prolactin, or adrenocorticotropic hormone [4, 6]. In the absence of medical intervention, MEN-1 tumors can lead to early mortality in patients.

The *MEN-1* Gene

History and Cloning

On the basis of the linkage analysis of MEN-1 families and studies on the loss of heterozygosity (LOH) in MEN-1 tumors, the causative gene for the MEN-1 syndrome was narrowed down to a location on the chromosome region 11q13, and proposed to function as a tumor-suppressor gene following Knudson's two-hit

S.K. Libutti (✉)
Professor of Surgery, Vice Chairman, Department of Surgery;
Director, Montefiore-Einstein Center for Cancer Care.Bronx, NY USA
e-mail: slibutti@montefiore.org

C. Sturgeon (ed.), *Endocrine Neoplasia*, Cancer Treatment and Research, vol 153,
DOI 10.1007/978-1-4419-0857-5_15, © Springer Science+Business Media, LLC 2010

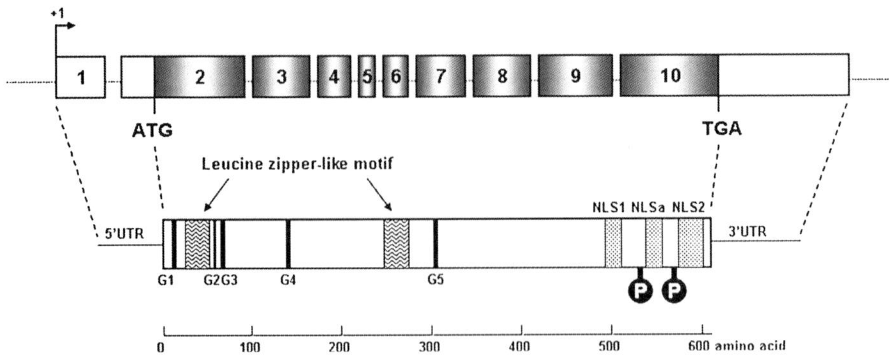

Fig. 15.1 Schematic representations of the human *MEN-1* genomic structure (top) and its encoded menin protein (bottom). The *MEN-1* gene contains 10 exons and encodes 610-amino acid protein. The transcriptional start site (+1) in exon 1, start codon (ATG) in exon 2, and stop codon (TGA) in exon 10 are as shown. The untranslated region in exon 1 and 5′ part of exon 2 (5′-UTR), and 3′ part of exon 10 (3′-UTR) are indicated by open boxes. The 1.83 kb coding region from exon 2 to exon 10 is denoted by shaded boxes. At the *N*-terminus, two leucine zipper-like motifs are as shown, and five consensus sequences for guanosine triphosphatase (GTPase) motifs are shown as G1–G5. At the *C*-terminus, three nuclear localization sequences (NLS) at codons 479-497 (NLS1), 546–572 (NLSa), and 588–608 (NLS2), and two phosphorylation sites (Ser543 and Ser 583) are as indicated

hypothesis [7, 8]. It was not until 1997 that the *MEN-1* gene was positionally cloned by two different groups [1, 2]. The *MEN-1* gene consists of 10 exons that span more than 9 kb of genomic DNA (Fig. 15.1). The first exon of the *MEN-1* gene is noncoding and constitutes a majority of the 5′-UTR region. The predominant transcript of the *MEN-1* gene is a 2.8 kb mRNA, which encodes a 610-amino acid, 68-kD novel protein termed menin.

The *MEN-1* homologues in other species have been identified for mouse, rat, zebrafish, and *Drosophila melanogaster* [9–11]; however, orthologs in yeast *S. cerevisiae* and round worm *C. elegans* have not been reported. Comparison of the mammalian menin amino acid sequences has revealed a high level of evolutionary conservation, as mouse and rat menin proteins share 96.7% and 97.2% identity with their human counterpart [12]. To date, three nuclear localization signals (NLSs, all transcribed from exon 10), NLS1, NLS2, and NLSa, are known for the *MEN-1* gene [13]. High similarity between the NLS1 and NLS2 is shared among the human, rat, mouse, zebrafish NLSs, confirming the significance of these evolutionarily conserved residues [12].

MEN-1 Mutations: Germline Vs. Somatic

In the first 10 years since the *MEN-1* gene was cloned, a wealth of *MEN-1* mutations have been identified in patients with germline and somatic *MEN-1* mutations. Detailed analyses utilizing the NCBI public database indicates that a total of 459 germline mutations and 167 somatic mutations have been reported for the *MEN-1* gene in the literature thus far [14]. A total of 565 different *MEN-1* mutations are determined since 61 of the mutations occur in both germline and somatic mutations. Following Knudson's two-hit hypothesis for a tumor suppressor gene, MEN-1 patients inherit the germline *MEN-1* mutation and harbor point mutations or a somatic LOH involving chromosome 11q13. In addition, the *MEN-1* gene has been implicated in tumorigenesis of 5–50% of sporadic endocrine tumors due to LOH on chromosome 11q13 in these tumors.

Germline mutations have been identified in 70–90% of typical MEN-1 families, and these mutations are found to be scattered throughout the entire coding region and splice sites of the *MEN-1* gene. While a majority of these germline mutations are frameshift deletions/insertions (41%), nonsense (23%), and missense (20%) mutations, splice site (9%), in-frame deletions/insertions (6%), whole or partial gene deletions (1%) all have been reported. Potential mutational hot spots were proposed since several mutations were found to occur in unrelated kindreds [14]. In studies reporting the lack of identifiable mutations in apparent MEN-1 patients, the mutations may reside in the promoter, untranslated region, or intron sequence, which are outside the tested open reading frame of the *MEN-1* gene [1, 2, 15–19]. To date, it has been difficult to establish a clear genotype-phenotype correlation in familial MEN-1 patients.

Among the somatic *MEN-1* mutations identified for nonhereditary patients, 40% are frameshift deletions/insertions, 29% are missense mutations, 18% are nonsense mutations, 7% are splice-site mutations, and 6% are in-frame deletions/insertions [14]. Sporadic tumors with high frequencies of *MEN-1* mutations include glucagonoma (~60%) [20], gastrinoma (~40%) [1, 21, 22], bronchial carcinoid tumors (~35%) [23–25], lipoma (~30%) [26], parathyroid adenoma (~20%) [21, 23, 27–30], and insulinoma (~15%) [1, 21, 31]. Tumors with lower *MEN-1* mutation frequencies include angiofibroma (~10%) and anterior pituitary adenoma (<5%) [32–34]. Similar to patients with germline MEN-1 mutations, no clear pattern of somatic mutation is associated with a particular tumor type or stage. Thus, *MEN-1* mutation testing of tumors is not used clinically since it has no implication in tumor type, stage, or aggressiveness.

Transcriptional Regulation of the MEN-1 gene

Little is known about how the *MEN-1* gene is transcriptionally regulated. The general promoter structure of the human *MEN-1* gene and the mouse *Men-1* gene appears similar, and contains an identical transcriptional start site [35]. The immediate upstream sequence is conserved between human and mouse by 60%, and exhibits promoter activity. Functional analysis of promoter regions in endocrine and non-endocrine cells indicated that the *MEN-1* gene is differentially regulated depending on the cellular context, and by the intracellular levels of the menin protein itself [35, 36].

Gene Expression

On the basis of the analyses of Northern, Western, and in situ hybridization techniques, expression of *MEN-1* appears to be ubiquitous despite the fact that the loss of the *MEN-1* gene results in tumorigenesis, primarily in endocrine tissues. Studies in human and rodent models demonstrate that *MEN-1* is expressed widely in adult and fetal tissues, including liver, brain, pancreas, spleen, heart, lung, testis, kidney, and in many fetal human tissue extracts [1, 9, 37, 38]. The ubiquitous expression of *MEN-1* does not appear to alter significantly at different stages of the cell cycle [10, 39], although transient decreases in the *MEN-1* expression levels have been reported at the G1/S phase [40, 41]. Quantitative PCR analysis suggested higher *MEN-1* expression in certain tissues and at different stages of development [11, 40]; however, these patterns of expression do not explain the endocrine-restrictive nature of the MEN-1 syndrome.

The Menin Protein

The protein product of the *MEN-1* gene, menin, is highly conserved among species; however, it does not display significant homology to any previously known family of proteins. Menin has been described predominantly as a nuclear protein based on identification of multiple NLSs at the *C*-terminus and menin's interaction with numerous nuclear proteins. Menin also contains five putative sequence motifs characteristic of guanosine triphosphatase (GTPase) or GTP-binding proteins, and two leucine zipper-like motifs within the *N*-terminus region. Two phosphorylation sites at serine residues (Ser543 and Ser583) for menin have also been reported (Fig. 15.1). Identification of these functional domains has not uncovered menin's role as a tumor suppressor in the MEN-1 syndrome. (Table 15.1)

Interactions with Transcriptional Regulators

In transcriptional regulation, JunD was the first protein to be recognized to interact with menin, and has been studied in great detail [42, 43]. JunD belongs to the family of activator protein 1 (AP1) transcription factors, which consists of Jun (cJun, JunB, and JunD) and Fos (c-Foc, FocB, Fra1, and Fra2) proteins. AP1 transcription factors are mediators of cellular pathways that involve tumorigenesis, differentiation, apoptosis, and immune response [44, 45]. Various techniques have demonstrated that menin directly binds to JunD, but not to the other Jun-Fos family members [42, 43]. Interaction between menin and JunD is shown to suppress the Jun-mediated transcriptional activation. Since "free" JunD protein is considered a growth promoter and menin is a tumor suppressor, menin-JunD interaction appears to reverse the effect of JunD on cell growth, forming a growth repressor complex [46, 47]. Menin's ability to repress JunD-activated transcription has also been attributed to the association between menin and Sin3A-histone deacetylase (HDAC) complex

Table 15.1 Menin-interacting proteins and proposed functions

Interacting proteins	Functions	References
Nuclear		
JunD	Transcriptional Regulation	[42, 43]
Sin3A and HDAC	Transcriptional Regulation	[48]
Smad1, Smad5, Runx2	Transcriptional Regulation	[87]
MLL histone methyltransferase	Transcriptional Regulation	[55, 70]
LEDGF	Transcriptional Regulation	[57]
ERα	Transcriptional Regulation	[58]
Pem	Transcriptional Regulation	[88]
RPA2	DNA replication and repair	[59]
FANCD2	DNA processing and repair	[60]
ASK	Cell cycle control	[61]
CHES1 (FOXN3)	DNA damage response	[89]
Double-stranded DNA	DNA stability	[66]
Cytoplasmic		
NMMHC IIA	Cytoskeletal organization	[64]
GFAP and Vimentin	Cytoskeletal organization, cell division	[65]
Nuclear and Cytoplasmic		
NF-kB (p50, p52, p65)	Transcriptional Regulation	[49]
Smad3	Transcriptional Regulation	[50]
Nm23	GTPase activity	[62]
Hsp70 and CHIP[a]	Protein degradation	[90]

[a]Interacting partners for mutant menin protein

[48]. Similar to menin's interaction with JunD, menin binds to p50, p52, and p65 of the nuclear factor κB (NF-κB) family, and acts as an inhibitor of p65-mediated transcriptional activation on NF-κB sites [49]. Members of the NF-κB family are major regulators of the cellular response to stress.

Menin has also been shown to interact with members of the Smad family in transforming the growth factor β (TGF-β) and bone morphogenic protein 2 (BMP-2) signaling pathways [50, 51]. TGF-β signaling is complex: it affects tumor cell invasion and metastasis, and has been shown to stimulate tumorigenesis but causes growth inhibition in normal cells [52, 53]. BMP signaling plays a critical role in heart, neural, and cartilage development, and postnatal bone formation. Menin interacts with Smad3 physically, and antisense inactivation of menin is shown to suppress Smad3/4-DNA binding, resulting in inhibition of TGF-β-induced, Smad3-mediated transcriptional activity. Thus, impaired TGF-β signaling might disrupt cellular homeostasis and push cells toward inappropriate growth and proliferation [50]. Similarly, direct association between menin and Smad1/5 has been reported, and menin inactivation inhibits BMP-2-induced transcriptional activity in Smad1/5. Menin also binds to Runx2, or cbfa1, in uncommitted mesenchymal stem cells, but not in well-differentiated osteoblasts [51, 54]. Together, these data suggest that menin might be involved in different stages of osteoblast differentiation during bone development.

Menin has been suggested to regulate transcription at a genomic level because it was identified as an integral part of histone methyltransferase complexes. Together with proteins from the mixed-lineage leukemia (MLL) and trithorax family, menin-MLL complexes can methylate the lysine 4 residue of histone H3 (H3K4), an epigenetic mark associated with transcriptionally active chromatin [55, 56]. More recently, lens epithelium-derived growth factor (LEDGF) is shown to critically associate with menin-MLL complexes to explain both the oncogenic and tumor suppressor functions of this large protein [57]. Direct interaction between menin and estrogen nuclear receptor (ERα) has also been reported, linking estrogen receptor activation to histone H3K4 trimethylation [58].

Interactions with Proteins to Regulate Genome Stability, Cell Cycle and Division

A role for menin in maintaining genome stability has been suggested based on its interaction with the 32 kDa subunit of replication protein A (RPA2), and the Fanconi anemia complementation group D2 (FANCD2) proteins. RPA2 is a heterotrimeric protein required for DNA replication, recombination, and repair [59]; whereas FANCD2 is involved in the repair of DNA damage [60]. Mutations in the *FANCD2* gene can lead to one subtype of Fanconi anemia, an inherited cancer-prone genetic disease associated with bone marrow failure and predisposition to acute myeloid leukemia.

Menin has also been implicated in cell cycle control as it interacts with activator of S-phase kinase (ASK) and rat nm23β. ASK is a component of the Cdc7/ASK kinase complex, and ASK-induced cell proliferation can be completely repressed by specific interaction between menin and ASK [61]. Nm23β is a putative tumor metastasis suppressor and nucleoside diphosphate kinase, which induces guanosine triphosphate (GTPase) activity [62]. Notably, menin contains five GTPase sequence motifs although menin alone exhibits no detectable GTPase activity, and shows low affinity binding to GTP/GDP [63]. However, menin effectively hydrolyzes GTP to GDP in the presence of nm23, suggesting menin is an atypical GTPase mediated by nm23.

Menin has been shown to mediate cell division as it associates with cytoskeleton proteins, such as non-muscle myosin-type II-A heavy chain (NMMHC IIA) and type III intermediate filament (IF) proteins. Co-localization of menin with NMMHC IIA implicates menin in mediating cytokinesis and cell shape during cell division [64]. Menin's association with IF proteins, glial fibrillary acidic protein (GFAP), and vimentin, suggest that this interaction may control nuclear transport of menin, and serve as a sequestering network for menin at the S-G2 phase of the cell cycle [65].

Menin Target Genes

Menin does not have any recognizable DNA binding motifs, and data are inconsistent as to whether menin can directly bind to DNA, and whether it binds in a sequence-specific manner [12, 66]. However, most of the menin-interacting proteins indicate menin's role in regulating gene transcription. Even if menin is not physically bound to a specific gene promoter, menin must have effects on the regulation of gene transcription that specify normal and tumor processes.

In cooperative interaction with MLL proteins, menin associates directly with the promoters of cyclin-dependent kinase (cdk) inhibitors, p27 and p18, resulting in an increase in histone H3K4 trimethylation on these promoters [67, 68]. Phenotypes observed in p27 and p18 double knockout mice further support menin in regulating these cdk inhibitors, as these mice develop a spectrum of endocrine tumors resembling those observed in the MEN-1 syndromes [69]. However, mice with individual knockout of p27 or p18 do not display these lesions, suggesting that these cdk inhibitors cooperatively serve as essential growth regulators in endocrine cells.

As part of the MLL nuclear protein complex, menin has also been shown to regulate homeobox (*HOX*) gene expression in leukemogenesis. *HOXA7*, *HOXA9*, and *HOXA10* are shown to be direct targets for menin in human HeLa cells or leukemia cells [56, 70]. Menin also positively regulates *Hoxc8* in mouse embryonic fibroblast (MEF) cells [55], and directly activates *Hoxa9* in mouse bone marrow cells [71]. Importantly, a genome-wide analysis of menin binding demonstrates that menin occupies intergenic and intragenic portions of *HOX* gene clusters in HeLa cells, confirming *HOX* as a class of menin target genes [72]. Expression studies utilizing MEN-1 tumors further suggest that menin might be a positive or negative regulator for *HOX* gene transcription depending on cellular context [73].

Independent from being part of the histone transferase complex, menin also targets a broad range of promoters in multiple tissues, implicating menin in maintaining stable gene expression by interacting with currently unknown proteins [72]. For instance, menin is shown to suppress endogenous insulin-like growth factor binding protein 2 (IGFBP-2) via alteration of the chromatin structure surrounding the *IGFBP-2* gene promoter [74]. By binding to the 5′-UTR of the caspase 8 locus, menin can activate caspase 8 and TNF-α-mediated apoptosis, suggesting that menin might suppresses MEN-1 tumorigenesis by upregulating caspase 8 expression [75, 76]. In summary, unraveling functional domains and target genes of menin has proven to be informative; yet, these studies have clearly demonstrated that the functions of menin are more complicated than was assumed based on its role as a tumor suppressor gene in the MEN-1 syndrome.

Animal Models of MEN-1 Tumorigenesis

Men-1 Knockout Mice

To better understand menin's role in MEN-1 tumorigenesis, several mouse models of MEN-1 have been generated through homologous recombination, as well as utilizing the Cre-LoxP system to generate tissue-specific knockouts of the *Men-1* gene (Table 15.2). The human *MEN-1* and mouse *Men-1* genes share highly conserved genomic structures and sequences at both nucleotide (89% identity) and amino acid (97% identity) levels; thus, allowing the development of animal models to investigate

Table 15.2 Genetically engineered MEN-1 mouse models

Reference	Background strain	Deleted exons	Model name	Tumor types
Crabtree JS, 2001 [78]	NIH Black Swiss	Exon 3-8	Men-1 tsm/tsm	Resorbed by E14.5
	129Sv/EvTacFBR		Men-1 tsm/+	Pancreatic islet cell tumor Parathyroid adenoma Pituitary adenoma Adrenal cortical carcinoma Bilateral pheochromocytoma Lung adenocarcinoma
			Men-1 ΔN3-8/ΔN3-8	Resorbed between E10.5-11.5
			Men-1 ΔN3-8/+	Pancreatic islet cell tumor
Bertolino P, 2003 [77]	129/Ola/Sv	Exon 3	Men-1 T/T	Resorbed between E11.5-13.5
			Men-1 +/T	Pancreatic islet tumor Parathyroid adenoma Pituitary adenoma/ carcinoma Adrenal gland adenoma/carcinoma Testis Leydig cell tumor Sex-cord stromal cell tumor Gastrinoma
Loffler KA, 2006 [80]	C57/129	Exon 2	Men-1 +/–	Pancreatic islet adenoma Parathyroid adenoma Pituitary adenoma Adrenal adenoma Testis Leydig cell tumor Sex-cord stromal cell tumor Thyroid tumor
Crabtress JS, 2003 [84]	B6/FVB/129Sv	Exon 3-8	Men-1 ΔN/ΔN;RIP2-Cre	Pancreatic islet cell tumor Pituitary adenoma
Bertolino P, 2003 [82]	NA	Exon 3	Men-1 F/F;Rip-Cre	Insulinoma
Biondi CA, 2004 [83]	C57BL/6J	Exon 2	Men-1 loxP/ loxP;Rip-Cre	Pancreatic insulinoma Prolactinoma
Libutti SK, 2003 [81]	FVB/129SvEvTac	Exon 3-8	Men-1 dN/ dN;PTH-Cre	Parathyroid neoplasia
Scacheri PC, 2004 [85]	FVB/N/129Sv	Exon 3-8	Men-1 loxP/ loxP;alb-cre	No tumor phenotype in liver pancreatic islet cell tumor due to leakiness of cre

basic functions of menin [9, 38]. Two studies, either deletion of exon 3 or exon 3–8 of the *Men-1* gene [77, 78], demonstrated that homozygous inactivation of both *Men-1* alleles resulted in embryonic lethality. These embryos appeared normal at E9.5, but were developmentally delayed and smaller than control genotype littermates at E11.5–12.5. Craniofacial abnormalities, failure to close the neural tube, myocardial hypotrophy, abnormal liver organization, and enhanced apoptosis were some of the phenotypes observed in menin-null fetuses, which were resorbed by E14.5 [78, 79]. Together, these reports suggest that menin is essential for the development of multiple organs during embryogenesis.

Heterozygous mice with one wild-type copy of the *Men-1* allele gestated and developed normally [77, 78, 80]. However, after the age of 9 months, they developed endocrine tumors commonly seen in human MEN-1 patients, including parathyroid adenoma, pancreatic insulinoma, and pituitary prolactinoma. While parathyroid adenoma was not associated with hypercalcemia, mice developing pancreatic islet cell tumors were found to have elevated serum insulin levels [77, 78]. Similar to tumors developed in MEN-1 patients, these tumors heterozygous for the *Men-1* allele exhibited loss of the remaining wild-type *Men-1* allele, further supporting MEN-1 as a tumor suppressor in these endocrine organs.

Conditional Inactivation of Men-1

Due to the fact that biallelic loss of the *Men-1* gene led to embryonic lethality, tissue-specific knockout of *Men-1* was generated utilizing the Cre-LoxP system to allow analysis of menin deficiency in adult mice. Mice with homozygous inactivation of *Men-1* in parathyroid were characterized by hypercalcemia and parathyroid neoplasia by as early as 7 months of age [81]. Homozygous deletion of the *Men-1* alleles in pancreatic islet beta cells led to the development of beta-cell hyperplasia at 2–5 months of age, which progress to pancreatic islet insulinomas by 12 months of age [82–84]. These pancreatic multiple insulinomas were physiologically coupled with elevated serum insulin levels and reduction in blood glucose levels. In two of these three reports on beta-cell specific loss of *Men-1*, mice also developed anterior pituitary tumors at maturity due to leakiness of the Rip-Cre transgene [83]. In summary, generation of conditional homozygous inactivation of *Men-1* succeeded in bypassing embryonic lethality observed in the total knockout of *Men-1*. Not only do these mouse models recapitulate different aspects of the human MEN-1 syndrome, they also demonstrate that menin is not required for the development of parathyroid, endocrine pancreas, and pituitary gland during embryogenesis.

On the basis of MEN-1 human patients and mouse models, *MEN-1* appears to act as a tumor suppressor gene only in the endocrine context. Mice, deficient of menin in liver hepatocytes, have no effects on liver development and function [85]. Homozygous loss of *Men-1* in pancreatic exocrine cells also results in a normal and functional exocrine pancreas [86]. Together these reports indicate that biallelic loss of *Men-1* is insufficient to cause tumorigenesis in every tissue.

The prevailing hypothesis to explain the endocrine restrictive nature of the MEN1 syndrome has been the proposal of cell- or tissue-specific cofactors for menin. Physical interaction among the nuclear protein, menin, and its cell-specific cofactors are thought to regulate gene expression only in tissue affected by MEN-1. However, it is also possible that protective mechanisms or redundant tumor suppressor systems exist in tissues unaffected by the loss of menin. Finally, menin may play completely distinct roles in different cell types, and in normal differentiation versus tumorigenesis.

Prospects and Future Directions

Identification of the *MEN-1* gene and menin-interacting partners has led to the rapid progress in elucidating the functional roles of *MEN-1* in normal tissues and during tumorigenesis. While the examples of menin-regulating transcription, genomic stability, and cell proliferation have provided molecular clues for menin's function, much is yet to be learned about the endocrine-based feature of the MEN-1 syndrome. Comparative evaluation of human MEN-1 tumors and mouse models of MEN-1 may facilitate the understanding of menin's molecular mechanisms of actions in endocrine tumorigenesis. Together, continued efforts to address molecular, physiological, and pathological roles of menin are crucial to the development of effective therapies for patients with the MEN-1 syndrome.

References

1. Zhuang Z, Vortmeyer AO, Pack S et al (1997) Somatic mutations of the MEN1 tumor suppressor gene in sporadic gastrinomas and insulinomas. Cancer Res 57:4682–4686
2. Lemmens I, Van de Ven WJ, Kas K et al (1997) Identification of the multiple endocrine neoplasia type 1 (MEN1) gene. The European Consortium on MEN1. Hum Mol Genet 6:1177–1183
3. Marx S, Spiegel AM, Skarulis MC, Doppman JL, Collins FS, Liotta LA (1998) Multiple endocrine neoplasia type 1: clinical and genetic topics. Ann Intern Med 129:484–494
4. Trump D, Farren B, Wooding C et al (1996) Clinical studies of multiple endocrine neoplasia type 1 (MEN1). Qjm 89:653–669
5. Stratakis CA, Schussheim DH, Freedman SM et al (2000) Pituitary macroadenoma in a 5-year-old: an early expression of multiple endocrine neoplasia type 1. J Clin Endocrinol Metab 85:4776–4780
6. Schussheim DH, Skarulis MC, Agarwal SK et al (2001) Multiple endocrine neoplasia type 1: new clinical and basic findings. Trends Endocrinol Metab 12:173–178
7. Larsson C, Skogseid B, Oberg K, Nakamura Y, Nordenskjold M (1988) Multiple endocrine neoplasia type 1 gene maps to chromosome 11 and is lost in insulinoma. Nature 332:85–87
8. Knudson AG (1996) Hereditary cancer: two hits revisited. J Cancer Res Clin Oncol 122: 135–140
9. Guru SC, Crabtree JS, Brown KD et al (1999) Isolation, genomic organization, and expression analysis of Men1, the murine homolog of the MEN1 gene. Mamm Genome 10:592–596

10. Guru SC, Prasad NB, Shin EJ et al (2001) Characterization of a MEN1 ortholog from Drosophila melanogaster. Gene 263:31–38
11. Manickam P, Vogel AM, Agarwal SK et al (2000) Isolation, characterization, expression and functional analysis of the zebrafish ortholog of MEN1. Mamm Genome 11:448–454
12. Chandrasekharappa SC, Teh BT (2003) Functional studies of the MEN1 gene. J Intern Med 253:606–615
13. La P, Desmond A, Hou Z, Silva AC, Schnepp RW, Hua X (2006) Tumor suppressor menin: the essential role of nuclear localization signal domains in coordinating gene expression. Oncogene 25:3537–3546
14. Lemos MC, Thakker RV (2008) Multiple endocrine neoplasia type 1 (MEN1): analysis of 1336 mutations reported in the first decade following identification of the gene. Hum Mutat 29:22–32
15. Agarwal SK, Kester MB, Debelenko LV et al (1997) Germline mutations of the MEN1 gene in familial multiple endocrine neoplasia type 1 and related states. Hum Mol Genet 6:1169–1175
16. Bassett JH, Forbes SA, Pannett AA et al (1998) Characterization of mutations in patients with multiple endocrine neoplasia type 1. Am J Hum Genet 62:232–244
17. Giraud S, Choplin H, Teh BT et al (1997) A large multiple endocrine neoplasia type 1 family with clinical expression suggestive of anticipation. J Clin Endocrinol Metab 82:3487–3492
18. Pannett AA, Thakker RV (1999) Multiple endocrine neoplasia type 1. Endocr Relat Cancer 6:449–473
19. Teh BT, Kytola S, Farnebo F et al (1998) Mutation analysis of the MEN1 gene in multiple endocrine neoplasia type 1, familial acromegaly and familial isolated hyperparathyroidism. J Clin Endocrinol Metab 83:2621–2626
20. Hessman O, Lindberg D, Skogseid B et al (1998) Mutation of the multiple endocrine neoplasia type 1 gene in nonfamilial, malignant tumors of the endocrine pancreas. Cancer Res 58:377–379
21. Shan L, Nakamura Y, Nakamura M et al (1998) Somatic mutations of multiple endocrine neoplasia type 1 gene in the sporadic endocrine tumors. Lab Invest 78:471–475
22. Wang EH, Ebrahimi SA, Wu AY, Kashefi C, Passaro E Jr, Sawicki MP (1998) Mutation of the MENIN gene in sporadic pancreatic endocrine tumors. Cancer Res 58:4417–4420
23. Heppner C, Kester MB, Agarwal SK et al (1997) Somatic mutation of the MEN1 gene in parathyroid tumours. Nat Genet 16:375–378
24. Fujii T, Kawai T, Saito K et al (1999) MEN1 gene mutations in sporadic neuroendocrine tumors of foregut derivation. Pathol Int 49:968–973
25. Gortz B, Roth J, Krahenmann A et al (1999) Mutations and allelic deletions of the MEN1 gene are associated with a subset of sporadic endocrine pancreatic and neuroendocrine tumors and not restricted to foregut neoplasms. Am J Pathol 154:429–436
26. Vortmeyer AO, Boni R, Pak E, Pack S, Zhuang Z (1998) Multiple endocrine neoplasia 1 gene alterations in MEN1-associated and sporadic lipomas. J Natl Cancer Inst 90:398–399
27. Carling T, Correa P, Hessman O et al (1998) Parathyroid MEN1 gene mutations in relation to clinical characteristics of nonfamilial primary hyperparathyroidism. J Clin Endocrinol Metab 83:2960–2963
28. Farnebo F, Teh BT, Kytola S et al (1998) Alterations of the MEN1 gene in sporadic parathyroid tumors. J Clin Endocrinol Metab 83:2627–2630
29. Ludwig L, Schleithoff L, Kessler H, Wagner PK, Boehm BO, Karges W (1999) Loss of wild-type MEN1 gene expression in multiple endocrine neoplasia type 1-associated parathyroid adenoma. Endocr J 46:539–544
30. Pannett AA, Thakker RV (2001) Somatic mutations in MEN type 1 tumors, consistent with the Knudson "two-hit" hypothesis. J Clin Endocrinol Metab 86:4371–4374
31. Cupisti K, Hoppner W, Dotzenrath C et al (2000) Lack of MEN1 gene mutations in 27 sporadic insulinomas. Eur J Clin Invest 30:325–329
32. Tanaka C, Kimura T, Yang P et al (1998) Analysis of loss of heterozygosity on chromosome 11 and infrequent inactivation of the MEN1 gene in sporadic pituitary adenomas. J Clin Endocrinol Metab 83:2631–2634

33. Zhuang Z, Ezzat SZ, Vortmeyer AO et al (1997) Mutations of the MEN1 tumor suppressor gene in pituitary tumors. Cancer Res 57:5446–5451
34. Prezant TR, Levine J, Melmed S (1998) Molecular characterization of the men1 tumor suppressor gene in sporadic pituitary tumors. J Clin Endocrinol Metab 83:1388–1391
35. Zablewska B, Bylund L, Mandic SA, Fromaget M, Gaudray P, Weber G (2003) Transcription regulation of the multiple endocrine neoplasia type 1 gene in human and mouse. J Clin Endocrinol Metab 88:3845–3851
36. Fromaget M, Vercherat C, Zhang CX et al (2003) Functional characterization of a promoter region in the human MEN1 tumor suppressor gene. J Mol Biol 333:87–102
37. Stewart C, Parente F, Piehl F et al (1998) Characterization of the mouse Men1 gene and its expression during development. Oncogene 17:2485–2493
38. Bassett JH, Rashbass P, Harding B, Forbes SA, Pannett AA, Thakker RV (1999) Studies of the murine homolog of the multiple endocrine neoplasia type 1 (MEN1) gene, men1. J Bone Miner Res 14:3–10
39. Wautot V, Khodaei S, Frappart L et al (2000) Expression analysis of endogenous menin, the product of the multiple endocrine neoplasia type 1 gene, in cell lines and human tissues. Int J Cancer 85:877–881
40. Ikeo Y, Sakurai A, Suzuki R et al (2000) Proliferation-associated expression of the MEN1 gene as revealed by in situ hybridization: possible role of the menin as a negative regulator of cell proliferation under DNA damage. Lab Invest 80:797–804
41. Kaji H, Canaff L, Goltzman D, Hendy GN (1999) Cell cycle regulation of menin expression. Cancer Res 59:5097–5101
42. Agarwal SK, Guru SC, Heppner C et al (1999) Menin interacts with the AP1 transcription factor JunD and represses JunD-activated transcription. Cell 96:143–152
43. Gobl AE, Berg M, Lopez-Egido JR, Oberg K, Skogseid B, Westin G (1999) Menin represses JunD-activated transcription by a histone deacetylase-dependent mechanism. Biochim Biophys Acta 1447:51–56
44. Jochum W, Passegue E, Wagner EF (2001) AP-1 in mouse development and tumorigenesis. Oncogene 20:2401–2412
45. Mechta-Grigoriou F, Gerald D, Yaniv M (2001) The mammalian Jun proteins: redundancy and specificity. Oncogene 20:2378–2389
46. Agarwal SK, Novotny EA, Crabtree JS et al (2003) Transcription factor JunD, deprived of menin, switches from growth suppressor to growth promoter. Proc Natl Acad Sci USA 100:10770–10775
47. Yazgan O, Pfarr CM (2001) Differential binding of the Menin tumor suppressor protein to JunD isoforms. Cancer Res 61:916–920
48. Kim H, Lee JE, Cho EJ, Liu JO, Youn HD (2003) Menin, a tumor suppressor, represses JunD-mediated transcriptional activity by association with an mSin3A-histone deacetylase complex. Cancer Res 63:6135–6139
49. Heppner C, Bilimoria KY, Agarwal SK et al (2001) The tumor suppressor protein menin interacts with NF-kappaB proteins and inhibits NF-kappaB-mediated transactivation. Oncogene 20:4917–4925
50. Kaji H, Canaff L, Lebrun JJ, Goltzman D, Hendy GN (2001) Inactivation of menin, a Smad3-interacting protein, blocks transforming growth factor type beta signaling. Proc Natl Acad Sci USA 98:3837–3842
51. Sowa H, Kaji H, Hendy GN et al (2004) Menin is required for bone morphogenetic protein 2- and transforming growth factor beta-regulated osteoblastic differentiation through interaction with Smads and Runx2. J Biol Chem 279:40267–40275
52. Dockray GJ (2003) Keeping neuroendocrine cells in check: roles for TGFbeta, Smads, and menin? Gut 52:1237–1239
53. Ratineau C, Bernard C, Poncet G et al (2004) Reduction of menin expression enhances cell proliferation and is tumorigenic in intestinal epithelial cells. J Biol Chem 279:24477–24484

54. Sowa H, Kaji H, Canaff L et al (2003) Inactivation of menin, the product of the multiple endocrine neoplasia type 1 gene, inhibits the commitment of multipotential mesenchymal stem cells into the osteoblast lineage. J Biol Chem 278:21058–21069
55. Hughes CM, Rozenblatt-Rosen O, Milne TA et al (2004) Menin associates with a trithorax family histone methyltransferase complex and with the hoxc8 locus. Mol Cell 13:587–597
56. Yokoyama A, Somervaille TC, Smith KS, Rozenblatt-Rosen O, Meyerson M, Cleary ML (2005) The menin tumor suppressor protein is an essential oncogenic cofactor for MLL-associated leukemogenesis. Cell 123:207–218
57. Yokoyama A, Cleary ML (2008) Menin critically links MLL proteins with LEDGF on cancer-associated target genes. Cancer Cell 14:36–46
58. Dreijerink KM, Mulder KW, Winkler GS, Hoppener JW, Lips CJ, Timmers HT (2006) Menin links estrogen receptor activation to histone H3K4 trimethylation. Cancer Res 66:4929–4935
59. Sukhodolets KE, Hickman AB, Agarwal SK et al (2003) The 32-kilodalton subunit of replication protein A interacts with menin, the product of the MEN1 tumor suppressor gene. Mol Cell Biol 23:493–509
60. Jin S, Mao H, Schnepp RW et al (2003) Menin associates with FANCD2, a protein involved in repair of DNA damage. Cancer Res 63:4204–4210
61. Schnepp RW, Hou Z, Wang H et al (2004) Functional interaction between tumor suppressor menin and activator of S-phase kinase. Cancer Res 64:6791–6796
62. Ohkura N, Kishi M, Tsukada T, Yamaguchi K (2001) Menin, a gene product responsible for multiple endocrine neoplasia type 1, interacts with the putative tumor metastasis suppressor nm23. Biochem Biophys Res Commun 282:1206–1210
63. Yaguchi H, Ohkura N, Tsukada T, Yamaguchi K (2002) Menin, the multiple endocrine neoplasia type 1 gene product, exhibits GTP-hydrolyzing activity in the presence of the tumor metastasis suppressor nm23. J Biol Chem 277:38197–38204
64. Obungu VH, Lee Burns A, Agarwal SK, Chandrasekharapa SC, Adelstein RS, Marx SJ (2003) Menin, a tumor suppressor, associates with nonmuscle myosin II-A heavy chain. Oncogene 22:6347–6358
65. Lopez-Egido J, Cunningham J, Berg M, Oberg K, Bongcam-Rudloff E, Gobl A (2002) Menin's interaction with glial fibrillary acidic protein and vimentin suggests a role for the intermediate filament network in regulating menin activity. Exp Cell Res 278:175–183
66. La P, Silva AC, Hou Z et al (2004) Direct binding of DNA by tumor suppressor menin. J Biol Chem 279:49045–49054
67. Karnik SK, Hughes CM, Gu X et al (2005) Menin regulates pancreatic islet growth by promoting histone methylation and expression of genes encoding p27Kip1 and p18INK4c. Proc Natl Acad Sci USA 102:14659–14664
68. Milne TA, Hughes CM, Lloyd R et al (2005) Menin and MLL cooperatively regulate expression of cyclin-dependent kinase inhibitors. Proc Natl Acad Sci USA 102:749–754
69. Franklin DS, Godfrey VL, O'Brien DA, Deng C, Xiong Y (2000) Functional collaboration between different cyclin-dependent kinase inhibitors suppresses tumor growth with distinct tissue specificity. Mol Cell Biol 20:6147–6158
70. Yokoyama A, Wang Z, Wysocka J et al (2004) Leukemia proto-oncoprotein MLL forms a SET1-like histone methyltransferase complex with menin to regulate Hox gene expression. Mol Cell Biol 24:5639–5649
71. Chen YX, Yan J, Keeshan K et al (2006) The tumor suppressor menin regulates hematopoiesis and myeloid transformation by influencing Hox gene expression. Proc Natl Acad Sci USA 103:1018–1023
72. Scacheri PC, Davis S, Odom DT et al (2006) Genome-wide analysis of menin binding provides insights into MEN1 tumorigenesis. PLoS Genet 2:e51
73. Shen HC, Rosen JE, Yang LM et al (2008) Parathyroid tumor development involves deregulation of homeobox genes. Endocr Relat Cancer 15:267–275
74. La P, Schnepp RW, Petersen CD, Silva AC, Hua X (2004) Tumor suppressor menin regulates expression of insulin-like growth factor binding protein 2. Endocrinology 145:3443–3450

75. La P, Yang Y, Karnik SK et al (2007) Menin-mediated caspase 8 expression in suppressing multiple endocrine neoplasia type 1. J Biol Chem 282:31332–31340
76. Schnepp RW, Mao H, Sykes SM et al (2004) Menin induces apoptosis in murine embryonic fibroblasts. J Biol Chem 279:10685–10691
77. Bertolino P, Tong WM, Galendo D, Wang ZQ, Zhang CX (2003) Heterozygous Men1 mutant mice develop a range of endocrine tumors mimicking multiple endocrine neoplasia type 1. Mol Endocrinol 17:1880–1892
78. Crabtree JS, Scacheri PC, Ward JM et al (2001) A mouse model of multiple endocrine neoplasia, type 1, develops multiple endocrine tumors. Proc Natl Acad Sci USA 98:1118–1123
79. Bertolino P, Radovanovic I, Casse H, Aguzzi A, Wang ZQ, Zhang CX (2003) Genetic ablation of the tumor suppressor menin causes lethality at mid-gestation with defects in multiple organs. Mech Dev 120:549–560
80. Loffler KA, Biondi CA, Gartside M et al (2007) Broad tumor spectrum in a mouse model of multiple endocrine neoplasia type 1. Int J Cancer 120:259–267
81. Libutti SK, Crabtree JS, Lorang D et al (2003) Parathyroid gland-specific deletion of the mouse Men1 gene results in parathyroid neoplasia and hypercalcemic hyperparathyroidism. Cancer Res 63:8022–8028
82. Bertolino P, Tong WM, Herrera PL, Casse H, Zhang CX, Wang ZQ (2003) Pancreatic beta-cell-specific ablation of the multiple endocrine neoplasia type 1 (MEN1) gene causes full penetrance of insulinoma development in mice. Cancer Res 63:4836–4841
83. Biondi CA, Gartside MG, Waring P et al (2004) Conditional inactivation of the MEN1 gene leads to pancreatic and pituitary tumorigenesis but does not affect normal development of these tissues. Mol Cell Biol 24:3125–3131
84. Crabtree JS, Scacheri PC, Ward JM et al (2003) Of mice and MEN1: Insulinomas in a conditional mouse knockout. Mol Cell Biol 23:6075–6085
85. Scacheri PC, Crabtree JS, Kennedy AL et al (2004) Homozygous loss of menin is well tolerated in liver, a tissue not affected in MEN1. Mamm Genome 15:872–877
86. Shen HC, He M, Powell A et al (2009) Recapitulation of pancreatic neuroendocrine tumors in human multiple endocrine neoplasia type I syndrome via Pdx1-directed inactivation of Men1. Cancer Res 69:1858–1866
87. Sowa H, Kaji H, Kitazawa R et al (2004) Menin inactivation leads to loss of transforming growth factor beta inhibition of parathyroid cell proliferation and parathyroid hormone secretion. Cancer Res 64:2222–2228
88. Lemmens IH, Forsberg L, Pannett AA et al (2001) Menin interacts directly with the homeobox-containing protein Pem. Biochem Biophys Res Commun 286:426–431
89. Busygina V, Kottemann MC, Scott KL, Plon SE, Bale AE (2006) Multiple Endocrine Neoplasia Type 1 Interacts with Forkhead Transcription Factor CHES1 in DNA Damage Response. Cancer Res 66:8397–8403
90. Yaguchi H, Ohkura N, Takahashi M, Nagamura Y, Kitabayashi I, Tsukada T (2004) Menin missense mutants associated with multiple endocrine neoplasia type 1 are rapidly degraded via the ubiquitin-proteasome pathway. Mol Cell Biol 24:6569–6580

Chapter 16
Multiple Endocrine Neoplasia Type 1: Clinical Manifestations and Management

Anathea C. Powell and Steven K. Libutti

Introduction

Multiple endocrine neoplasia type I (MEN-1) is an autosomal dominant syndrome associated with anterior pituitary, parathyroid, and enteropancreatic endocrine tumors as well as other endocrine and nonendocrine tumors [1]. MEN-1 is defined as the presence of two of three main MEN-1-related manifestations, or at least one manifestation plus a first degree relative with at least one MEN-1-related manifestation [1,2]. The estimated prevalence of MEN-1 ranges from 1 in 10,000 to 1 in 100,000 [3], with 43 and 94% penetrance of MEN-1 by ages 20 and 50, respectively [4].

The *MEN-1* gene was first mapped to chromosome 11q13 by linkage analysis [5] and then identified in 1997 [3]. The 610-amino acid protein product, menin, was also identified; its normal function remains under investigation [1,3]. Despite a lack of specifics regarding its function, it is believed to convey tumor suppression when present. Patients with MEN-1 inherit an inactivated copy of *MEN-1* in all cells; a second inactivation occurs postnatally in certain cells and neoplasia results from clonal expansion in the cells with dual inactivation [1]. Individual tumors and their penetrance at age 40 are shown in Table 16.1.

In several series, the percentage of patients with MEN-1 who died of a complication of the disease ranges from 28% to 56% [6–9]. In these series, patients who died of MEN-1-related causes died at earlier ages than the general population [6,8], or kindred members who died of non-MEN-1-related causes [7,9]. Malignant islet cell tumor accounted for the most frequent cause of MEN-1-related deaths in the American series [6,7], while complications of hypercalcemia were the most frequent cause in the Tasmanian series [9].

A.C. Powell
Clinical Fellow, Tumor Angiogenesis Section, Surgery Branch,
National Cancer Institute, Bethesda, MD
e-mail: powela01@nyumc.org

S.K. Libutti (✉)
Professor of Surgery, Vice Chairman, Department of Surgery;
Director, Montefiore-Einstein Center for Cancer Care.Bronx, NY USA
e-mail: slibutti@montefiore.org

C. Sturgeon (ed.), *Endocrine Neoplasia*, Cancer Treatment and Research, vol 153,
DOI 10.1007/978-1-4419-0857-5_16, © Springer Science+Business Media, LLC 2010

Table 16.1 Expression of MEN-1 endocrine features with estimated penetrance (in parentheses) at age 40 years

Parathyroid adenoma (90%)
Enteropancreatic tumor (10%)
Gastrinoma (40%)
Insulinoma (10%)
NF (20%)
Other (2%)
Foregut carcinoid
Thymic NF (2%)
Bronchial NF (2%)
Gastric NF (10%)
Anterior pituitary tumor
Prolactinoma (20%)
Growth Hormone + Prolactinoma (5%)
Growth Hormone (5%)
NF (5%)
ACTH (2%)
Adrenal cortex NF (25%)

NF = non-functioning
Adapted from [1]

Screening for MEN-1 carrier state is recommended for index case patients who meet the clinical criteria or have manifestations suspicious for MEN-1 as well as for family members of a patient with a known *MEN-1* mutation [1]. Periodic screening for MEN-1 manifestations in MEN-1 carriers has not been shown to improve the outcome [1]; however, biochemical evidence of neoplasia has been found as much as 10 years before clinical evidence [10]. Biochemical screening is recommended yearly with tumor imaging every 3–5 years, beginning once carrier status is established, or at age 8 if already established, and continuing for life [1] (Table 16.2).

Parathyroid Disease

Primary hyperparathyroidism (PHPT) is the most frequent and earliest onset manifestation of MEN-1, with a penetrance of 90–99% [4,6,11,12]. The age of onset is usually between 20 and 30 years [1,11,12]. In contrast, only 2–5% of patients with PHPT have MEN-1 [13,14], and the onset of PHPT in patients with sporadic disease is approximately 20–30 years after the onset in patients with MEN-1 [1,12]. Parathyroid disease is multiglandular in MEN-1 patients, and all parathyroid tissues are considered abnormal [15]. The expected pathology is an asymmetric hyperplasia involving all parathyroid glands, with an average size ratio of 10:1 between the largest and smallest glands [16].

Symptoms and signs of MEN-1-related PHPT are similar to those of sporadic PHPT [17]. Decreased bone mineral density has been reported in women with MEN-1-related PHPT as early as age 35; this is thought to be due to uncontrolled hyper-

Table 16.2 Clinical Management Recommendations for MEN1

Issue/Manifestation	Management recommendations
Screening	
MEN-1 carrier state	• For index patients who meet clinical criteria or have suspicious manifestations • For family members of a patient with a known familial *MEN-1* mutation
Known carriers	• Biochemical screening yearly • Tumor imaging every 3–5 years once carrier state is established or at age 8 if already established; continue for life
Parathyroid	• 3.5 gland resection with IOPTH monitoring and cryopreservation of parathyroid tissue • Selective transcervical thymectomy if <4 glands found during operation
Enteropancreatic	
Gastrinoma	• Abdominal exploration with palpation via extended Kocher maneuver intraoperative ultrasound (IOUS) duodenotomy with intraoperative endoscopy selective pancreatic resection as dictated by operative findings
Insulinoma	• Localize lesion with noninvasive imaging and intraarterial calcium stimulation as necessary • Abdominal exploration with IOUS palpation fine needle aspirate/ insulin assay to determine functionality • Resect insulin positive lesions and any lesion over 3 cm via Enucleation if safe distal pancreatectomy as necessary
Pituitary	• Pharmacologic suppression first line for prolactinoma • If suppression fails or other lesions resect via transsphenoidal approach

parathyroidism and correlates more closely with elevations in parathyroid hormone than serum calcium [18]. Nephrolithiasis has been reported in up to 51% of patients with MEN-1-related PHPT [11,17,19,20]. MEN-1 patients who have both Zollinger–Ellison syndrome (ZES) and PHPT have been found to have a more severe form of PHPT than those who have PHPT alone, with a higher frequency of nephrolithiasis, higher serum PTH levels, and higher recurrence rates after subtotal parathyroid resections [21]. The onset of hyperparathyroidism generally predates the onset of ZES. Hypercalcemia is a potent stimulus for gastrin secretion, and it has been observed that serum gastrin levels and gastric acid output can be reduced, and in some cases even normalized, by parathyroidectomy that restores eucalcemia. Because of this, most experts agree that parathyroidectomy should be performed before gastrinoma resection. Furthermore, many experts consider coexistent PHPT and ZES to be an indication for parathyroidectomy and recommend early parathyroidectomy in order to facilitate non-operative management of hypergastrinemia. Conversely, due to the success of antisecretory pharmacotherapy, some authors contend that concomitant ZES and PHPT may not be an absolute indication for parathyroidectomy [1,22].

The biochemical findings in MEN-1-related PHPT are identical to those of sporadic PHPT. The diagnosis is confirmed by documenting the elevated serum calcium concurrently with an inappropriately elevated serum PTH [11]. Familial hypocalciuric hypercalcemia (FHH) is unrelated to MEN-1 and may be ruled out by a normal 24 h urinary calcium clearance value [22]. Most experts agree that the surgical indications for parathyroid resection should mirror those for sporadic disease. Any patient with symptomatic PHPT should be offered surgery. Surgery should also be offered to apparently asymptomatic patients with marked hypercalcemia (total serum calcium ≥1mg/dL over the upper limit of normal), nephrolithiasis, decreased glomerular filtration rate, fracture, or decreased bone mineral density. Patients with symptoms that are more subjective or difficult to quantify, such as musculoskeletal complaints, psychiatric or cognitive changes, cardiovascular disease, or alterations in gastrointestinal function, may also benefit from parathyroidectomy [23].

Due to the multiglandular nature of the disease, parathyroid imaging and localization is rarely helpful and often misleading prior to the initial exploration [12,24]. However, imaging studies such as neck ultrasound, neck and mediastinal CT/MRI, and sestamibi scintigraphy are useful to localize a recurrence. Invasive studies such as selective arteriography, venous sampling for PTH, or percutaneous fine-needle aspiration for PTH may be used if noninvasive localization fails. The National Institutes of Health (NIH)'s approach is to accept the results of localization studies if two or more provide concordant data consistent with a parathyroid lesion and none show discordant data [25].

The goal of parathyroid resection is to remove as much abnormal parathyroid tissue as possible while minimizing the risk of permanent hypoparathyroidism [20]. The two current approaches are subtotal parathyroidectomy or total parathyroidectomy with immediate autotransplantation. Rates of recurrent hyperparathyroidism after initial operation for subtotal and total parathyroidectomy have been reported to range from 30 to 56% and 0 to 38%, respectively, while rates of severe hypoparathyroidism have ranged from 4 to 24% and 22 to 38%, respectively [18,26–29].

In a 42-year review of 92 patients with MEN-1-related PHPT seen at the NIH, hyperparathyroidism recurred in 33% of patients overall; 33% of patients after subtotal resection (3 or more glands; median follow up 5.7 years) and 23% of patients after total resection (median follow up 10.9 years) with no difference in time to recurrence. Resections of 2.5 glands or less resulted in a recurrence rate of 46% and a shorter time to recurrence than more extensive resections (7.0 vs. 16.5 years, $p=0.03$). Severe hypoparathyroidism was seen in 46% and 26% of patients after total and subtotal resections, respectively [20]. A similar study reviewed the reoperative NIH data; although reoperations were successful in 91% of cases, hyperparathyroidism eventually recurred in 36% of patients [25].

A routine four-gland exploration with subtotal parathyroidectomy is mandatory for patients with MEN-1. Intraoperative parathormone (IOPTH) assay can be useful in determining the adequacy of the resection that has been performed. Similar to sporadic PHPT, a 50% drop from baseline has been reported to correlate with effective resection in MEN-1 [25,30], although there is some debate regarding this due to the concerns on length of follow up and potentially suppressed remaining glands [29,30].

Protocols for cryopreservation of parathyroid tissue and immediate or delayed forearm implantation have been described [31]. In a study of 46 autografts placed at the NIH for both MEN-1 and non-MEN-1 patients, 35% of grafts placed immediately were successful, while 55 and 45% of grafts placed after less than 12 months of cryopreservation and more than 12 months were successful, respectively. There was no statistical difference between the success rates for MEN-1 versus non-MEN-1 patients [31].

Transcervical thymectomy (TCT) has been advocated to be included with parathyroid resection in MEN-1 patients. TCT is usually performed by dissecting as much thymic tissue as possible down to the innominate vein and below if safe, resulting in an estimated removal of 30–40% of the thymus [19]. The rationale for this procedure has been a concern for ectopic or supernumerary parathyroid tissue in the thymus as well as thymic carcinoid tumors [32–34]. A recent retrospective review of 66 patients with MEN-1-related PHPT investigated the benefit of routine TCT. No carcinoids were found in any of the specimens. When four parathyroid glands were found in the initial neck exploration, only 2 (6%) thymectomy specimens contained additional parathyroid tissue. In contrast, when less than four glands were found in the initial neck exploration, 17 (53%, $p<0.0001$) thymectomy specimens contained additional parathyroid tissue [19].

A prospective study of 128 patients with MEN-1 at the NIH investigated the incidence of thymic carcinoid. Seven patients (8%) developed thymic carcinoid and at least one patient had undergone previous TCT. Six of the seven patients remained alive; ranging from 0.3–8.8 years after discovery. One patient died of a cause unrelated to thymic carcinoid or MEN-1 disease [32]. Despite the indolent course of thymic carcinoid demonstrated in this series, other reports have described aggressive behavior of thymic carcinoids in MEN-1 patients [33,35].

Given the data regarding recurrence, hypoparathyroidism, thymectomy, and autograft success rates, we recommend a 3.5 gland resection with intraoperative PTH monitoring and cryopreservation of parathyroid tissue, and a selective TCT based on the number of glands found at neck exploration (Table 16.2).

Enteropancreatic Disease

Enteropancreatic disease is present in an estimated 30–80% of patients with MEN-1 [1,4,11,12]. Gastrinomas account for the largest percentage of these tumors, 40–63% in several series. Insulinomas account for 10–27%, while nonfunctioning tumors range from 1 to 20%, depending on the series. Tumors producing the clinical syndromes of glucagon, somatostatin, and VIP excess account for 2–4% [1,4,12]. The age of onset of enteropancreatic disease is later than parathyroid disease; tumors will usually cause symptoms related to excess hormone production in the fourth decade [1].

Enteropancreatic lesions are usually multiple and small (<1 cm), although they may occasionally be larger [36,37]. Microadenomas, macroadenomas, and metastatic lesions may be seen [36]. In a study of 100 pancreatic tumors from 28 MEN-1 patients, 60% were located in the tail, 30% in the body, and 10% in the head of the pancreas [36]. Many enteropancreatic lesions stain positive for more than one peptide on immunohistochemistry; however, patients are either asymptomatic or demonstrate a single clinical syndrome [36,38]. Only one case in the literature has clearly demonstrated two clinically recognizable syndromes arising from a single pancreatic lesion (ZES and insulinoma), but this patient did not meet the criteria for MEN-1 [39].

All of the clinical syndromes resulting as a consequence of excess hormone secretion by enteropancreatic lesions, including gastrinoma, VIPoma, glucagonoma, and somatostatinoma, may be treated with pharmacotherapy, except for insulinomas [1]. Gastrinoma and insulinoma are discussed in detail below.

Gastrinoma/ZES

Zollinger–Ellison syndrome (ZES) is the eponym for the clinical syndrome due to autonomous and excess gastrin production by a gastrinoma. Since gastrinomas are common in patients with MEN-1, the incidence of MEN-1 in patients who present with ZES is also common; estimated between 20 and 60% [11,37].

MEN-1 gastrinomas usually range in size from 1 mm to 2 cm, and are almost always multiple. They are most frequently located in the mucosa and submucosa of the duodenum [37,40]; however, not all MEN-1 patients have duodenal gastrinomas [41]. In one series of 38 patients with MEN-1 ZES, 33 patients (87%) had duodenal gastrinomas and all patients had a palpable neuroendocrine tumor in the body or tail of the pancreas [42]. Between 60 and 90% of MEN-1 gastrinomas are reported to be malignant [43] and approximately half will have metastasized to lymph nodes or beyond by the time of diagnosis [37,40]. Both pancreatic and duodenal gastrinomas can metastasize to lymph nodes; however, liver metastases are more often associated with pancreatic gastrinomas [44]. Primary lymph node gastrinomas have also been described, but these have almost all been found in patients with sporadic ZES [45]. Liver metastases have been correlated with a primary tumor ≥ 3 cm [44,46].

Aggressive and non-aggressive forms of MEN-1 gastrinoma have also been described. In a series of 57 patients with MEN-1 gastrinoma, followed prospectively for a mean of 8 years, 14% of patients had aggressive growth of the gastrinoma as defined by an increase in tumor volume of 25% or more per month or the appearance of a new lesion in follow up. Twenty-three percent of patients had or developed liver metastases. Aggressive tumor growth, and not liver metastases alone, correlated with decreased survival (88% 5-year survival for patients with aggressive growth vs. 100% for those without aggressive growth, with or without liver metastases). Factors predictive of aggressive growth include young age at diagnosis and ZES onset (<35 and ≤27 years, respectively), fasting gastrin levels ≥ 10,000 pg mL^{-1}, pancreatic tumor size greater than 3 cm, and the presence of bone and/or liver metastases as well as the presence of gastric carcinoid [47].

Symptoms of excess gastrin production include peptic ulcer disease (PUD): epigastric pain, diarrhea, heartburn, nausea, vomiting, weight loss, and bleeding. Complications of PUD, such as obstruction, perforation, and esophageal stricture, may be seen rarely [43]. Peptic ulcers are most commonly found in the duodenal bulb [12]. In a series of 107 patients with MEN-1 and ZES, pain, diarrhea, and heartburn were the most common presenting symptoms [43]. Hypercalcemia from hyperparathyroidism can increase the gastrin secretion, and can also increase the resistance to antisecretory therapy and decrease the lower esophageal sphincter pressure [48].

The diagnosis of ZES is made biochemically. Recent recommendations for fasting and provocative serum gastrin testing were made based on analysis of approximately 300 NIH patients [49,50]. Fasting serum gastrin (FSG) values 10 times greater than the normal correlate with ZES. However, two thirds of patients have a non-diagnostic FSG level (elevated, but less than 10 times the normal) and will require further provocative testing; these patients often have more common conditions than ZES. Of note, MEN-1 ZES patients were not found to have higher FSG levels than non-MEN-1 ZES patients [49].

Antisecretory therapy became available in 1981. From the period of 1981–1989, H_2-antagonists were used. Since 1990, proton pump inhibitors (PPIs) have been the mainstay of therapy. In a study at the NIH, 261 patients with both sporadic and MEN-1-related ZES seen from 1974 to 1999 were analyzed for the effects of antisecretory therapy. Patients reported less pain with PPIs than H_2-antagonists (70% vs. 83%, $p<0.02$). The percentage of patients who had undergone previous gastric acid-reducing surgery prior to NIH admission decreased from 44% before 1981 to 11% during the period 1990–1999 ($p<0.01$). The percentage of patients with perforation did not change during these time periods, but was a small number (6%) [51].

Preoperative imaging and localization studies for gastrinomas include computed tomography (CT), magnetic resonance imaging (MRI), portal venous sampling (PVS; now rarely performed), endoscopic ultrasound (EUS), selective angiography, and somatostatin receptor scintigraphy (SRS) [52]. Somatostatin receptors located on gastrinomas bind octreotide and, therefore, highlight the lesion on SRS [53]. SRS has been shown to be more sensitive than all other conventional imaging studies combined at detecting both intra- and extra-hepatic gastrinomas [40,54]. SRS is usually combined with CT or MRI in order to provide information on tumor size and location [53], and to increase the imaging sensitivity; reports on the magnitude of the increase vary [54,55]. However, SRS has been shown to miss small extra-hepatic lesions, and in one study, detected only 30% of duodenal gastrinomas found at operation [56]. Despite the improvement in sensitivity of SRS, a study of 37 patients did not show an improvement in the disease-free rate after operation either immediately or at 2 years [56]. Given the inability of SRS to detect small gastrinomas, a negative SRS should not preclude surgical exploration [56]. EUS may be useful in localizing additional pancreatic neuroendocrine tumors or nodal disease [53,57].

Regardless of intraoperative imaging and technical improvements for identifying duodenal lesions, patients with MEN-1-related ZES are probably never cured by surgical resection. Prior to the late 1990s, patients routinely underwent extensive exploratory laparotomy, but postoperative cure was not demonstrated in MEN-1 ZES patients [58–60]. After 1982, intraoperative ultrasound (IOUS) was performed, and after 1987, intraoperative endoscopy (IOE) with transillumination with or without duodenotomy was performed [61]. These methods were compared prospectively in a study of 35 sporadic and MEN-1 ZES patients. Duodenotomy was superior to all other methods, identifying 100% of duodenal tumors versus 61% with standard palpation, 64% with IOE, and 26% with IOUS. The postoperative complication rate was 17%, with pancreatitis and duodenal leak occurring in 2 (5.7%) and 1 (2.8%)

patients, respectively. No deaths occurred as a result of the operation. On the basis of these findings, duodenotomy with IOE to guide placement of the incision, was recommended in ZES operations [62]. However, a study of resection in 10 MEN-1 ZES patients, 7 of which had duodenal gastrinomas, did not reveal any cures with the improved intraoperative localization techniques. This was thought to be due to high percentages of lymph node metastases and multiple tumors [41].

Considering the lack of cures following operation for MEN-1 ZES and survival data, the indications for routine surgical exploration in these patients remain controversial [53]. Some groups advocate exploration with enucleation of lesions less than 2 cm, in order to provide an early, curative resection, combined with routine distal pancreatectomy [42,63]. In contrast, a series of 81 consecutive MEN-1 ZES patients at our institution showed excellent survival data with selective use of resection [64]. The 15-year survival rate was 100% for 25 patients with primary gastrinoma less than 2.5 cm who did not undergo surgery. In comparison, the 15-year survival of patients undergoing resection for larger tumors was 89%. Resection was offered to patients with a primary gastrinoma 2.5–6 cm in size or with 2 or more tumors measuring between 2.5 and 6 cm each or a single lesion larger than 6 cm. The operation consisted of abdominal exploration, palpation via an extended Kocher maneuver, IOUS, and duodenotomy with IOE. Enucleation was performed if safe; otherwise resection was performed as directed by operative findings. Lymph nodes, indicated by clinical suspicion, were inspected and dissected. With these methods, there were no deaths at 5 years, but the patients were not cured either [64].

Given these data for MEN-1 ZES patients and the success of antisecretory therapy, we recommend exploration be reserved for patients with primary tumors ≥ 2.5 cm. The operation should consist of exploration with palpation via extended Kocher, IOUS, and duodenotomy, and selective pancreatic resection as dictated by operative findings [53,65] (Table 16.2).

Insulinoma

Although insulinoma is rarer than gastrinoma in MEN-1 patients [1,4], insulinoma has been reported to be the dominant functional enteropancreatic tumor in patients under 25 years [66]. MEN-1-related insulinomas are often multiple [67,68], and cases have been reported with 14 or more tumors in a single patient [68]. Malignancy rates, usually described as metastases present at resection, have been reported to be between 8 and 11% [67,68], although one small series reported 3 out of 8 cases (38%) to have malignant disease [67].

Symptoms of insulinoma are due to hypoglycemia caused by excess insulin secretion. Neuroglycopenic symptoms include confusion, fatigue, headache, abnormal behavior, lightheadedness, seizures, syncope, and adrenergic symptoms, such as sweating, tremor, and palpitations [69,70]. The standard diagnostic maneuver for insulinoma is the 48 h supervised fast [71]. Patients fast under close supervision, with blood glucose, insulin, C peptide, and proinsulin samples drawn every 4–6 h. The supervised fast is described in detail in Chap. 13. In the face of hypoglycemia, patients with insulinoma will have elevated insulin and proinsulin levels [71]. C-peptide levels are measured to exclude exogenous insulin administration, and should be elevated in patients with insulinoma [72].

Unlike other excess hormonal syndromes from MEN-1 enteropancreatic lesions, insulinomas are not well controlled with non-operative management [73]. Cure rates with resection approach almost 100%, depending on the series, but may be accompanied by diabetes, depending on the extent of resection [67,73,74].

Many imaging studies have been investigated for their utility in preoperative localization of insulinoma. Unlike gastrinomas, insulinomas have a low density of somatostatin receptors; therefore, SRS has little utility in insulinoma localization [75]. Preoperative imaging studies used currently include non-invasive modalities such as computed tomography (CT, Figure 1), magnetic resonance imaging (MRI), and transabdominal ultrasound (US), as well as invasive modalities including endoscopic ultrasound (EUS), portal venous sampling (PVS), angiography, and intra-arterial calcium stimulation with hepatic vein sampling.

CT and MRI technology have improved in recent decades, and have been reported recently to localize insulinoma correctly in 80% (28/35) of sporadic and 70% (14/20) of MEN-1 patients, respectively [70]. Transabdominal ultrasonography has not been shown to be useful for insulinoma localization in most institutions [70,76]. Endoscopic ultrasound is being used increasingly for pancreatic neuroendocrine

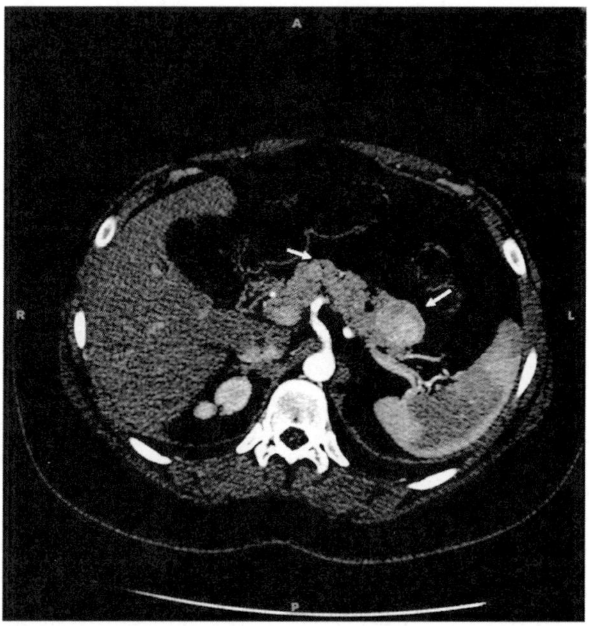

Fig. 16.1 Computed Tomography (CT) image of MEN-1 patient with two pancreatic insulinomas; one in the uncinate and one in the body (arrows)

tumors (PNETs). In a study of 82 patients with PNETs at the University of Michigan, EUS detected 85% (29/34) of insulinomas [77].

Angiography, portal venous sampling, and intra-arterial calcium stimulation have all been used to localize insulinomas not seen on noninvasive imaging. The utility of angiography alone is variable [70,78], and has been reported to be 35% for insulinomas smaller than 2 cm [76]. PVS does not depend on the size of the tumor [76] and has been shown to localize insulinomas correctly in 75–100% of cases [70,78]. However, PVS has been shown to have small but significant morbidity associated with the procedure [79] and is used rarely. Intraarterial calcium stimulation with hepatic vein sampling was developed to overcome the morbidity of PVS [76]. In a series of 25 patients with insulinoma, two of which had MEN-1, intra-arterial calcium stimulation was shown to localize the insulinoma to the correct region of the pancreas (determined intraoperatively) in 22/25 (87%) of patients with no morbidity [76].

Intraoperative localization techniques can facilitate identification of insulinomas. IOUS has been shown to locate previously occult insulinomas and to allow for less extensive operations [80]. IOUS can be performed effectively in both laparoscopic and open approaches. Surgeons blinded to preoperative localization studies used laparoscopic or open IOUS to localize the insulinoma successively in 12/14 (87%) of cases in both approaches [81,82]. Palpation alone has been shown to be of lesser value than IOUS in several series [80]. Fine needle aspirate for a rapid insulin assay has also been described as another means to identify functionally active insulinomas [83].

Intraoperative techniques for resecting insulinomas include enucleation if located safely away from the pancreatic or common bile duct, or standard resections (pancreaticoduodenectomy or distal pancreatectomy) [72]. Due to the frequent multiplicity of insulinomas in MEN-1 patients, many groups advocate routine subtotal pancreatectomy with enucleation of tumors in the head [67,74,84,85]. However, due to the combined accuracies of pre- and intraoperative localization techniques, we recommend a step-wise approach to selective MEN-1 insulinoma resection.

In our approach, we localize the lesion(s) with noninvasive imaging and intra-arterial calcium stimulation as necessary. We then explore the patient using IOUS, palpation, and FNA/insulin assay to determine the functionality of the lesion as necessary. All insulin-positive lesions and any lesion over 3 cm are resected. Enucleation, if safe, is preferred to spare normal pancreas; distal pancreatectomy may be performed as necessary [73] (Table 16.2).

Pituitary Disease

The incidence of pituitary disease in patients with MEN-1 has been reported to vary between 22% and 47% [4,12,66,86]. The majority of these lesions are reported to be prolactinomas [4,12,86]. In one of these series, growth hormone-producing lesions were the next most frequent [4], while in the other, nonfunctioning tumors accounted for the next most frequently seen lesion after prolactinoma [12]. Other pituitary lesions may produce adrenocorticotropic hormone (ACTH) but these are rare, representing 4–7% of MEN-1 pituitary lesions [4,12,86]. The age of onset of prolactinoma varies based on the series, from around age 30 in one series [12] to 38 in another [86]. The prevalence of MEN-1 among patients with pituitary tumors has been shown to be as high as 14.3% in patients with prolactinoma, and these patients should be screened for MEN-1 at the time of prolactinoma diagnosis [87].

Pituitary tumors from 136 MEN-1 patients were recently compared to non-MEN-1 pituitary tumors. Eighty-five percent of these MEN-1 tumors were macroadenomas versus 42% in non-MEN-1 tumors ($p<0.001$), and 43 (32%) of the MEN-1 tumors were considered invasive. Further, the functional MEN-1 tumors were more resistant to treatment; only 42% of patients showed normalization of pituitary hypersecretion versus 90% of functional non-MEN-1 tumors [86]. Pathologic analysis of these tumors confirmed these results [88]. These results suggest that MEN-1 pituitary lesions have a more aggressive phenotype than nonMEN-1 pituitary lesions.

Symptoms of functioning pituitary tumors depend on the syndrome of hormonal excess. Prolactinoma may present as amenorrhea, infertility, and/or galactorrhea in women and impotence in men. Acromegaly will accompany excess growth hormone secretion, and Cushing's disease will be seen with excess ACTH and secondary adrenal hyperplasia [11]. Diagnosis of pituitary tumors may be made by biochemical assessment and imaging with CT and/or MRI [11]. Treatment of MEN-1 pituitary tumors is similar to that of nonMEN-1 tumors. Bromocriptine, a dopamine agonist, may be used to manage prolactinoma nonoperatively. If pharmacologic suppression fails for prolactinoma, or for other lesions, surgical resection via transsphenoidal approach may be offered [11]. However, pharmacologic suppression is less effective for macroadenomas than microadenomas, and given the larger phenotype of MEN-1 pituitary tumors, resection may be used more frequently [89] (Table 16.2). In addition, given the frequent resistance of MEN-1-related pituitary tumors to therapy [86], these patients should be followed closely after resection [1,89]

Other manifestations of MEN-1

Foregut carcinoids were seen in 21 of 130 patients (16%) with MEN-1 investigated at the NIH. Of these carcinoids, 11 were bronchial, 9 gastric, and 1 thymic in origin [12]. Foregut carcinoids produce syndromes of hormonal excess rarely, and their prognosis is relatively unknown [1]. Adrenocortical tumors were seen in 21 (16%) of the 130 NIH MEN-1 patients; 14 of these were non-functioning and 7 were functioning [12]. Adrenal lesions in MEN-1 patients are associated with concomitant pancreatic lesions, and are usually bilateral, hyperplastic, and nonfunctional [90,91], with an indolent course [90]. Adrenocortical carcinoma has been seen rarely [90]. There is currently no consensus on clinical management of MEN-1 adrenocortical lesions [1].

Cutaneous abnormalities are also common in MEN-1 patients. In a series of 32 MEN-1 patients examined specifically for cutaneous lesions, a variety of lesions were seen [92]. Multiple facial angiofibromas, similar to those of tuberous sclerosis, were seen in 28 (88%) patients. Other lesions included collagenomas (23 patients,

72%), café au lait macules (12 patients, 38%), lipomas (11 patients, 34%), confetti-like hypopigmented macules (2 patients, 6%), and multiple gingival papules (2 patients, 6%) [92]. Angiofibromas observed in patients without tuberous sclerosis is an indication for MEN-1 screening [91]. MEN-1 angiofibromas, collagenomas, and lipomas have been shown to have allelic loss of the MEN-1 gene, suggesting that these lesions are benign neoplasms arising from clonal expansion [93].

Thyroid tumors were seen in 16 (12%) of the 130 NIH MEN-1 patients; 10 of these were found to be follicular adenomas and 6 (5%) were papillary carcinomas [12]. It is not clear whether there is a true association between thyroid disease and MEN-1; the prevalence of thyroid disease may be due to scrutiny of the gland during parathyroid surgery in these patients [94]. Pheochromocytoma has only been reported in a small number of MEN-1 cases, but DNA testing, when done, did show germline MEN-1 mutations [94].

Conclusion

Patients with MEN-1 present specific management issues. Due to the hereditary basis of the disease, all tissues in the affected organs, primarily the pituitary, parathyroid, and enteropancreatic region, may be at risk for tumor, and tumors may develop throughout the patient's lifespan. Therefore, a high index of suspicion for MEN-1 must be maintained when patients present with a cluster of tumors suggestive of the syndrome, or with single tumors or manifestations with a high correlation with MEN-1, such as prolactinoma or multigland parathyroid hyperplasia. These patients should be screened for MEN-1 at the time of initial presentation. Once patients are identified as known carriers of MEN-1, regular screening for manifestations should be carried out according to consensus guidelines [1], and patients who have undergone resection of MEN-1 lesions must be monitored for recurrence.

Non-operative management of MEN-1 tumors has limited utility, and resection is usually indicated. For pituitary lesions not amenable to bromocriptine, we recommend transsphenoidal resection. Three-and-a-half gland parathyroid resection with selective transcervical thymectomy is recommended for parathyroid disease. Resection of enteropancreatic lesions should be guided by pre- and intraoperative localization techniques. Given the multiplicity of tumors and the frequency of recurrence, the overall goals of resection in any location should be removal of as much disease as feasible while preserving as much functional normal tissue as possible.

References

1. Brandi ML, Gagel RF, Angeli A et al (2001) Guidelines for diagnosis and therapy of MEN type 2 and type 2. J Clin Endocrinol Metab 86(12):5658–5671
2. Marx SJ, Agarwal SK, Kester MB et al (1999) Multiple endocrine neoplasia type I: Clinical and genetic features of the hereditary endocrine neoplasias. Recent Prog Horm Res 54:397–438

3. Chandrasekharappa SC, Siradanahalli CG, Manickam P et al (1997) Positional cloning of the gene for multiple endocrine neoplasia-type 1. Science 276(5311):404–407
4. Trump D, Farren B, Wooding C et al (1996) Clinical studies of multiple endocrine neoplasia type 1. Q J Med 89:653–669
5. Larsson C, Skogseid B, Oberg K et al (1988) Multiple endocrine neoplasia type 1 gene maps to chromosome 11 and is lost in insulinoma. Nature 332(6159):85–87
6. Dean PG, van Heerden JA, Farley DR et al (2000) Are patients with multiple endocrine neoplasia type 1 prone to premature death? World J Surg 24(11):1437–1441
7. Doherty GM, Olson JA, Frisella MM et al (1998) Lethality of multiple endocrine neoplasia type I. World J Surg 22(6):581–586
8. Geerdink EA, Van der Luijt RB, Lips CJ (2003) Do patients with multiple endocrine neoplasia syndrome type 1 benefit from periodical screening? Eur J Endocrinol 149(6):577–582
9. Wilkinson S, The BT, Davey KR et al (1993) Cause of death in multiple endocrine neoplasia type 1. Arch Surg 128(6):683–690
10. Lairmore TC, Piersall LD, DeBenedetti MK et al (2004) Clinical genetic testing and early surgical intervention in patients with multiple endocrine neoplasia type 1 (MEN 1). Ann Surg 239(5):637–647
11. Brandi ML, Marx SK, Aurbach GD, Fitzpatrick LA (1987) Familial multiple endocrine neoplasia type I: a new look at pathophysiology. Endocr Rev 8(4):391–405
12. Marx S, Spiegel AM, Skarulis MC et al (1998) Multiple endocrine neoplasia type 1: clinical and genetic topics. Ann Intern Med 129(6):484–494
13. Marx SJ (2001) Multiple endocrine neoplasia type 1. In: Beaudet SCR, AL SWS, Valle D (eds) The metabolic and molecular bases of inherited disease, 8th edn. McGraw-Hill, New York, pp 943–966
14. Uchino S, Noguchi S, Sato M et al (2000) Screening of the *MEN-1* gene and discovery of germ-line and somatic mutations in apparently sporadic parathyroid tumors. Cancer Res 60(19):5553–5557
15. Rizzoli R, Green J, Marx SJ (1985) Primary hyperparathyroidism in familial multiple endocrine neoplasia type I. Am J Med 78(3):467–474
16. Marx SJ, Menczel J, Campbell G et al (1991) Heterogenous size of the parathyroid glands in familial multiple endocrine neoplasia type 1. Clin Endocrinol 35(6):521–526
17. Lamers CB, Froeling PG (1979) Clinical significance of hyperparathyroidism in familial multiple endocrine adenomatosis type I (MEA I). Am J Med 66(3):422–424
18. Burgess JR, David R, Parameswaran V et al (1998) The outcome of subtotal parathyroidectomy for the treatment of hyperparathyroidism in multiple endocrine neoplasia type 1. Arch Surg 133(2):126–129
19. Powell AC, Alexander HR, Pingpank JF et al (2008) The utility of routine transcervical thymectomy for MEN-1 related hyperparathyroidism. Surgery 144(6):878–883
20. Elaraj DM, Skarulis MC, Libutti SK et al (2003) Results of initial operation for hyperparathyroidism in patients with multiple endocrine neoplasia type 1. Surgery 134(6):858–864
21. Norton JA, Venzon DJ, Berna MJ et al (2008) Prospective study of surgery for primary hyperparathyroidism (HPT) in multiple endocrine neoplasia-type 1 and Zollinger-Ellison syndrome. Ann Surg 247(3):501–510
22. Marx SJ, Simonds WF, Agarwal SK et al (2002) Hyperparathyroidism in hereditary syndromes: special expressions and special managements. J Bone Miner Res 17(Suppl 2):N37–N43
23. Udelsman R, Pasieka JL, Sturgeon C et al (2009) Surgery for Asymptomatic Primary Hyperparathryoidism: Proceedings of the Third International Workshop. J Clin Endocrinol Metab 94(2):366–372
24. Doppman JL, Miller DL (1991) Localization of parathyroid tumors in patients with asymptomatic hyperparathyroidism and no previous surgery. J Bone Miner Res 6(Suppl 2): S153–S158
25. Kivlen MH, Bartlett DL, Libutti SK et al (2001) Reoperation for hyperparathyroidism in multiple endocrine neoplasia type 1. Surgery 130(6):991–998
26. Malmaeus J, Benson L, Johansson H et al (1986) Parathyroid surgery in the multiple endocrine neoplasia type I syndrome: choice of surgical procedure. World J Surg 10:668–672

27. Hellman P, Skogseid B, Juhlin C et al (1992) Findings and long term results of parathyroid surgery in multiple endocrine neoplasia type 1. World J Surg 16:718–723
28. Hellman P, Skogseid B, Oberg K et al (1998) Primary and reoperative parathyroid operations in hyperparathyroidism of multiple endocrine neoplasia type 1. Surgery 124:993–999
29. Tonelli F, Marcucci T, Fratini G et al (2007) Is total parathyroidectomy the treatment of choice for hyperparathyroidism in multiple endocrine neoplasia type 1? Ann Surg 246(6):1075–1082
30. Arnalsteen LC, Alesina PF, Quiereux JL et al (2002) Long-term results of less than total parathyroidectomy for hyperparathyroidism in multiple endocrine neoplasia type 1. Surgery 132:1119–1125
31. Feldman AL, Sharaf RN, Skarulis MC et al (1999) Results of heterotopic parathyroid autotransplantation: a 13-year experience. Surgery 126:1042–1048
32. Gibril F, Chen Y-J, Schrump D et al (2003) Prospective study of thymic carcinoids in patients with multiple endocrine neoplasia type 1. J Clin Endocrinol Metab 88(3):1066–1081
33. Ferolla P, Falchetti A, Filosso P et al (2005) Thymic neuroendocrine carcinoma (carcinoid) in multiple endocrine neoplasia type 1 syndrome: the Italian series. J Clin Endocrinol Metab 90:2603–2609
34. Teh BT, Zedenius J, Kytola S et al (1998) Thymic carcinoids in multiple endocrine neoplasia type 1. Ann Surg 228(1):99–105
35. Manes JL, Taylor HB (1973) Thymic carcinoid in familial multiple endocrine adenomatosis. Arch Pathol 95:252–255
36. LeBodic M-F, Heymann M-F, Lecomte M et al (1996) Immunohistochemical study of 100 pancreatic tumors in 28 patients with multiple endocrine neoplasia, type 1. Am J Surg Pathol 20(11):1378–1384
37. Pipeleers-Marichal M, Somers G, Willems G et al (1990) Gastrinomas in the duodenums of patients with multiple endocrine neoplasia type 1 and the Zollinger-Ellison syndrome. N Engl J Med 322(11):723–727
38. Chiang H-C, O'Dorisio TM, Huang SC et al (1990) Multiple hormone elevations in Zollinger-Ellison syndrome. Gastroenterology 99(6):1565–1575
39. Lodish MB, Powell AC, Abu-Asab M et al (2008) Insulinoma and gastrinoma syndromes from a single intrapancreatic neuroendocrine tumor. J Clin Endocrinol Metab 93(4):1123–1128
40. Norton JA, Fraker DL, Alexander HR et al (1999) Surgery to cure the Zollinger-Ellison syndrome. N Engl J Med 341(9):635–644
41. MacFarlane MP, Fraker DL, Alexander HR et al (1995) Prospective study of surgical resection of duodenal and pancreatic gastrinomas in multiple endocrine neoplasia type 1. Surgery 118: 973–980
42. Thompson NW (1998) Management of pancreatic endocrine tumors in patients with multiple endocrine neoplasia type 1. Surg Oncol Clin N Am 7(4):881–891
43. Gibril F, Schumann M, Pace A, Jensen RT (2004) Multiple endocrine neoplasia type 1 and Zollinger-Ellison syndrome. Medicine (Baltimore) 83(1):43–83
44. Weber HC, Venzon DJ, Lin JT et al (1995) Determinants of metastatic rate and survival in patients with Zollinger-Ellison syndrome: a prospective long-term study. Gastroenterology 108(6):1637–1649
45. Norton JA, Alexander HR, Fraker DL et al (2003) Possible primary lymph node gastrinoma: occurrence, natural history, and predictive factors. Ann Surg 237(5):650–659
46. Cadiot G, Vuagnat A, Doukjan I et al (1999) Prognostic factors in patients with Zollinger-Ellison syndrome and multiple endocrine neoplasia type 1. Gastroenterology 116:286–293
47. Gibril F, Venzon DJ, Ojeaburu JV (2001) Prospective study of the natural history of gastrinoma in patients with MEN-1: definition of an aggressive and a nonaggressive form. J Clin Endocrinol Metab 86(11):5282–5293
48. Hoffman KM, Gibril F, Entsuah LK et al (2006) Patients with multiple endocrine neoplasia type 1 with gastrinomas have an increased risk of severe esophageal disease including stricture and the premalignant condition, Barrett's esophagus. J Clin Endocrinol Metab 91(1):204–212
49. Berna MJ, Hoffmann M, Serrano J et al (2006) Serum gastrin in Zollinger-Ellison syndrome I. Medicine 85:295–330

50. Berna MJ, Hoffmann M, Long SH et al (2006) Serum gastrin in Zollinger-Ellison syndrome II. Medicine 85:331–364
51. Roy PK, Venzon DJ, Shojamenesh H (2000) Zollinger-Ellison syndrome. Medicine 79(6):379–411
52. Alexander HR, Fraker DL, Norton JA et al (1998) Prospective study of somatostatin receptor scintigraphy and its effect on operative outcome in patients with Zollinger-Ellison syndrome. Ann Surg 228(2):228–238
53. Norton JA, Jensen RT (2004) Resolved and unresolved controversies in the surgical management of patients with Zollinger-Ellison syndrome. Ann Surg 240(5):757–773
54. Gibril F, Reynolds JC, Doppman JL et al (1996) Somatostatin receptor scintigraphy: its sensitivity compared with that of other imaging methods in detecting primary and metastatic gastrinomas. Ann Intern Med 125(1):26–34
55. Cadiot G, Lebtahi R, Sarda L et al (1996) Preoperative detection of duodenal gastrinomas and peripancreatic lymph nodes by somatostatin receptor scintigraphy. Gastroenterology 111:845–854
56. Alexander HR, Bartlett DL, Venzon DJ et al (1998) Analysis of factors associated with long-term (five or more years) cure in patients undergoing operation for Zollinger-Ellison syndrome. Surgery 124:1160–1166
57. Wamsteker EJ, Gauger PG, Thompson NW, Scheiman JM (2003) EUS detection of pancreatic endocrine tumors in asymptomatic patients with type 1 multiple endocrine neoplasia. Gastroinest Endosc 58(4):531–535
58. Thompson JC, Lewis BG, Wiener I, Townsend CM Jr (1983) The role of surgery in Zollinger-Ellison syndrome. Ann Surg 197(5):594–607
59. Sheppard BC, Norton JA, Doppman JL et al (1989) Management of islet cell tumors in patients with multiple endocrine neoplasia: a prospective study. Surgery 106:1108–1118
60. van Heerden JA, Smith SL, Miller LJ (1986) Management of the Zollinger-Ellison syndrome in patients with multiple endocrine neoplasia type I. Surgery 100(6):971–975
61. Norton JA, Doppman JL, Jensen RT (1992) Curative resection in Zollinger-Ellison syndrome. Ann Surg 215(1):8–18
62. Sugg SL, Norton JA, Fraker DL et al (1993) A prospective study of intraoperative methods to diagnose and resect duodenal gastrinomas. Ann Surg 218(2):138–144
63. Bartsch DK, Langer P, Wild A et al (2000) Pancreaticoduodenal endocrine tumors in multiple endocrine neoplasia type 1: surgery or surveillance. Surgery 128:958–966
64. Norton JA, Alexander HR, Fraker DL et al (2001) Comparison of surgical results in patients with advanced and limited disease with multiple endocrine neoplasia type 1 and Zollinger-Ellison syndrome. Ann Surg 234(4):495–506
65. Libutti SK, Alexander HR Jr (2006) Gastrinoma: sporadic and familial disease. Surg Oncol Clin N Am 15(3):479–496
66. Shepherd JJ (1991) The natural history of multiple endocrine neoplasia type 1. Highly uncommon or highly unrecognized? Arch Surg. 126(8):935–952
67. Demeure MJ, Klonoff DC, Karam JH et al (1991) Insulinomas associated with multiple endocrine neoplasia type I: the need for a different surgical approach. Surgery 110:998–1005
68. Rasbach DA, van Heerden JA, Telander RL et al (1985) Surgical management of hyperinsulinism in the multiple endocrine neoplasia, type 1 syndrome. Arch Surg 120:584–589
69. Dizon AM, Kowalyk S, Hoogwerf B (1999) Neuroglycopenic and other symptoms in patients with insulinomas. Am J Med 106:307–310
70. Nikfarjam M, Warshaw AL, Axelrod L et al (2008) Improved contemporary surgical management of insulinomas. Ann Surg 247(1):165–172
71. Hirshberg B, Livi A, Bartlett DL et al (2000) Forty-eight-hour fast: the diagnostic test for insulinoma. J Clin Endocrinol Metab 85:3222–3226
72. Doherty GM, Doppman JL, Shawker TH et al (1991) Results of a prospective strategy to diagnose, localize, and resect insulinomas. Surgery 110:989–997
73. Norton JA, Fang TD, Jensen RT (2006) Surgery for gastrinoma and insulinoma in multiple endocrine neoplasia type 1. J Natl Compr Canc Netw 4(2):148–153
74. O'Riordain DS, O'Brien T, van Heerden JA et al (1994) Surgical management of insulinoma associated with multiple endocrine neoplasia type I. World J Surg 18:488–494

75. Hiramoto JS, Feldstein VA, LaBerge J, Norton JA (2001) Intraoperative ultrasound and preoperative localization detects all occult insulinomas. Arch Surg 136:1020–1026
76. Doppman JL, Chang R, Fraker DL et al (1995) Localization of insulinomas to regions of the pancreas by intra-arterial stimulation with calcium. Ann Intern Med 123:269–273
77. Anderson MA, Carpenter S, Thompson NW et al (2000) Endoscopic ultrasound is highly accurate and directs management in patients with neuroendocrine tumors of the pancreas. Am J Gastroenterol 95(9):2271–2277
78. Norton JA, Shawker TH, Doppman JL et al (1990) Localization and surgical treatment of occult insulinomas. Ann Surg 212(5):615–620
79. Miller DL, Doppman JL, Metz DC et al (1992) Zollinger-Ellison syndrome: technique, results and complications of portal venous sampling. Radiology 182(1):235–241
80. Zeiger MA, Shawker TH, Norton JA (1993) Use of intraoperative ultrasonography to localize islet cell tumors. World J Surg 17:448–454
81. Brown CK, Bartlett DL, Doppman JL et al (1997) Intraarterial calcium stimulation and intraoperative ultrasonography in the localization and resection of insulinomas. Surgery 122:1188–1193
82. Grover AC, Skarulis M, Alexander HR et al (2005) A prospective evaluation of laparoscopic exploration with intraoperative ultrasound as a technique for localizing sporadic insulinomas. Surgery 138:1033–1038
83. Albright SA, McCart JA, Libutti SK, et al. (2002) Rapid measurement of insulin using the Abbott IMx: application to the management of insulinoma. Ann Clin Biochem 39(Pt5):513–515
84. Jordan PH Jr (1999) A personal experience with pancreatic and duodenal neuroendocrine tumors. J Am Coll Surg 189(5):470–482
85. Lo CY, Lam KY, Fan ST (1998) Surgical strategy for insulinomas in multiple endocrine neoplasia type I. Am J Surg 175(4):305–307
86. Verges B, Boureille F, Goudet P (2002) Pituitary disease in MEN Type 1 (MEN-1): data from the France-Belgium MEN-1 multicenter study. J Clin Endocrinol Metab 87(2):457–465
87. Corbetta S, Pizzocaro A, Peracchi M et al (1997) Multiple endocrine neoplasia type 1 in patients with recognized pituitary tumours of different types. Clin Endocrinol 47(5):507–512
88. Trouillas J, Labat-Moleur F, Sturm N et al (2008) Pituitary tumors and hyperplasia in multiple endocrine neoplasia type 1 syndrome (MEN-1): a case-control study in a series of 77 patients versus 2509 non-MEN-1 patients. Am J Surg Pathol 32(4):534–543
89. Marx SJ, Nieman LK (2002) Aggressive pituitary tumors in MEN-1: do they refute the two-hit model of tumorigenesis. J Clin Endocrinol Metab 87(2):453–456
90. Skogseid B, Larsson C, Lindgren P-G et al (1992) Clinical and genetic features of adrenocortical lesions in multiple endocrine neoplasia type 1. J Clin Endocrinol Metab 75(1):76–81
91. Burgess JR, Harle RA, Rucker P et al (1996) Adrenal lesions in a large kindred with multiple endocrine neoplasia type 1. Arch Surg 131(7):699–702
92. Darling TN, Skarulis MC, Steinberg SM et al (1997) Multiple facial angiofibromas and collagenomas in patients with multiple endocrine neoplasia type 1. Arch Dermatol 133(7):853–857
93. Pack S, Turner ML, Zhuang Z et al (1998) Cutaneous tumors in patients with multiple endocrine neoplasia type 1 show allelic deletion of the *MEN-1* gene. J Invest Dermatol 110:438–440
94. Schussheim DM, Skarulis MC, Agarwal SK et al (2001) Multiple endocrine neoplasia type 1: new clinical and basic findings. Trends Endocrinol Metab 12(4):173–178

Chapter 17
The *RET* Protooncogene

Amber L. Traugott and Jeffrey F. Moley

The *RET* Protooncogene

The *RET* protooncogene encodes a transmembrane receptor tyrosine kinase (RTK) with affinity for multiple ligands, including glial cell line-derived neurotrophic factor (GDNF). It was first described in 1985 by Takahashi and others, who identified rearrangements in the gene from human lymphoma DNA with transforming activity in a transfected cell line [1]. Over the next few years, the gene was mapped to its location on chromosome 10q11.2 [2]. RET signaling activates a number of downstream pathways implicated in cell survival and differentiation. RET knockout mice demonstrate a phenotype that includes renal agenesis and aberrant gut neurophysiology. Many effects of normal and abnormal RET proteins have been characterized in human development, physiology, and disease. Somatic mutations or rearrangements involving *RET* have been implicated in sporadic thyroid carcinomas. Germline activating mutations in the *RET* gene cause the multiple endocrine neoplasia type 2 (MEN-2) syndromes. This discovery has fundamentally changed the clinical approach and management of these patients and their at-risk family members, and provides insight into RET structure and function.

Normal Structure and Function of RET

The *RET* gene comprises 21 exons over a span of 60 kb, encoding a transmembrane RTK with several conserved domains that encode protein regions that mediate signaling function. Extracellular regions include four cadherin-like domains and a cysteine-rich domain. Additional regions of importance include a transmembrane domain, an intracellular juxtamembrane domain, and two intracellular tyrosine kinase domains.

J.F. Moley (✉)
Endocrine and Oncologic Surgery Section, Siteman Cancer Center, Washington University School of Medicine, St. Louis, MO USA
e-mail: moleyj@wustl.edu

C. Sturgeon (ed.), *Endocrine Neoplasia*, Cancer Treatment and Research, vol 153,
DOI 10.1007/978-1-4419-0857-5_17, © Springer Science+Business Media, LLC 2010

The RET protein has four known ligands that induce its activation: GDNF, artemin, persephin, and neurturin, known collectively as the GDNF family ligands (GFLs) [3–7]. RET activation by each of these GFLs is mediated through one of four ligand-specific coreceptors, belonging to the GDNF family receptors α (GFRα). These GFRα coreceptors are anchored to the plasma membrane by a glycosylphosphatidylinositol (GPI) residue, likely facilitating their interaction with the membrane-bound RET protein. Normal RET activation occurs with an assembly of a dimeric complex, including two RET proteins, two ligand molecules, and two GFRα coreceptors. (Fig. 17.1)

Current evidence indicates that the entire complex is necessary for RET signaling, and that ligand binding and downstream activation require the coreceptor [6, 8, 9].

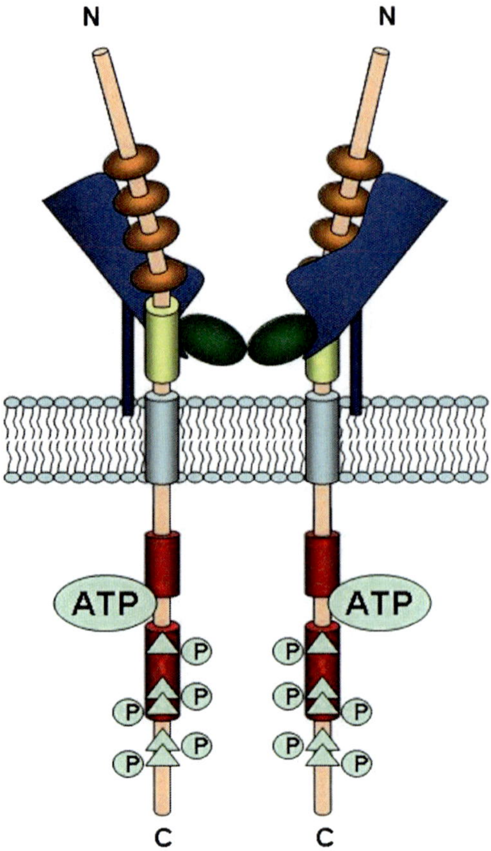

Fig. 17.1 The RET-GFRα-GFL dimeric signaling complex. The RET protein is a transmembrane receptor tyrosine kinase, represented here in its normal activated form. Two RET proteins associate with two GPI-anchored GFRα coreceptors (dark blue) and two GDNF-family ligands (dark green). Each RET molecule contains four extracellular cadherin-like domains (orange ovals), a cysteine-rich domain (yellow), a transmembrane domain (light blue), and two intracellular tyrosine kinase domains (red). Light green triangles represent the five autophosphorylated tyrosine residues known to be essential for normal RET signaling. Light green circles illustrate phosphorylation at these sites when RET is activated. The approximate position of the ATP binding site is also illustratedd

Studies investigating the molecular interactions of the GDNF-GFRα1-RET signaling complex suggest that GDNF does not directly bind RET at all [6, 9, 10]. Binding of the GDNF-GFRα1 complex appears to be mediated through interactions of the GFRα molecule with the first cadherin-like domain and the cysteine-rich domain of RET [10, 11]. The order in which these molecules associate with each other and the role of each functional domain in normal dimerization are not yet fully described. However, the cysteine-rich domain is thought to play a role in stabilizing the tertiary structure of RET with disulfide bonds [8].

Studies of the RET-coreceptor signaling complex have shown that in normal activation, the RET molecule is recruited to specialized regulatory regions of the plasma membrane, called lipid rafts, where the RET-coreceptor complex is formed and/or stabilized [12–14]. Lipid rafts are thought to promote specific protein–protein interactions over others, and have a regulatory role in numerous signal transduction pathways [15]. The GFRα coreceptors are located within these rafts and mediate the recruitment of RET to these sites, which seems to be required for normal RET signaling [12–14]. This localization also protects activated RET from proteasome-mediated degradation, which readily occurs outside of the raft environment [16]. Recently, an endogenous inhibitor of RET, Lrig1, was identified which appears to act by sequestering the RET molecule outside of the lipid rafts and decreasing its overall signaling activity [17].

The dimerized RET receptor complex activates a number of intracellular signaling pathways. Autophosphorylation of intracellular tyrosine residues is necessary for the activation of downstream effectors. Five phosphorylated tyrosine residues, at codons 905, 981, 1015, 1062, and 1096, have demonstrated importance for RET signaling, as docking sites for adaptor or effector molecules [18–34]. Other intracellular tyrosine residues are also autophosphorylated (806, 809, 900, 1090), but their biological significance is not yet understood [35]. RET activates the Ras/ERK and PI3K/Akt pathways, which are important in cell proliferation, differentiation, and survival [36–38]. Additional pathways activated by RET include p38MAPK, phospholipase C-γ (PLCγ), JNK, and ERK5, suggesting additional roles for RET in cell differentiation, migration, and cytokine production [26, 36, 39, 40]. Activated RET also has a phosphorylated serine residue (S696) in the juxtamembrane domain. This site has been implicated in Rac-mediated migration of enteric neural crest cells during normal development [41]. An inactivating mutation at this site in mice resulted in a lack of enteric neurons in the distal colon, similar to the phenotype of Hirschsprung's disease (HSCR) in humans [42].

There is evidence that the different GFL-GFRα complexes result in different patterns of intracellular signaling by the RET molecule. One study examined the differential effects of neurturin versus GDNF on RET signaling in a cell line expressing RET and GFRα1 [43]. Neurturin stimulation resulted in maximal autophosphorylation at Y1015, though other residues were phosphorylated to a lesser degree. Conversely, GDNF stimulation resulted in greater phosphorylation of Y1062 compared to the other residues. Neurturin and GDNF had different kinetics of autophosphorylation, with maximal activity at 15 min for neurturin versus 5 min for GDNF. In vitro, neurturin produced a more sustained activation of MAPK, and greater activation of PLCγ than GDNF. Neurturin, and not GDNF, promoted neuronal differentiation of the cell line through the PLCγ pathway; however, GDNF and not neurturin promoted cell survival through the MAPK pathway. In contrast, a second study showed no difference in phosphorylation patterns or kinetics between different GFLs, but did not examine differences in downstream signaling [34]. A third study showed that GDNF activates the MAPK pathway more rapidly than artemin [44]. Crystallographic studies demonstrate that the bend angle of the GDNF-GFRα1 homodimer is more acute, or v-shaped, than the relatively planar artemin-GFRα3 homodimer [44]. The investigators suggested that these differences may result in subtle changes in the conformation of activated RET for GDNF versus artemin, exposing different phosphorylated tyrosines for adaptor protein docking, and accounting for some signaling differences not related to phosphorylation pattern.

In addition to the variable effects of specific ligand-GFRα interactions on RET signaling, there are differential signaling effects based on the isoform of RET that is expressed. Alternative splicing results in three RET isoforms that differ by the number of amino acids in the C-terminus: RET9, RET43, and RET51. RET9 and RET51 are the best characterized isoforms. One of the phosphorylated tyrosines important for signaling, Y1096, is contained in RET51 but not in RET9. Several studies have demonstrated that the downstream effects of signaling through RET51 versus RET9 are different [23, 45–47]. Mice lacking RET9, but not RET51, exhibit defects in development of the kidneys and enteric nervous system [48]. This phenotype is only rescued by RET9, not RET51, suggesting that RET9 has a more important role in the normal early development of these systems [49, 50]. However, RET51, and not RET9, appears to be necessary for later differentiation and survival of mouse renal collecting duct system cells [51].

RET is expressed in multiple tissues from the neural crest, including the thyroid parafollicular cells, parathyroid glands, adrenal chromaffin cells, enteric ganglia, and other peripheral and central neurons. On the basis of studies in animal models, RET signaling is necessary for the normal development of thekidney, theparasympathetic nervous system, gut-associated lymphoid tissue, and the enteric nervous system [48, 52–58]. In humans, inactivating mutations in *RET* are associated with HSCR, a defect in migration and development of enteric neurons, which causes megacolon in infancy. Activating germline mutations in *RET* have been associated with the MEN-2 syndrome, while activating somatic mutations are associated with sporadic thyroid carcinomas.

Abnormal RET Activation in MEN-2 Syndromes

Activating germline mutations in the *RET* protooncogene are responsible for the MEN-2 syndromes, which include MEN-2A, MEN-2B, and familial medullary thyroid carcinoma (FMTC). These rare syndromes have an autosomal dominant pattern of inheritance. All MEN-2 syndromes include medullary thyroid carcinoma (MTC), which occurs with near complete penetrance. Additional manifestations include variably penetrant pheochromocytoma in MEN-2A and MEN-2B, and hyperparathyroidism in MEN-2A. MEN-2B patients also develop skeletal abnormalities, mucosal neuromas, and enteric gangliomas, with symptoms of megacolon or other derangements of gut motility. During the late 1980s and early 1990s, investigators in the U.S. and U.K. performed genetic mapping studies in kindreds with MEN-2A and FMTC, ultimately associating mutations in the *RET* protooncogene with these syndromes [59, 60]. Subsequent studies confirmed this finding in MEN-2B [61]. Understanding the genetic basis of MEN-2 syndromes has led to a paradigm shift in the screening and treatment of affected patients and their families. Treatment now focuses on the early identification of *RET* mutation carriers and early thyroidectomy to prevent MTC, when possible.

Genotype-Phenotype Correlations in MEN-2 Syndromes

The clinical features and aggressiveness of MEN-2 syndromes correlate with the codon and functional domain of the mutation within the RET protein (Fig. 17.2). For example, a patient with MEN-2A due to a mutation in codon 634 is more likely

Codon	Risk Level	MEN 2B	MEN 2A			FMTC	HSCR
			MTC	Pheo	HPT		
533	I		X	X		X	
9-bp ins	I*					X	
606	I*		X				
609	II*		X	X	X	X	X
611	II		X	X	X	X	X
618	II		X	X	X	X	X
620	II		X	X		X	X
630	II*		X		X	X	
631	I*		X	X		X	
634	II		X	X	X	X	
768	I		X	X		X	
777	I*					X	
790	I		X	X		X	
791	I		X	X	X	X	
804	I		X	X	X	X	
804 +806	III*	X					
883	III	X					
891	I		X	X		X	
912	I*					X	
918	III	X					

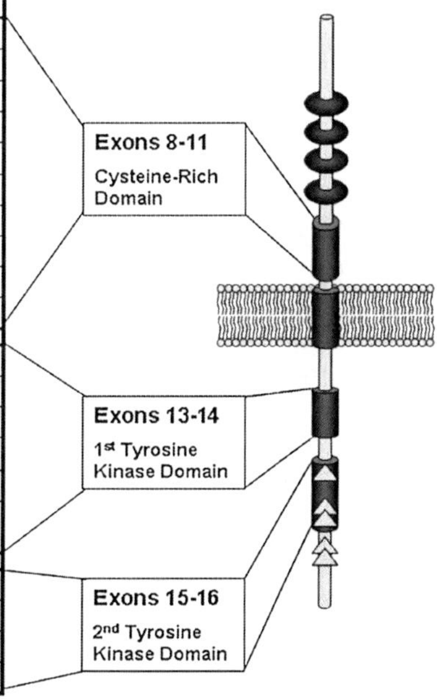

Fig. 17.2 RET mutation sites associated with MEN-2 syndromes. Codons previously reported in association with MEN-2 syndromes are listed by structural domain within the RET protein. Risk level is based on consensus guidelines or more recent clinical reports. Previously reported phenotypes for each codon are shown (MTC = medullary thyroid carcinoma, Pheo = pheochromocytoma, HPT = hyperparathyroidism, FMTC = familial medullary thyroid carcinoma, HSCR = Hirschsprung's disease). * indicates risk level based on recent clinical reports, not available at publication of the consensus guidelines

to develop MTC in early childhood than a patient with a codon 804 mutation. On the basis of clinical observations, consensus guidelines released in 2001 stratified the affected codons into three risk levels for clinical management of MTC [62]. Risk level III (highest risk) denotes patients at risk of MTC in infancy, with mutations that cause MEN-2B at codons 918, 883, or dual mutations at 804 and 806. Risk level II (high risk) includes specific codons associated with MEN-2A (634, 620, 618, 611, and possibly 609 and 630), where MTC has been seen in young children. Risk level I is the lowest risk group, and includes all other *RET* mutations associated with MEN-2A or FMTC. Patients with level I mutations typically develop MTC in their teens or in adulthood, though some of these are rare mutations with poorly characterized phenotypes.

Pheochromocytoma occurs with incomplete penetrance in MEN-2A, but the prevalence is highly variable between kindreds. Higher penetrance has been seen in association with some *RET* mutations as compared with others. Nearly all MEN-2B patients have the same M918T mutation, and their penetrance of pheochromocytoma has been estimated at about 50% [63]. A number of studies have shown that among MEN-2A patients, the lifetime prevalence of pheochromocytoma appears to be highest for those with codon 634 mutations [64–68]. One recent retrospective study from a large MEN-2A database reported an incidence of 50% in patients with codon 634 mutations versus 22% for codon 618, 9% for codon 620, and 4% for codon 609 [66]. Even within a single codon, the incidence of pheochromocytoma differed by the specific mutation. For example, 80% of patients with a C634W mutation and 48% of patients with a C634R mutation developed pheochromocytoma, but no cases occurred in patients with C634G mutations [66]. The earliest age of pheochromocytoma diagnosis is seen in patients with codon 634 and 918 mutations, with previous reports as early as 12 years of age, presenting either with symptoms or abnormal screening tests [68]. Recently, an 8-year-old with a codon 634 mutation and pheochromocytoma underwent an adrenalectomy at our institution, likely the youngest known case to date (as yet unpublished). For codons 618 and 620, the youngest reported presentation was at age 19 [66]. For other mutations, the earliest age at presentation was later, ranging from 22 to 59, depending on the codon [66, 68]. Specific modifiers of pheochromocytoma expression beyond *RET* mutation have not yet been identified.

Not much data are available on the *RET* genotype–phenotype correlations for hyperparathyroidism in MEN-2A. Retrospective studies indicate that the penetrance of hyperparathyroidism varies widely, from 0%–100%, between kindreds; on an average, 20%–30% of MEN-2A patients will develop parathyroid hyperplasia [69, 70]. Limited data suggest that this phenotype is more common among patients with codon 634 mutations (19%–46%) than those with mutations at other codons (0%–12%) [71, 72]. However, the penetrance also varies widely by kindred even when all the carriers bear codon 634 mutations (0%–66%) [72]. Additional studies will be needed to clarify the genetic factors responsible for this variable penetrance.

In MEN-2 syndromes, endocrine neoplasms result from constitutive activation of RET, most commonly due to missense mutations. The functional consequences of these mutations are most significant when the kinase or cysteine-rich domains are involved. Animal and in vitro studies have shown that the mechanism and downstream effects of RET activation are different in MEN-2A versus MEN-2B.

MEN-2B and Alterations in the Kinase Domain

MEN-2B patients have the most aggressive form of MTC and can develop metastatic disease in infancy or early childhood if untreated. Approximately 50% of MEN-2B patients will develop pheochromocytoma during their lifetime. They often have disorders of gut motility, mucosal neuromas, and skeletal abnormalities, which present as early as birth. MEN-2B is caused by mutations in the intracellular tyrosine kinase domain of RET. Most cases (~95%) result from a substitution of the methionine at codon 918 with a threonine, and the other 5% are associated with A883F. There also has been a case report of MEN-2B caused by dual mutations at codons 804 and 806 [73].

The M918T mutation changes the conformation of a region of the kinase domain important for binding of ATP substrate, and demonstrates increased affinity for ATP relative to wild-type RET [74]. RET molecules in MEN-2B are constitutively highly activated in monomeric and dimeric forms, unlike wild-type RET molecules which require a dimeric complex to maintain activation [74, 75] (Fig. 17.3b). In the presence

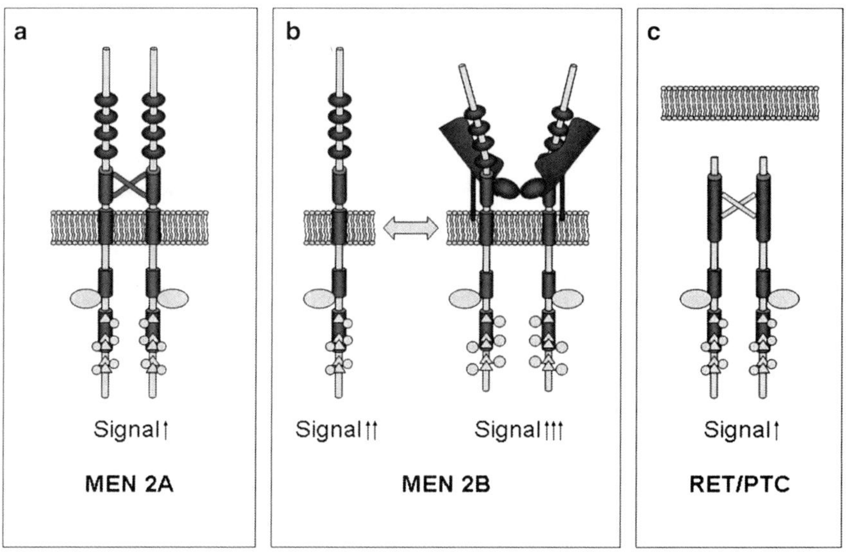

Fig. 17.3 Mechanisms of abnormal RET activation. (**a**) In MEN-2A, mutations of cysteine residues in the cysteine-rich domain of RET result in ligand-independent dimerization, likely by disulfide bond formation between unpaired cysteines on two abnormal RET molecules. (**b**) In MEN-2B, mutations in the tyrosine kinase domain result in constitutive activation in monomeric form. Abnormal RET molecules can still dimerize in association with ligand and coreceptor, resulting in even higher levels of phosphorylation and signaling. (**c**) RET/PTC molecules result from chromosomal rearrangements of the portion of the *RET* gene encoding the tyrosine kinase domains with other activating genes encoding a dimerization domain. The resulting fusion proteins exhibit dysregulated dimerization and activation of the RET kinase. RET/PTC proteins lack a transmembrane domain and are localized to the cytosol

of ligand, M918T mutant RET demonstrates even greater activity, and this effect is most pronounced for the RET9 isoform versus the RET51 isoform [76]. This suggests that the formation of GFL-GFRα-RET dimeric complex stabilizes and enhances the signaling activity of the M918T mutant RET to a level beyond its highly elevated baseline, which may account for some of the aggressive characteristics of MEN-2B.

Methionine at the position corresponding to codon 918 is highly conserved in RTKs, whereas cytoplasmic tyrosine kinases have a threonine at that position [77]. Based on this observation, the M918T mutation has been speculated to alter the substrate specificity for downstream signaling, possibly involving pathways known to be activated by cytoplasmic rather than transmembrane kinases, including SRC-dependent pathways involved in cell cycle regulation. Some differences in patterns of autophosphorylation and downstream effector activation have been reported, including differential binding of adaptor proteins Grb2 and Crk and increased phosphatidylinositol-3 (PI-3) kinase activity, for wild-type versus M918T mutant RET in vitro [77–80]. However, some recent studies found no differences between SRC kinase activation by wild-type and M918T mutant RET [74, 75]. Based on this mixed evidence, it is unclear to what degree qualitative versus quantitative signaling differences play a role in the development of the MEN-2B phenotype.

MEN-2A, FMTC, and Mutations in the Cysteine-Rich Region

All MEN-2A patients develop MTC during their lifetime, though the age of onset varies from early childhood to adulthood, depending on the specific mutation and kindred. Forty to fifty percent of MEN-2A patients will develop pheochromocytoma, which may or may not be synchronous with MTC in its presentation. Primary hyperparathyroidism occurs in 20%–35% of these patients overall. Patients who inherit FMTC also develop MTC, but do not have pheochromocytoma or parathyroid hyperplasia. There is considerable overlap in the codons and mutations that cause MEN-2A and FMTC, and they are thought to involve the same general mechanisms of constitutive RET activation.

The most common mutations associated with MEN-2A/FMTC occur in exons 10 and 11, within the extracellular cysteine-rich domain of the RET protein. Cysteine residues at codons 609, 611, 618, 620, 630, and 634 fall within this region, and germline mutations at these sites correspond to risk level II for thyroid management as per the consensus guidelines [62]. The cysteine-rich domain is considered to stabilize the normal tertiary structure of the RET protein, through formation of disulfide bonds between the cysteine residues in this region. Changing one of these cysteine residues to another amino acid results in an unpaired cysteine, which may form aberrant bonds with other cysteines within the same molecule or between abnormal RET molecules [81, 82]. This results in ligand-independent dimerization and persistent intracellular signaling by RET [75]. (Fig. 17.3a)

In addition to constitutive signaling effects, mutations in the cysteine-rich domain may alter the patterns of downstream effector activation. RET molecules with cysteine mutations associated with MEN-2A do not need to form a complex with the coreceptor or localize to lipid rafts in order to dimerize and become activated. This raft-independent signaling is associated with sustained activation of the AKT pathway compared to wild-type RET, and may result in other qualitative signaling changes which are not yet characterized, in addition to an overall increase in signaling activity [12].

Other Mutations

Numerous other activating mutations in *RET* have been identified in association with MEN-2A or FMTC, though these are less common than the cysteine mutations previously discussed. These include non-cysteine mutations within the cysteine-rich domain (encoded by exons 8–11), as well as mutations within the tyrosine kinase domains (encoded by exons 13–18). To date, other identified mutation sites include codons 533, 606, 631, 768, 777, 790, 791, 804, 891, 912, and a 9 base-pair duplication in exon 8 [36, 83–86]. The phenotypes from these mutations include MEN-2A and FMTC with a later age of onset of MTC and pheochromocytoma, and lower penetrance of pheochromocytoma, than the risk level II cysteine mutations [68, 87]. Because these are seen infrequently in practice, the phenotypes have not been well characterized. As more clinical experience with these kindreds is reported, the appropriate ages for preventive thyroidectomy and pheochromocytoma screening for carriers of these mutations may become more refined.

RET Mutations in Sporadic Thyroid Carcinomas

Somatic mutations or rearrangements involving *RET* have been identified in 40%–50% of sporadic MTCs and up to 70% of sporadic papillary thyroid carcinomas (PTCs) [36, 88]. Most of the mutations identified in sporadic MTCs are point mutations involving the same codons associated with the MEN-2 syndromes, including 918, 634, and 883 [88]. Of sporadic MTCs with alterations of *RET*, 60%–80% are found to have the M918T mutation [88–91]. Patients with sporadic MTCs bearing a *RET* mutation (particularly M918T) have a more advanced stage at diagnosis, increased rates of recurrent or persistent disease after resection, and poorer long-term survival (10–20 years) than those without a *RET* mutation [88, 90, 91]. In addition, sporadic MTCs are heterogeneous with regard to the distribution of *RET* mutations. Molecular studies of sporadic MTCs demonstrate that some cell subpopulations within a given primary tumor or its metastases have a *RET* mutation, while others do not [92]. This suggests that the *RET* mutation may be a later event in tumorigenesis, occurring in subclonal populations of an already established MTC. It is unclear what survival advantage, if any, is conferred on these subgroups of cells by the presence of a *RET* mutation. Because of this, it is unclear whether *RET* mutations are actually responsible for the poorer prognosis seen clinically, or whether this observation reflects an association due to some other cause.

Chromosomal rearrangements of *RET*, rather than point mutations, are associated with sporadic or radiation-associated PTCs. A number of rearrangements have been reported which result from the fusion of the *RET* tyrosine kinase domain to activating portions of other genes. Collectively, these fusion genes are referred to as RET/PTC, and to date 13 distinct variants, resulting from rearrangement events from different genes, have been described [36, 93]. These are designated RET/PTC1 through RET/PTC9, PCM1-RET, ELKS-RET, RFP-RET, and HOOK3-RET [36, 93]. Of these, RET/PTC1 (a rearrangement with CCDC6) and RET/PTC3 (a rearrangement with NcoA4) are the most common, representing over 90% of the RET/PTC variants identified [94]. The prevalence of RET/PTC rearrangements in sporadic PTCs varies widely between studies, from 3% to 85%. Some of the differences in the reported findings may be due to large differences in the ability of different laboratory methods to detect RET/PTC [95].

These fusion genes result in dysregulated expression and activation of the RET kinase domain within thyroid follicular cells, the cell type which gives rise to PTCs. Although the activating genes that participate in this rearrangement have somewhat divergent, and in most cases poorly understood normal functions within the cell, they have several characteristics in common. All seem to be normally expressed within thyroid follicular cells. In addition, they all encode structural domains which are thought to facilitate dimerization, based on their sequence homology to well-characterized proteins [36]. (Fig. 17.3c) Because the sequence of the RET tyrosine kinase domain is normal within the fusion protein, dimerization is probably required for its activation, as it is for normal RET. RET/PTC proteins are not membrane-bound or localized to lipid rafts, but are contained within the cytosolic compartment, where their interactions with downstream effectors and membrane-bound regulatory proteins are likely to be altered relative to normal RET function [94].

RET/PTC rearrangements have been found in clonal and subclonal populations of tumor cells [94, 95]. This implies that for some tumors, it may be an early or initiating event in carcinogenesis, while it is a later, perhaps non-essential event in others. Radiation exposure, a strong risk factor for the development of thyroid carcinoma, appears to be related to RET/PTC expression. There is a high frequency of RET/PTC in radiation-induced PTCs among patients exposed to radiation during the Chernobyl disaster or nuclear testing, and those who have received external beam radiation to the neck [96–104]. In vitro studies also show that radiation induces the specific chromosomal rearrangements of the RET/PTC fusion genes and results in expression of RET/PTC in cell lines [105–107]. Overexpression of RET/PTC in cell lines induces histopathologic cellular changes consistent with PTC [108]. However, RET/PTC has also been identified in non-neoplastic thyroid tissue associated with Hashimoto's thyroiditis, a finding of unclear significance and some controversy [94].

Targeting RET in Chemotherapeutics

Due to its prominence in the pathogenesis of hereditary and sporadic thyroid carcinomas, RET has become an attractive target for new therapeutics. No effective chemotherapeutic treatment is currently known for metastatic MTC or for metastatic PTC unresponsive to radioactive iodine. A number of RTK inhibitors have been identified over the past 20 years. Several of these, including imatinib, ZD6474, sunitinib, and sorafenib, have demonstrated decreased phosphorylation of activating RET point mutants and/or RET/PTC proteins in vitro, as well as decreased growth of cell lines transfected with these activated forms of RET [109–113]. Another compound, 17-allylaminogeldanamycin (17-AAG), inhibits heat shock protein 90 (HSP-90) [114]. HSP-90 is a chaperone protein that interacts with RET/PTC1 and promotes proper protein folding, without which ubiquitin-mediated degradation of RET/PTC1 takes place. In vitro, 17-AAG resulted in decreased levels of RET/PTC1 [114]. 17-AAG also increased the accumulation of radioactive iodine in thyroid cell lines, independent of RET/PTC1 expression [114]. All of these compounds are being evaluated in clinical trials for patients with advanced MTC and/or PTC. If they prove to be efficacious, these compounds have the potential to fundamentally change the medical management of metastatic MTC and/or PTC, where current effective chemotherapeutic options are limited or nonexistent.

Conclusions

Over the past two decades, the structure and function of the *RET* protooncogene has been extensively studied in vitro and in vivo. Experiments in animal models have highlighted the importance of RET function in normal development. Inactivating mutations in RET are a known cause of HSCR in humans. Insights into the relationship between activating *RET* mutations and the MEN-2 syndromes has fundamentally changed the approach to risk assessment and preventive care for families affected by these rare inherited diseases. Somatic activating mutations or rearrangements of RET are associated with sporadic thyroid carcinomas. Chemotherapeutics that target inappropriately activated RET may prove to be effective in clinical trials. Hopefully, these new modalities for diagnosis and treatment will translate into better outcomes for patients with RET-related diseases.

References

1. Takahashi M, Ritz J, Cooper GM (1985) Activation of a novel human transforming gene, ret, by DNA rearrangement. Cell 42:581–588
2. Ishizaka Y, Itoh F, Tahira T et al (1989) Human ret proto-oncogene mapped to chromosome 10q11.2. Oncogene 4:1519–1521

3. Baloh RH, Tansey MG, Lampe PA et al (1998) Artemin, a novel member of the GDNF ligand family, supports peripheral and central neurons and signals through the GFRalpha3-RET receptor complex. Neuron 21:1291–1302
4. Kotzbauer PT, Lampe PA, Heuckeroth RO et al (1996) Neurturin, a relative of glial-cell-line-derived neurotrophic factor. Nature 384:467–470
5. Milbrandt J, de Sauvage FJ, Fahrner TJ et al (1998) Persephin, a novel neurotrophic factor related to GDNF and neurturin. Neuron 20:245–253
6. Treanor JJ, Goodman L, de Sauvage F et al (1996) Characterization of a multicomponent receptor for GDNF. Nature 382:80–83
7. Trupp M, Arenas E, Fainzilber M et al (1996) Functional receptor for GDNF encoded by the c-ret proto-oncogene. Nature 381:785–789
8. Runeberg-Roos P, Saarma M (2007) Neurotrophic factor receptor RET: structure, cell biology, and inherited diseases. Ann Med 39:572–580
9. Jing S, Wen D, Yu Y et al (1996) GDNF-induced activation of the ret protein tyrosine kinase is mediated by GDNFR-alpha, a novel receptor for GDNF. Cell 85:1113–1124
10. Amoresano A, Incoronato M, Monti G, Pucci P, de Franciscis V, Cerchia L (2005) Direct interactions among Ret, GDNF and GFRalpha1 molecules reveal new insights into the assembly of a functional three-protein complex. Cell Signal 17:717–727
11. Kjaer S, Ibanez CF (2003) Identification of a surface for binding to the GDNF-GFR alpha 1 complex in the first cadherin-like domain of RET. J Biol Chem 278:47898–47904
12. Freche B, Guillaumot P, Charmetant J et al (2005) Inducible dimerization of RET reveals a specific AKT deregulation in oncogenic signaling. J Biol Chem 280:36584–36591
13. Paratcha G, Ledda F, Baars L et al (2001) Released GFRalpha1 potentiates downstream signaling, neuronal survival, and differentiation via a novel mechanism of recruitment of c-Ret to lipid rafts. Neuron 29:171–184
14. Tansey MG, Baloh RH, Milbrandt J, Johnson EM Jr (2000) GFRalpha-mediated localization of RET to lipid rafts is required for effective downstream signaling, differentiation, and neuronal survival. Neuron 25:611–623
15. Lucero HA, Robbins PW (2004) Lipid rafts-protein association and the regulation of protein activity. Arch Biochem Biophys 426:208–224
16. Pierchala BA, Milbrandt J, Johnson EM Jr (2006) Glial cell line-derived neurotrophic factor-dependent recruitment of Ret into lipid rafts enhances signaling by partitioning Ret from proteasome-dependent degradation. J Neurosci 26:2777–2787
17. Ledda F, Bieraugel O, Fard SS, Vilar M, Paratcha G (2008) Lrig1 is an endogenous inhibitor of Ret receptor tyrosine kinase activation, downstream signaling, and biological responses to GDNF. J Neurosci 28:39–49
18. Donatello S, Fiorino A, Degl'Innocenti D et al (2007) SH2B1beta adaptor is a key enhancer of RET tyrosine kinase signaling. Oncogene 26:6546–6559
19. Alberti L, Borrello MG, Ghizzoni S, Torriti F, Rizzetti MG, Pierotti MA (1998) Grb2 binding to the different isoforms of Ret tyrosine kinase. Oncogene 17:1079–1087
20. Arighi E, Alberti L, Torriti F et al (1997) Identification of Shc docking site on Ret tyrosine kinase. Oncogene 14:773–782
21. Asai N, Murakami H, Iwashita T, Takahashi M (1996) A mutation at tyrosine 1062 in MEN2A-Ret and MEN2B-Ret impairs their transforming activity and association with shc adaptor proteins. J Biol Chem 271:17644–17649
22. De Vita G, Melillo RM, Carlomagno F et al (2000) Tyrosine 1062 of RET-MEN2A mediates activation of Akt (protein kinase B) and mitogen-activated protein kinase pathways leading to PC12 cell survival. Cancer Res 60:3727–3731
23. Degl'Innocenti D, Arighi E, Popsueva A et al (2004) Differential requirement of Tyr1062 multidocking site by RET isoforms to promote neural cell scattering and epithelial cell branching. Oncogene 23:7297–7309
24. Encinas M, Crowder RJ, Milbrandt J, Johnson EM Jr (2004) Tyrosine 981, a novel ret autophosphorylation site, binds c-Src to mediate neuronal survival. J Biol Chem 279:18262–18269

25. Hayashi H, Ichihara M, Iwashita T et al (2000) Characterization of intracellular signals via tyrosine 1062 in RET activated by glial cell line-derived neurotrophic factor. Oncogene 19:4469–4475
26. Hayashi Y, Iwashita T, Murakamai H et al (2001) Activation of BMK1 via tyrosine 1062 in RET by GDNF and MEN2A mutation. Biochem Biophys Res Commun 281:682–689
27. Iwashita T, Asai N, Murakami H, Matsuyama M, Takahashi M (1996) Identification of tyrosine residues that are essential for transforming activity of the ret proto-oncogene with MEN2A or MEN2B mutation. Oncogene 12:481–487
28. Kurokawa K, Iwashita T, Murakami H, Hayashi H, Kawai K, Takahashi M (2001) Identification of SNT/FRS2 docking site on RET receptor tyrosine kinase and its role for signal transduction. Oncogene 20:1929–1938
29. Lopez-Ramirez MA, Dominguez-Monzon G, Vergara P, Segovia J (2008) Gas1 reduces Ret tyrosine 1062 phosphorylation and alters GDNF-mediated intracellular signaling. Int J Dev Neurosci 26:497–503
30. Pandey A, Duan H, Di Fiore PP, Dixit VM (1995) The Ret receptor protein tyrosine kinase associates with the SH2-containing adapter protein Grb10. J Biol Chem 270:21461–21463
31. Pandey A, Liu X, Dixon JE, Di Fiore PP, Dixit VM (1996) Direct association between the Ret receptor tyrosine kinase and the Src homology 2-containing adapter protein Grb7. J Biol Chem 271:10607–10610
32. Salvatore D, Barone MV, Salvatore G et al (2000) Tyrosines 1015 and 1062 are in vivo autophosphorylation sites in ret and ret-derived oncoproteins. J Clin Endocrinol Metab 85: 3898–3907
33. Wong A, Bogni S, Kotka P et al (2005) Phosphotyrosine 1062 is critical for the in vivo activity of the Ret9 receptor tyrosine kinase isoform. Mol Cell Biol 25:9661–9673
34. Coulpier M, Anders J, Ibanez CF (2002) Coordinated activation of autophosphorylation sites in the RET receptor tyrosine kinase: importance of tyrosine 1062 for GDNF mediated neuronal differentiation and survival. J Biol Chem 277:1991–1999
35. Kawamoto Y, Takeda K, Okuno Y et al (2004) Identification of RET autophosphorylation sites by mass spectrometry. J Biol Chem 279:14213–14224
36. Arighi E, Borrello MG, Sariola H (2005) RET tyrosine kinase signaling in development and cancer. Cytokine Growth Factor Rev 16:441–467
37. Trupp M, Scott R, Whittemore SR, Ibanez CF (1999) Ret-dependent and -independent mechanisms of glial cell line-derived neurotrophic factor signaling in neuronal cells. J Biol Chem 274:20885–20894
38. van Weering DH, Medema JP, van Puijenbroek A, Burgering BM, Baas PD, Bos JL (1995) Ret receptor tyrosine kinase activates extracellular signal-regulated kinase 2 in SK-N-MC cells. Oncogene 11:2207–2214
39. Borrello MG, Alberti L, Arighi E et al (1996) The full oncogenic activity of Ret/ptc2 depends on tyrosine 539, a docking site for phospholipase Cgamma. Mol Cell Biol 16:2151–2163
40. Chiariello M, Visconti R, Carlomagno F et al (1998) Signalling of the Ret receptor tyrosine kinase through the c-Jun NH2-terminal protein kinases (JNKS): evidence for a divergence of the ERKs and JNKs pathways induced by Ret. Oncogene 16:2435–2445
41. Fukuda T, Kiuchi K, Takahashi M (2002) Novel mechanism of regulation of Rac activity and lamellipodia formation by RET tyrosine kinase. J Biol Chem 277:19114–19121
42. Asai N, Fukuda T, Wu Z et al (2006) Targeted mutation of serine 697 in the Ret tyrosine kinase causes migration defect of enteric neural crest cells. Development 133:4507–4516
43. Lee RH, Wong WL, Chan CH, Chan SY (2006) Differential effects of glial cell line-derived neurotrophic factor and neurturin in RET/GFRalpha1-expressing cells. J Neurosci Res 83:80–90
44. Parkash V, Leppanen VM, Virtanen H et al (2008) The structure of the glial cell line-derived neurotrophic factor-coreceptor complex: insights into RET signaling and heparin binding. J Biol Chem 283:35164–35172
45. Borrello MG, Mercalli E, Perego C et al (2002) Differential interaction of Enigma protein with the two RET isoforms. Biochem Biophys Res Commun 296:515–522

46. Tsui-Pierchala BA, Ahrens RC, Crowder RJ, Milbrandt J, Johnson EM Jr (2002) The long and short isoforms of Ret function as independent signaling complexes. J Biol Chem 277: 34618–34625
47. Schuetz G, Rosario M, Grimm J, Boeckers TM, Gundelfinger ED, Birchmeier W (2004) The neuronal scaffold protein Shank3 mediates signaling and biological function of the receptor tyrosine kinase Ret in epithelial cells. J Cell Biol 167:945–952
48. Schuchardt A, D'Agati V, Larsson-Blomberg L, Costantini F, Pachnis V (1994) Defects in the kidney and enteric nervous system of mice lacking the tyrosine kinase receptor Ret. Nature 367:380–383
49. de Graaff E, Srinivas S, Kilkenny C et al (2001) Differential activities of the RET tyrosine kinase receptor isoforms during mammalian embryogenesis. Genes Dev 15:2433–2444
50. Srinivas S, Wu Z, Chen CM, D'Agati V, Costantini F (1999) Dominant effects of RET receptor misexpression and ligand-independent RET signaling on ureteric bud development. Development 126:1375–1386
51. Lee DC, Chan KW, Chan SY (2002) RET receptor tyrosine kinase isoforms in kidney function and disease. Oncogene 21:5582–5592
52. Pichel JG, Shen L, Sheng HZ et al (1996) Defects in enteric innervation and kidney development in mice lacking GDNF. Nature 382:73–76
53. Schuchardt A, D'Agati V, Pachnis V, Costantini F (1996) Renal agenesis and hypodysplasia in ret-k- mutant mice result from defects in ureteric bud development. Development 122:1919–1929
54. Enomoto H, Araki T, Jackman A et al (1998) GFR alpha1-deficient mice have deficits in the enteric nervous system and kidneys. Neuron 21:317–324
55. Enomoto H, Heuckeroth RO, Golden JP, Johnson EM, Milbrandt J (2000) Development of cranial parasympathetic ganglia requires sequential actions of GDNF and neurturin. Development 127:4877–4889
56. Taraviras S, Marcos-Gutierrez CV, Durbec P et al (1999) Signalling by the RET receptor tyrosine kinase and its role in the development of the mammalian enteric nervous system. Development 126:2785–2797
57. Veiga-Fernandes H, Coles MC, Foster KE et al (2007) Tyrosine kinase receptor RET is a key regulator of Peyer's patch organogenesis. Nature 446:547–551
58. Marcos C, Pachnis V (1996) The effect of the ret- mutation on the normal development of the central and parasympathetic nervous systems. Int J Dev Biol Suppl. 1:137S–138S
59. Donis-Keller H, Dou S, Chi D et al (1993) Mutations in the RET proto-oncogene are associated with MEN 2A and FMTC. Hum Mol Genet 2:851–856
60. Mulligan LM, Kwok JB, Healey CS et al (1993) Germ-line mutations of the RET proto-oncogene in multiple endocrine neoplasia type 2A. Nature 363:458–460
61. Carlson KM, Dou S, Chi D et al (1994) Single missense mutation in the tyrosine kinase catalytic domain of the RET protooncogene is associated with multiple endocrine neoplasia type 2B. Proc Natl Acad Sci USA 91:1579–1583
62. Brandi ML, Gagel RF, Angeli A et al (2001) Guidelines for diagnosis and therapy of MEN type 1 and type 2. J Clin Endocrinol Metab 86:5658–5671
63. Miller CA, Ellison EC (2005) Multiple Endocrine Neoplasia Type 2B. In: Clark OH, Duh Q-Y, Kebebew E (eds) Textbook of endocrine surgery, 2nd edn. W.B. Saunders, Philadelphia, pp 757–763
64. Eng C, Clayton D, Schuffenecker I et al (1996) The relationship between specific RET proto-oncogene mutations and disease phenotype in multiple endocrine neoplasia type 2. International RET mutation consortium analysis. JAMA 276:1575–1579
65. Frank-Raue K, Hoppner W, Frilling A et al (1996) Mutations of the ret protooncogene in German multiple endocrine neoplasia families: relation between genotype and phenotype. German medullary thyroid carcinoma study group. J Clin Endocrinol Metab 81:1780–1783
66. Quayle FJ, Fialkowski EA, Benveniste R, Moley JF (2007) Pheochromocytoma penetrance varies by RET mutation in MEN 2A. Surgery 142:800–805 Discussion 5 e1
67. Rodriguez JM, Balsalobre M, Ponce JL et al (2008) Pheochromocytoma in MEN 2A syndrome. Study of 54 patients. World J Surg 32:2520–2526

68. Machens A, Brauckhoff M, Holzhausen HJ, Thanh PN, Lehnert H, Dralle H (2005) Codon-specific development of pheochromocytoma in multiple endocrine neoplasia type 2. J Clin Endocrinol Metab 90:3999–4003
69. Howe JR, Norton JA, Wells SA Jr (1993) Prevalence of pheochromocytoma and hyperparathyroidism in multiple endocrine neoplasia type 2A: results of long-term follow-up. Surgery 114:1070–1077
70. Kraimps JL, Denizot A, Carnaille B et al (1996) Primary hyperparathyroidism in multiple endocrine neoplasia type IIa: retrospective French multicentric study. Groupe d'Etude des Tumeurs a Calcitonine (GETC, French Calcitonin Tumors Study Group), French Association of Endocrine Surgeons. World J Surg 20:808–812 Discussion 12–13
71. Herfarth KK, Bartsch D, Doherty GM, Wells SA Jr, Lairmore TC (1996) Surgical management of hyperparathyroidism in patients with multiple endocrine neoplasia type 2A. Surgery 120:966–973 Discussion 73–74
72. Schuffenecker I, Virally-Monod M, Brohet R et al (1998) Risk and penetrance of primary hyperparathyroidism in multiple endocrine neoplasia type 2A families with mutations at codon 634 of the RET proto-oncogene. Groupe D'etude des Tumeurs a Calcitonine. J Clin Endocrinol Metab 83:487–491
73. Miyauchi A, Futami H, Hai N et al (1999) Two germline missense mutations at codons 804 and 806 of the RET proto-oncogene in the same allele in a patient with multiple endocrine neoplasia type 2B without codon 918 mutation. Jpn J Cancer Res 90:1–5
74. Gujral TS, Singh VK, Jia Z, Mulligan LM (2006) Molecular mechanisms of RET receptor-mediated oncogenesis in multiple endocrine neoplasia 2B. Cancer Res 66:10741–10749
75. Santoro M, Carlomagno F, Romano A et al (1995) Activation of RET as a dominant transforming gene by germline mutations of MEN2A and MEN2B. Science 267:381–383
76. Bongarzone I, Vigano E, Alberti L et al (1998) Full activation of MEN2B mutant RET by an additional MEN2A mutation or by ligand GDNF stimulation. Oncogene 16:2295–2301
77. Songyang Z, Carraway KL 3rd, Eck MJ et al (1995) Catalytic specificity of protein-tyrosine kinases is critical for selective signalling. Nature 373:536–539
78. Bocciardi R, Mograbi B, Pasini B et al (1997) The multiple endocrine neoplasia type 2B point mutation switches the specificity of the Ret tyrosine kinase towards cellular substrates that are susceptible to interact with Crk and Nck. Oncogene 15:2257–2265
79. Liu X, Vega QC, Decker RA, Pandey A, Worby CA, Dixon JE (1996) Oncogenic RET receptors display different autophosphorylation sites and substrate binding specificities. J Biol Chem 271:5309–5312
80. Murakami H, Iwashita T, Asai N et al (1999) Enhanced phosphatidylinositol 3-kinase activity and high phosphorylation state of its downstream signalling molecules mediated by ret with the MEN 2B mutation. Biochem Biophys Res Commun 262:68–75
81. Asai N, Iwashita T, Matsuyama M, Takahashi M (1995) Mechanism of activation of the ret proto-oncogene by multiple endocrine neoplasia 2A mutations. Mol Cell Biol 15:1613–1619
82. Kjaer S, Kurokawa K, Perrinjaquet M, Abrescia C, Ibanez CF (2006) Self-association of the transmembrane domain of RET underlies oncogenic activation by MEN2A mutations. Oncogene 25:7086–7095
83. D'Aloiso L, Carlomagno F, Bisceglia M et al (2006) Clinical case seminar: in vivo and in vitro characterization of a novel germline RET mutation associated with low-penetrant nonaggressive familial medullary thyroid carcinoma. J Clin Endocrinol Metab 91:754–759
84. Jimenez C, Dang GT, Schultz PN et al (2004) A novel point mutation of the RET protooncogene involving the second intracellular tyrosine kinase domain in a family with medullary thyroid carcinoma. J Clin Endocrinol Metab 89:3521–3526
85. Pigny P, Bauters C, Wemeau JL et al (1999) A novel 9-base pair duplication in RET exon 8 in familial medullary thyroid carcinoma. J Clin Endocrinol Metab 84:1700–1704
86. Ercolino T, Lombardi A, Becherini L et al (2008) The Y606C RET mutation causes a receptor gain of function. Clin Endocrinol (Oxf) 69:253–258
87. Machens A, Dralle H (2007) Genotype-phenotype based surgical concept of hereditary medullary thyroid carcinoma. World J Surg 31:957–968

88. Elisei R, Cosci B, Romei C et al (2008) Prognostic significance of somatic RET oncogene mutations in sporadic medullary thyroid cancer: a 10-year follow-up study. J Clin Endocrinol Metab 93:682–687
89. Marsh DJ, Learoyd DL, Andrew SD et al (1996) Somatic mutations in the RET proto-oncogene in sporadic medullary thyroid carcinoma. Clin Endocrinol (Oxf) 44:249–257
90. Zedenius J, Larsson C, Bergholm U et al (1995) Mutations of codon 918 in the RET proto-oncogene correlate to poor prognosis in sporadic medullary thyroid carcinomas. J Clin Endocrinol Metab 80:3088–3090
91. Schilling T, Burck J, Sinn HP et al (2001) Prognostic value of codon 918 (ATG–>ACG) RET proto-oncogene mutations in sporadic medullary thyroid carcinoma. Int J Cancer 95:62–66
92. Eng C, Mulligan LM, Healey CS et al (1996) Heterogeneous mutation of the RET proto-oncogene in subpopulations of medullary thyroid carcinoma. Cancer Res 56:2167–2170
93. Ciampi R, Giordano TJ, Wikenheiser-Brokamp K, Koenig RJ, Nikiforov YE (2007) HOOK3-RET: a novel type of RET/PTC rearrangement in papillary thyroid carcinoma. Endocr Relat Cancer 14:445–452
94. Santoro M, Melillo RM, Fusco A (2006) RET/PTC activation in papillary thyroid carcinoma: European Journal of Endocrinology Prize Lecture. Eur J Endocrinol 155:645–653
95. Zhu Z, Ciampi R, Nikiforova MN, Gandhi M, Nikiforov YE (2006) Prevalence of RET/PTC rearrangements in thyroid papillary carcinomas: effects of the detection methods and genetic heterogeneity. J Clin Endocrinol Metab 91:3603–3610
96. Bounacer A, Wicker R, Caillou B et al (1997) High prevalence of activating ret proto-oncogene rearrangements, in thyroid tumors from patients who had received external radiation. Oncogene 15:1263–1273
97. Collins BJ, Chiappetta G, Schneider AB et al (2002) RET expression in papillary thyroid cancer from patients irradiated in childhood for benign conditions. J Clin Endocrinol Metab 87:3941–3946
98. Fugazzola L, Pilotti S, Pinchera A et al (1995) Oncogenic rearrangements of the RET proto-oncogene in papillary thyroid carcinomas from children exposed to the Chernobyl nuclear accident. Cancer Res 55:5617–5620
99. Ito T, Seyama T, Iwamoto KS et al (1994) Activated RET oncogene in thyroid cancers of children from areas contaminated by Chernobyl accident. Lancet 344:259
100. Klugbauer S, Jauch A, Lengfelder E, Demidchik E, Rabes HM (2000) A novel type of RET rearrangement (PTC8) in childhood papillary thyroid carcinomas and characterization of the involved gene (RFG8). Cancer Res 60:7028–7032
101. Nikiforov YE, Rowland JM, Bove KE, Monforte-Munoz H, Fagin JA (1997) Distinct pattern of ret oncogene rearrangements in morphological variants of radiation-induced and sporadic thyroid papillary carcinomas in children. Cancer Res 57:1690–1694
102. Rabes HM, Demidchik EP, Sidorow JD et al (2000) Pattern of radiation-induced RET and NTRK1 rearrangements in 191 post-chernobyl papillary thyroid carcinomas: biological, phenotypic, and clinical implications. Clin Cancer Res 6:1093–1103
103. Alipov G, Ito M, Prouglo Y, Takamura N, Yamashita S (1999) Ret proto-oncogene rearrangement in thyroid cancer around Semipalatinsk nuclear testing site. Lancet 354:1528–1529
104. Thomas GA, Bunnell H, Cook HA et al (1999) High prevalence of RET/PTC rearrangements in Ukrainian and Belarussian post-Chernobyl thyroid papillary carcinomas: a strong correlation between RET/PTC3 and the solid-follicular variant. J Clin Endocrinol Metab 84:4232–4238
105. Ito T, Seyama T, Iwamoto KS et al (1993) In vitro irradiation is able to cause RET oncogene rearrangement. Cancer Res 53:2940–2943
106. Mizuno T, Iwamoto KS, Kyoizumi S et al (2000) Preferential induction of RET/PTC1 rearrangement by X-ray irradiation. Oncogene 19:438–443
107. Mizuno T, Kyoizumi S, Suzuki T, Iwamoto KS, Seyama T (1997) Continued expression of a tissue specific activated oncogene in the early steps of radiation-induced human thyroid carcinogenesis. Oncogene 15:1455–1460

108. Fischer AH, Bond JA, Taysavang P, Battles OE, Wynford-Thomas D (1998) Papillary thyroid carcinoma oncogene (RET/PTC) alters the nuclear envelope and chromatin structure. Am J Pathol 153:1443–1450
109. Carlomagno F, Anaganti S, Guida T et al (2006) BAY 43–9006 inhibition of oncogenic RET mutants. J Natl Cancer Inst 98:326–334
110. Carlomagno F, Vitagliano D, Guida T et al (2002) ZD6474, an orally available inhibitor of KDR tyrosine kinase activity, efficiently blocks oncogenic RET kinases. Cancer Res 62:7284–7290
111. Cohen MS, Hussain HB, Moley JF (2002) Inhibition of medullary thyroid carcinoma cell proliferation and RET phosphorylation by tyrosine kinase inhibitors. Surgery 132:960–966 Discussion 6–7
112. de Groot JW, Plaza Menacho I, Schepers H et al (2006) Cellular effects of imatinib on medullary thyroid cancer cells harboring multiple endocrine neoplasia Type 2A and 2B associated RET mutations. Surgery 139:806–814
113. Kim DW, Jo YS, Jung HS et al (2006) An orally administered multitarget tyrosine kinase inhibitor, SU11248, is a novel potent inhibitor of thyroid oncogenic RET/papillary thyroid cancer kinases. J Clin Endocrinol Metab 91:4070–4076
114. Marsee DK, Venkateswaran A, Tao H et al (2004) Inhibition of heat shock protein 90, a novel RET/PTC1-associated protein, increases radioiodide accumulation in thyroid cells. J Biol Chem 279:43990–43997

Chapter 18
Multiple Endocrine Neoplasia Type 2: Clinical Manifestations and Management

Amber L. Traugott and Jeffrey F. Moley

In the 1950s and 1960s, an increasing association was reported between medullary thyroid carcinoma (MTC) and pheochromocytoma, two relatively rare conditions. Identification of kindreds affected by the constellation of MTC, pheochromocytoma, and hyperparathyroidism led to the recognition of multiple endocrine neoplasia type 2 (MEN-2) as a distinct syndrome in the 1960s [1]. Three distinct, but related, MEN-2 syndromes are now recognized: MEN-2A, MEN-2B, and familial medullary thyroid carcinoma (FMTC).

The MEN-2 syndromes are caused by germline activating missense mutations in the *RET* oncogene, a transmembrane receptor tyrosine kinase. These are rare syndromes, with an estimated prevalence of 1 per 40,000 in the United States. Transmission is autosomal dominant. All of these syndromes share the clinical feature of MTC, a malignancy of thyroid parafollicular cells (C cells) (Fig. 18.1). In patients with MEN-2A, MEN-2B, or FMTC, MTC occurs with nearly complete penetrance, is multifocal and bilateral, and occurs at an earlier age than sporadic cases. Development of hereditary MTC is preceded by multicentric C-cell hyperplasia, with an age-related progression to cancer [2–4]. Other clinical features of MEN-2 are variably expressed and the presentation differs between the specific syndromes.

Clinical Features of MEN-2 Syndromes

MEN-2A

MEN-2A is characterized by MTC, pheochromocytoma, and primary hyperparathyroidism. These patients develop multifocal, bilateral MTC (Fig. 18.2). Pheochromocytoma occurs in 42–46% of MEN-2A patients overall, though the prevalence varies from

J.F. Moley (✉)
Endocrine and Oncologic Surgery Section, Washington University School of Medicine, St. Louis, MO, USA
e-mail: moleyj@wustl.edu

C. Sturgeon (ed.), *Endocrine Neoplasia*, Cancer Treatment and Research, vol 153,
DOI 10.1007/978-1-4419-0857-5_18, © Springer Science+Business Media, LLC 2010

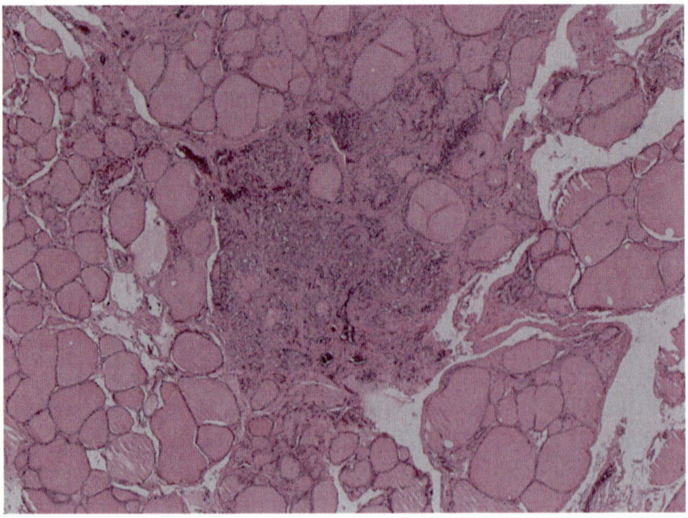

Fig. 18.1 Medullary thyroid cancer histology. A hematoxylin-eosin stained section showing a focus of medullary thyroid cancer surrounded by normal-appearing thyroid follicles

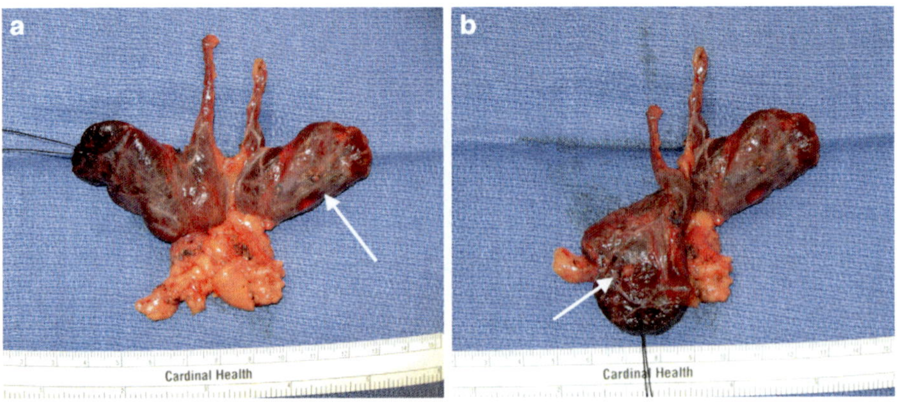

Fig. 18.2 Medullary thyroid cancer in MEN-2 syndromes. This thyroidectomy and central lymphadenectomy specimen from a patient with MEN-2A demonstrates multifocal, bilateral MTC (*arrows*) [5]

0 to 100% in different kindreds [6, 7]. The degree of penetrance for pheochromocytoma in MEN-2A correlates with specific *RET* mutations, with the highest expression in carriers of mutations at codon 634 [8]. Parathyroid hyperplasia in one or multiple glands results in primary hyperparathyroidism in 20–35% of MEN-2A patients overall; however, even this varies between kindreds [6, 9].

Cutaneous lichen amyloidosis (CLA) has been described in several kindreds and patients with MEN-2A [10–15]. CLA is a rare disorder characterized by amyloid deposition in the papillary dermis, resulting in pruritic cutaneous plaques, often localized to the interscapular region or extensor surfaces of the extremities (Fig. 18.3). In these MEN-2A kindreds, CLA phenotype co-segregates with the clinical features of MEN-2A. To date, all reported *RET* mutations in kindreds with combined MEN-2A/CLA features have been in codon 634 [11, 13, 15].

Hirschsprung disease (HSCR) is associated with MEN-2A and FMTC. This relatively common disease (1 in 5,000 births) is characterized by the congenital absence of ganglion cells within the myenteric and submucosal plexus of the distal colon.

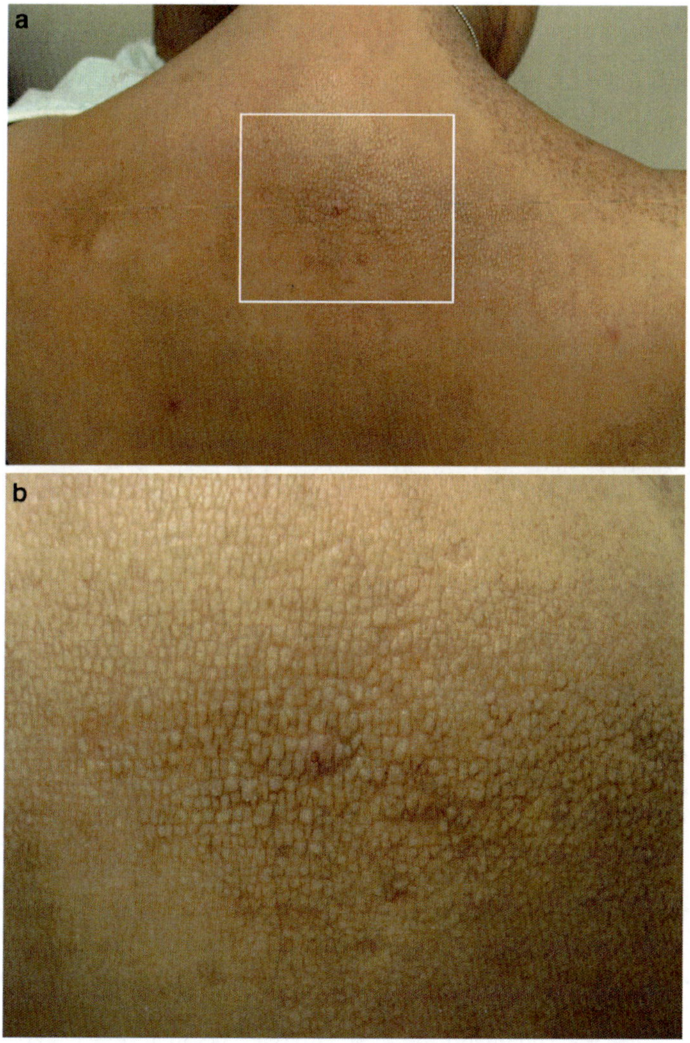

Fig. 18.3 Cutaneous lichen amyloidosis. (**a**) Interscapular CLA in a patient with MEN-2A. (**b**) Higher magnification view of thickened skin plaque typical of CLA

Newborn HSCR patients present with distal bowel obstruction and megacolon [16]. HSCR has been reported in 2.5–5% of patients with MEN-2A and FMTC, and co-segregates with mutations in *RET* codons 609, 611, 618, and 620 [17–19]. Within the affected MEN-2 kindreds, reported penetrance of HSCR is 16–50% among carriers [18]. Other forms of familial Hirschsprung's disease may be associated with inactivating *RET* mutations, rather than the constitutively active forms seen in MEN-2.

FMTC

FMTC is characterized by MTC but no other endocrine neoplasms. MTC in these patients tends to be the least aggressive, with a later age of onset and earlier stage at diagnosis. Middle-aged or, less commonly, elderly patients with FMTC may be encountered without clinical symptoms, despite the detection of MTC by the pathologist at the time of thyroidectomy. As with MEN-2A, HSCR has been reported in association with FMTC in a few kindreds [20]. Conservative criteria are used to diagnose FMTC, due to the potential overlap with MEN-2A if a kindred has low penetrance of pheochromocytoma and hyperparathyroidism. The most recent consensus guidelines recommend documentation of more than ten carriers in the kindred, multiple carriers or affected members over the age of 50 years, and an adequate medical history to exclude symptoms of other endocrine neoplasias [21]. These stringent criteria may result in the classification of small FMTC kindreds as MEN-2A, but they ensure that members of these families are appropriately screened for pheochromocytoma until their phenotype is well characterized.

MEN-2B

Patients with MEN-2B also develop MTC and pheochromocytomas, but do not develop primary hyperparathyroidism, in contrast to MEN-2A patients. All MEN-2B patients develop MTC, often in infancy or early childhood. Of the hereditary MTCs, those in the setting of MEN-2B present in the youngest patients and are most likely to have an advanced stage at diagnosis [22]. Pheochromocytoma occurs in approximately 50% of MEN-2B cases [23]. Many patients have skeletal abnormalities, including scoliosis, slipped capital femoral epiphyses, and club foot deformity.

Mucosal neuromas are another characteristic of MEN-2B. These proliferative lesions of nerves and Schwann cells develop in numerous mucosa-lined organs, and exhibit a plexiform pattern by histology. Most commonly, they are seen on the lips, tongue, and conjunctivae, though the gingiva, buccal mucosa, nasal mucosa, and vocal cords may also be involved. Clinically, these present as nodules and/or thickening of the lips and eyelids, with an enlarged, nodular, notched appearance of the tongue (Fig. 18.4). Thickening of the corneal nerves may be detected on ophthalmologic examination [24]. Ganglioneuromas may develop in the myenteric and

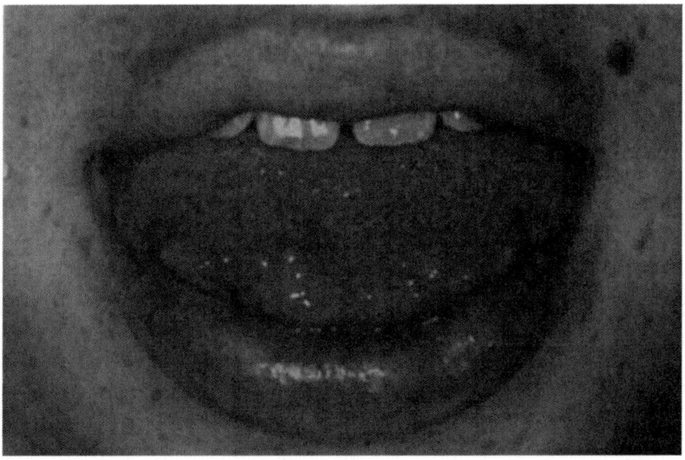

Fig. 18.4 Mucosal neuromas resulting in a nodular appearance of the tongue in a patient with MEN-2B

submucosal plexus of the gastrointestinal tract. Autopsy specimens have demonstrated diffuse involvement of the esophagus, stomach, and intestine [25]. As a result, these patients may present with symptoms of abnormal gut motility, including dysphagia, constipation, obstruction, vomiting, diarrhea, or megacolon [25–28]. These symptoms usually present at birth or in early childhood, in most cases preceding the other clinical manifestations of MEN-2B or MTC [28]. Megacolon arising in the setting of intestinal ganglioneuromatosis and MEN-2B should be distinguished from the association of MEN-2A with HSCR, which also presents with megacolon. There is no reported association between MEN-2B and HSCR. Rectal biopsies in MEN-2B patients with megacolon demonstrate neuromas, but not the aganglionosis diagnostic of HSCR.

Screening for MEN-2 and the Impact of *RET* Mutation Testing

Germline gain-of-function mutations in the *RET* oncogene are responsible for the development of MEN-2 syndromes. Prior to the genetic basis of MEN-2 being well characterized, pentagastrin-stimulated calcitonin testing was used to screen for MEN-2 and MTC in patients at risk for inheriting a MEN-2 syndrome. Calcitonin is produced by thyroid C cells, and is well-established as a tumor marker for MTC. Pentagastrin-stimulated calcitonin screening is highly sensitive and specific for MTC. However, the false positive rate is estimated at 5–10%, which previously led to a low rate of thyroidectomies in patients who had not inherited the disease [21, 29]. In addition, small foci of early stage MTC have been reported in MEN-2 carriers with negative stimulated calcitonin tests [29]. Sequencing of the *RET* gene to detect germline mutations is now the standard screening test for MEN-2 syndromes.

RET mutation testing can identify young carriers at an earlier stage of disease, often before they develop cancer, and it has lower false positive and false negative rates than calcitonin testing for MEN-2 screening.

Testing for germline *RET* mutations is indicated in a number of clinical settings. *RET* mutation testing should be performed routinely for at-risk family members of MEN-2 and FMTC patients. If possible, testing should be done at birth, because carrier status determines the need for clinical screening and preventive surgery. When an index case is identified, all family members at risk should undergo testing, regardless of their age. In families where the transmitted allele is already known, *RET* sequencing can be limited to the site of the known mutation [21]. Those family members who are negative for their kindred's known mutation have the same risk for MEN-2 as the general population, and they need no other screening. Patients who have negative genetic testing should consider a second test to verify the result, because of the serious potential consequences of a false negative test or laboratory error.

RET mutation testing is also indicated for adult or pediatric patients who present with MTC or pheochromocytoma, regardless of any family history of endocrine tumors. Approximately 5–7% of patients thought to have sporadic MTC are found to have a germline *RET* mutation [30–32]. Up to 24% of pheochromocytomas are hereditary, with 5% resulting from *RET* mutations [33]. Routine sequencing is performed first on exons 10, 11, 13, 14, 15, and 16; these are the most common sites for mutations which cause MEN-2. If the initial results are negative, the other 15 exons should then be sequenced. The estimated false-negative rate for complete *RET* sequencing to detect MEN-2, given a diagnosis of MTC or pheochromocytoma, is 0.18% [21]. Because pheochromocytoma can be associated with a number of genetic syndromes, patients with this diagnosis should undergo genetic testing for mutations in the *VHL*, *NF1*, *SDHD*, and *SDHB* genes in addition to *RET*.

Infants presenting with HSCR should undergo *RET* mutation testing. All reported cases of MEN-2A associated with HSCR have occurred in patients with mutations in exon 10 of *RET*, at codons 609, 611, 618, and 620, hence targeted sequencing limited to the regions of exons 10 and 11 may be more cost-effective and clinically relevant than extensive *RET* sequencing [18, 21, 34]. We recently reported two new MEN-2A kindreds that were identified by *RET* mutation testing of members diagnosed with HSCR [34]. Identification of other carriers in these two families resulted in thyroidectomies for a number of relatives, all of whom had C-cell hyperplasia or MTC identified on pathology.

Hereditary Medullary Thyroid Carcinoma

MTC arises from thyroid C cells, which produce, store, and secrete calcitonin. In the normal thyroid, C cells make up a small fraction of the total thyroid mass, and are dispersed throughout the interstitium, adjacent to the thyroid follicles. They are more densely concentrated in the posterior upper third of the thyroid lobes bilaterally, also the most common site for MTC [35]. Though not always present, amyloid deposits are characteristic of MTC. Immunohistochemical stains for calcitonin are usually positive. Positive carcinoembryonic antigen (CEA) and chromogranin-A staining are also consistent with the diagnosis. Only 1–3% of all thyroid cancers are diagnosed as MTC, but approximately 25% of MTCs are hereditary, associated with germline *RET* mutations [36].

Patients with MTC may present with a palpable thyroid mass or nodule. Associated symptoms of dysphagia, shortness of breath, or hoarseness are present in approximately 15% of cases. Although most MTCs are slow-growing tumors, metastases to regional cervical lymph nodes are present in >70% of patients who present with palpable disease [37]. The clinical course is often indolent, even in the setting of lymph node metastases. The most frequent sites of lymphatic spread are to the central compartment of the neck (levels VI and VII), followed by the ipsilateral jugular nodes (levels II–V), and the contralateral cervical nodes. Other typical metastatic sites include the upper and anterior mediastinum, as well as the lungs, liver, and bone [37].

Unlike sporadic cases, hereditary MTCs are often multifocal and bilateral. Multicentric C-cell hyperplasia has been shown to precede the development of hereditary MTC; this represents a precursor lesion along a stepwise progression to malignancy [2–4]. The time course of this progression is variable and the *RET* genotype accounts for some of the variation in aggressiveness. While the age of onset and rate of disease progression may differ, the lifetime penetrance of MTC is near 100% in carriers of *RET* mutations associated with MEN-2 syndromes. For this reason, all patients diagnosed with MEN-2 should undergo total thyroidectomy. Resection of cervical lymph nodes with transplantation of parathyroid glands is recommended for patients with basal calcitonin levels over 40 pg/ml (basal calcitonin levels are typically higher in infants than adults, and this should be considered in evaluating newborns and infants). Recommendations for the timing and extent of surgery differ based on the patient's age at diagnosis, clinical presentation, and the risk level of their *RET* mutation.

Preventive Surgery

The best option for cure or prevention of MTC in MEN-2 patients is thyroidectomy early in life, ideally before MTC develops. A number of studies have demonstrated improved biochemical cure rates and/or decreased recurrence rates from early thyroidectomy, performed after positive screening by calcitonin testing or *RET* mutation testing [38–41]. Those who undergo surgery later in life have a higher risk of metastatic disease. A truly preventive procedure can be achieved most reliably in infancy or early childhood, underlying the importance of screening family members of known carriers at birth. Even in young MEN-2 patients with normal calcitonin levels, MTC and/or C-cell hyperplasia may be detected in thyroidectomy specimens [29].

RET mutations have been stratified into three risk levels for ease of management, as per the consensus guidelines published in 2001 [21]. Patients with MEN-2B have the most aggressive form of MTC, with invasive disease reported in patients less than one year of age [21, 26, 42]. MEN-2B is most commonly caused by a mutation at codon 918 (>95%), but has also been associated with mutations at codons 883, 922, or dual mutations at codon 804 plus either 806 or 904. These mutations are considered to be the highest risk level, and are designated level III. Patients with level III mutations should undergo a total thyroidectomy as early in life as is possible [21]. As mentioned, calcitonin levels may be higher in infants than in adults, and should be considered in evaluating these babies. Central node dissection and parathyroidectomy should be considered in infants with high calcitonin levels. Identification of the parathyroid glands in infants, however, may be difficult. These procedures are best performed by a surgeon experienced in pediatric thyroidectomy. Hypoparathyroidism in a baby is a very serious complication, and we strongly recommend that these procedures should be performed by surgeons experienced in endocrine surgery and pediatric thyroidectomy.

Patients with MEN-2A have variably aggressive MTC. Mutations in codons 634, 620, 618, and 611 are considered high risk (level II) [21]. MTC has been found in thyroidectomies from patients with codon 634 mutations as young as 1 year of age [32]. The youngest reported child to date with a codon 634 mutation and cervical lymph node metastasis was 5 years old [43]. Patients with level II mutations should undergo a total thyroidectomy prior to 5 years of age. Central lymph node dissection is controversial in these patients. Rates of hypoparathyroidism and recurrent laryngeal nerve injury increase with more extensive resection, and complications of thyroidectomy are higher overall for children under 7 years of age than for other patients [2, 44, 45]. Calcitonin levels should be checked preoperatively in these young patients. The risk of lymph node metastasis is very low in MEN-2A with normal calcitonin levels [46, 47]. For these patients, total thyroidectomy alone, with attempted preservation of the parathyroid glands in situ, is sufficient [48].

A larger subset of *RET* mutations, associated with MEN-2A and/or FMTC, are considered lowest risk (level I). These include mutations at codons 768, 790, 791, 804, and 891 [21]. Codon 609 was also included as level I in the consensus guidelines, but since their publication a case report described focal MTC in a 5-year-old with a normal stimulated calcitonin level and a mutation at this site [49]. Based on this data, some authors now advocate managing patients with codon 609 mutations as risk level II. For patients with low risk, level I mutations, total thyroidectomy is recommended, but there are no established guidelines regarding the timing; surgery before age 5–10 is considered appropriate. Some advocate serial pentagastrin-stimulated calcitonin testing, with thyroidectomy at the first positive test [21]. However, pentagastrin is not available for clinical use in the United States, and basal or calcium-stimulated calcitonin assays may not be as sensitive for early MTC. As with level II mutations, the need for central lymph node dissection should be guided by calcitonin levels and clinical features of the patient and kindred.

Since publication of the consensus guidelines, a number of new mutations have been described in association with MEN-2 syndromes, at codons 912, 630, 631, 606, 533, and a 9-bp duplication in exon 8 [50–55]. These are uncommon mutations, and due to lack of clinical experience, their penetrance and aggressiveness are not well characterized. A recent report described a mutation in codon 630 associated with multifocal MTC in a patient of age 1 year and metastatic disease in a 15-year-old [56]. On the basis of this case, some authors now treat it as a high-risk codon, advocating stimulated calcitonin screening from infancy and surgery by 5 years of age [56]. However, with the exception of codon 630, these are generally thought to be comparable to level I mutations, and principles used for low-risk mutations should guide these patients' management.

Central lymph node dissection and four-gland parathyroidectomy with autotransplantation should be performed in patients of any age, regardless of their mutation risk level, if the basal calcitonin level is elevated (> 40 pg/ml in adults), or if there is intraoperative concern for lymphadenopathy. Parathyroidectomy with autotransplantation should also be done if the blood supply to the parathyroids is disrupted. Primary hyperparathyroidism does not typically develop in MEN-2A patients until adulthood, making it unlikely that they would need this procedure for treatment of parathyroid hyperplasia in childhood. Some surgeons may elect to perform four-gland parathyroidectomy with autotransplantation to a forearm muscle for selected asymptomatic MEN-2A patients at the time of thyroidectomy, if their mutation or kindred has a high rate of hyperparathyroidism. This may prevent a potentially morbid future neck reoperation if they develop parathyroid hyperplasia later in life. Reoperation at the forearm implantation site can usually be done under local anesthesia on an outpatient basis. MEN-2B or FMTC patients will not develop hyperparathyroidism as part of their syndrome, thus the sternocleidomastoid muscle can be used for autotransplantation if the parathyroids are removed. In the autotransplantation procedure, the excised parathyroids should be minced into small (1 by 3 mm) fragments and placed in individual muscle pockets, closed with a suture; the practice of transplanting large fragments, or an entire parathyroid, into a single muscle pocket is, however, discouraged.

Surgical Management of MTC in Adults with MEN-2 Syndromes

Ideally, patients with MEN-2 syndromes are diagnosed in childhood, based on early *RET* mutation screening. However, many present in adulthood as index cases, or with clinical symptoms of MTC or pheochromocytoma, while others are found by *RET* mutation screening after a relative's diagnosis with MEN-2. One large retrospective study found that index cases, presenting with symptoms of MTC or pheochromocytoma, had poorer 10-year survival and biochemical cure rates than asymptomatic patients identified by screening alone [57]. Index cases also tended to be older at the time of thyroidectomy, which was associated with a poorer prognosis.

Surgical strategy for older patients with established disease is dictated by their clinical picture and the specific *RET* mutation. Over 70% of patients presenting with palpable MTC, hereditary or sporadic, have central cervical lymph node metastases, with a similar rate of spread to ipsilateral jugular nodes (in unilateral disease), and a high rate of spread to the contralateral jugular nodes [37]. At a minimum, patients with palpable MTC should undergo total thyroidectomy with central lymph node dissection and unilateral dissection of level II–V nodes. Bilateral dissection of level II–V nodes should be done in patients with extensive disease, or with imaging studies that indicate bilateral nodal involvement. Preoperative ultrasound imaging to identify nodes with apparent metastatic spread is helpful in determining the extent of surgery.

Asymptomatic adult or teenage patients with positive *RET* mutation screening will often require a central lymph node dissection in addition to thyroidectomy. Calcitonin levels should be obtained preoperatively. A basal calcitonin level <40 pg/ml may be associated with lymph node metastases, and is an indication for central lymph node dissection. Patients with codon 634 (level II) mutations are at an increased risk of lymph node metastasis, beginning in the mid-teens, with over 40% cumulative risk by age 20 [46]. The data is less clear for patients with level I mutations, hence their surgical approach should be individualized based on calcitonin level, presence of palpable disease, and family history.

The same principles govern parathyroid management for adult MEN-2 patients as for children. If the parathyroids are devascularized, as usually occurs as a consequence of central lymph node dissection, parathyroidectomy with autotransplantation should be done. Some surgeons routinely remove and autotransplant the lower parathyroids during a central node dissection, but preserve the upper glands. Adult MEN-2A patients with primary hyperparathyroidism or enlarged parathyroids should also undergo this procedure. For MEN-2A patients, the forearm is the appropriate autotransplantation site, while the sternocleidomastoid muscle may be used for MEN-2B and FMTC patients.

Postoperative Surveillance and Long-Term Management

The postoperative management of MEN-2 patients with MTC diagnosis is similar to that for sporadic MTC patients. Thyroid hormone replacement is required for life. Patients who undergo four-gland parathyroidectomy and autotransplantation will need supplementation with oral calcium and vitamin D for at least 4–8 weeks postoperatively. This is gradually withdrawn as the function of the parathyroid autotransplant grafts improves. Serial calcitonin testing is used to monitor persistent or recurrent MTC. In the immediate postoperative period, calcitonin levels may be unreliable or falsely elevated. In most cases, these stabilize after about 72 h, but they may take up to weeks or months to normalize in some patients [58, 59].

The term "biochemical cure" is used to refer to patients with normal calcitonin levels after surgery for MTC. Complete postoperative normalization of calcitonin has been associated with decreased long-term risk of MTC recurrence, though the evidence is less clear for a survival benefit [57, 60, 61]. All patients who have undergone thyroidectomy and central lymph node dissection for MTC should have a basal calcitonin level measured two weeks postoperatively, and annual serial measurements thereafter. A persistent or recurrent elevation in calcitonin indicates residual or recurrent MTC, and warrants additional investigation by imaging, at a minimum. However, as most MTC has a fairly indolent course, patients with biochemical evidence of recurrent disease may not have corollary imaging findings for some time. Patients with findings indicating recurrent disease localized to the neck should undergo reoperation with the goal of removing all remaining disease. These operations may result in long-term survival benefit and prevent complications of recurrence in the neck [62].

Data are limited regarding the long-term risk of recurrence or metastasis in *RET* mutation carriers with normal preoperative calcitonin, who undergo preventive surgery based on genetic testing alone. Thyroidectomy in these patients is likely curative, especially if no MTC is detected in the surgical resection specimen. Annual serial calcitonin measurements are currently recommended indefinitely. Outcomes for these patients will be better characterized as more patients undergo treatment based on genetic screening.

Pheochromocytoma

Pheochromocytomas are neoplasms arising from chromaffin cells in the adrenal medulla, which synthesize and secrete catecholamines. Patients with pheochromocytoma may present with symptoms of catecholamine excess, including headache, hypertension, palpitations, tremors, and anxiety. This unregulated catecholamine secretion can have devastating consequences if unrecognized or untreated, including stroke, arrhythmias, myocardial infarction, malignant hypertension, and sudden death.

Approximately, 40–50% of all patients with MEN-2A or MEN-2B develop pheochromocytomas, with a mean age of diagnosis between 30 and 40 years of age. Younger patients have been reported, and we recently treated an 8-year-old patient with a codon 634 MEN-2A mutation who had a symptomatic 5-cm pheochromocytoma. The age of onset may also be earlier in patients with MEN-2B [21]. Two studies indicate that penetrance and age at diagnosis differ between kindred and correlate somewhat with specific *RET* mutations, with the highest penetrance associated with mutations at codons 918 or 634 [8, 63].

Unlike sporadic presentations of pheochromocytoma, which may be malignant or in an extra-adrenal location (paraganglioma), cases associated with MEN-2 are almost always benign and confined to the adrenal medulla. In hereditary pheochromocytomas, adrenal chromaffin cells undergo progressive hyperplastic changes leading to the development of nodular disease and eventually, pheochromocytoma. These tumors are usually multifocal in MEN-2 patients, and are bilateral in more than half the cases [64].

Screening for pheochromocytomas should be done in all patients diagnosed with MEN-2A or MEN-2B. Numerous studies show that measurement of plasma and/or 24-h urine metanephrines is more sensitive and specific than measurement of catecholamines or other metabolites for detecting pheochromocytoma [65–73]. Pheochromocytoma screening should begin at the age when thyroidectomy would be considered, based on the risk level of the patient's *RET* mutation and family history [21]. If negative, testing should be done annually thereafter. Positive or borderline results mandate additional investigation by imaging, usually adrenal CT or MRI. Benign incidental adrenal masses can occur in MEN-2 patients just as in the general population, where the prevalence of adrenal adenoma may be up to 9%. Opposed-phase or T2-weighted MRI may be able to distinguish pheochromocytoma from an adenoma. Core needle biopsies should not be performed on any adrenal lesion in a MEN-2 patient, even if imaging is inconclusive, due to the likelihood of pheochromocytoma in this population and the risk of catecholamine release during the procedure. ^{131}I-metaiodobenzylguanidine scanning, used to localize paraganglioma in sporadic cases, is not often helpful for MEN-2 patients due to the extreme rarity of extra-adrenal disease.

MEN-2 patients with pheochromocytoma should undergo partial or total unilateral adrenalectomy. The surgical management of unilateral disease has been the subject of some controversy, since many eventually develop pheochromocytoma on the contralateral side. Some authors had previously advocated bilateral adrenalectomies for all MEN-2 patients with pheochromocytoma. Patients with MEN-2 and unilateral pheochromocytoma, who undergo unilateral adrenalectomy and later develop contralateral disease, do so at a mean of 7–12 years after surgery [64, 74, 75]. Patients who have had both adrenals removed carry a substantial risk of adrenal insufficiency and Addisonian crisis, even with corticoid supplementation. In addition, the risk of malignant pheochromocytoma is extremely low for this population. Most surgeons now recommend removing only the affected adrenal in the setting of unilateral pheochromocytoma in MEN-2 patients, with annual screening thereafter. The remaining adrenal can be removed later if screening results become positive.

Laparoscopic adrenalectomy has gained favor as a preferred surgical approach for many MEN-2 patients, in part because the risk of malignancy is low. The conversion rate to an open procedure is less than 10% [64, 74, 75]. It is considered appropriate for lesions confined to the adrenal and less than 9–10 cm, depending on the capabilities of the surgeon. Laparoscopic adrenalectomy has been associated with shorter hospital stay, decreased postoperative pain, and faster recovery compared to open adrenalectomy [75].

Primary Hyperparathyroidism

The overall reported prevalence of primary hyperparathyroidism in MEN-2A patients is between 10 and 35%, though this is highly variable between kindreds [6, 76]. This is not a clinical feature of FMTC or MEN-2B. The age of onset tends to be later than MTC, so hyperparathyroidism is rarely the initial presenting complaint that leads to a diagnosis of MEN-2A. In over 80% of cases, parathyroid hyperplasia will be identified in multiple glands. Inappropriate secretion of parathyroid hormone (PTH) leads to hypercalcemia and can result in osteoporosis, kidney stones, musculoskeletal pain, depression, and a host of non-specific symptoms.

Patients known to have MEN-2A should be screened using a serum calcium measurement annually. If the calcium is elevated, a PTH level should be measured. Inappropriate elevation of PTH is diagnostic for parathyroid hyperplasia in a patient with MEN-2A.

The treatment for hyperparathyroidism in MEN-2A has traditionally been four-gland parathyroidectomy with autotransplantation to the non-dominant forearm muscle at the time of thyroidectomy. Management of this problem in the era of intraoperative parathyroid hormone monitoring may be less radical, with removal of abnormal glands only, based on the PTH response, or four-gland excision and autotransplantation. Patients with a new diagnosis of MEN-2A should be screened for hyperparathyroidism before undergoing thyroidectomy, because a positive finding will preclude preservation of the parathyroids in situ. Many MEN-2A patients who underwent preventive thyroidectomy in childhood had their parathyroids removed and autotransplanted at the time of the previous surgery. If hyperparathyroidism manifests in a patient with a forearm graft, sestamibi imaging should be done to rule out residual hyperfunctioning parathyroid tissue in the neck. The grafts can be explored and excised with intraoperative parathyroid hormone monitoring and viable cryopreservation of excised parathyroid tissue, if available. Patients who previously underwent thyroidectomy without removal of the parathyroids will need imaging and re-exploration of the neck.

Conclusions

The management of MEN-2 syndromes has changed significantly since the syndromes were first characterized in the mid-twentieth century. The advent of mutation testing in the RET protooncogene, and our growing understanding of the relationship between genotype and phenotype, has refined our diagnostic and prognostic capabilities for MEN-2 syndromes. Preventive surgery based on mutation analysis may prove to be a cure for MTC in young MEN-2 patients. More accurate identification of those at risk has reduced the need for screening in many members of MEN-2 kindreds. As more is learned about the pathogenesis of this disease, treatment can be further tailored to improve outcomes for individual patients.

References

1. Steiner AL, Goodman AD, Powers SR (1968) Study of a kindred with pheochromocytoma, medullary thyroid carcinoma, hyperparathyroidism and Cushing's disease: multiple endocrine neoplasia, type 2. Medicine (Baltimore) 47:371–409
2. Dralle H, Gimm O, Simon D et al (1998) Prophylactic thyroidectomy in 75 children and adolescents with hereditary medullary thyroid carcinoma: German and Austrian experience. World J Surg 22:744–750 discussion 50–51

3. Hinze R, Holzhausen HJ, Gimm O et al (1998) Primary hereditary medullary thyroid carcinoma – C-cell morphology and correlation with preoperative calcitonin levels. Virchows Arch 433:203–208
4. Wolfe HJ, Melvin KE, Cervi-Skinner SJ et al (1973) C-cell hyperplasia preceding medullary thyroid carcinoma. N Engl J Med 289:437–441
5. Fialkowski EA, Moley JF (2006) Current approaches to medullary thyroid carcinoma, sporadic and familial. J Surg Oncol 94(8):737–747
6. Howe JR, Norton JA, Wells SA Jr (1993) Prevalence of pheochromocytoma and hyperparathyroidism in multiple endocrine neoplasia type 2A: results of long-term follow-up. Surgery 114:1070–1077
7. Frank-Raue K, Kratt T, Hoppner W et al (1996) Diagnosis and management of pheochromocytomas in patients with multiple endocrine neoplasia type 2-relevance of specific mutations in the RET proto-oncogene. Eur J Endocrinol 135:222–225
8. Quayle FJ, Fialkowski EA, Benveniste R et al (2007) Pheochromocytoma penetrance varies by RET mutation in MEN 2A. Surgery 142:800–805 discussion 5 e1
9. Kraimps JL, Denizot A, Carnaille B et al (1996) Primary hyperparathyroidism in multiple endocrine neoplasia type IIa: retrospective French multicentric study. Groupe d'Etude des Tumeurs a Calcitonine (GETC, French Calcitonin Tumors Study Group), French Association of Endocrine Surgeons. World J Surg 20:808–812 discussion 12–13
10. Bugalho MJ, Limbert E, Sobrinho LG et al (1992) A kindred with multiple endocrine neoplasia type 2A associated with pruritic skin lesions. Cancer 70:2664–2667
11. Ceccherini I, Romei C, Barone V et al (1994) Identification of the Cys634–>Tyr mutation of the RET proto-oncogene in a pedigree with multiple endocrine neoplasia type 2A and localized cutaneous lichen amyloidosis. J Endocrinol Invest 17:201–204
12. Gagel RF, Levy ML, Donovan DT et al (1989) Multiple endocrine neoplasia type 2a associated with cutaneous lichen amyloidosis. Ann Intern Med 111:802–806
13. Lemos MC, Carrilho F, Rodrigues FJ et al (2002) Early onset of medullary thyroid carcinoma in a kindred with multiple endocrine neoplasia type iia associated with cutaneous lichen amyloidosis. Endocr Pract 8:19–22
14. Nunziata V, di Giovanni G, Lettera AM et al (1989) Cutaneous lichen amyloidosis associated with multiple endocrine neoplasia type 2A. Henry Ford Hosp Med J 37:144–146
15. Seri M, Celli I, Betsos N et al (1997) A Cys634Gly substitution of the RET proto-oncogene in a family with recurrence of multiple endocrine neoplasia type 2A and cutaneous lichen amyloidosis. Clin Genet 51:86–90
16. Sijmons RH, Hofstra RM, Wijburg FA et al (1998) Oncological implications of RET gene mutations in Hirschsprung's disease. Gut 43:542–547
17. Eng C, Clayton D, Schuffenecker I et al (1996) The relationship between specific RET proto-oncogene mutations and disease phenotype in multiple endocrine neoplasia type 2. International RET mutation consortium analysis. JAMA 276:1575–1579
18. Moore SW, Zaahl MG (2008) Multiple endocrine neoplasia syndromes, children, Hirschsprung's disease and RET. Pediatr Surg Int 24:521–530
19. Nishikawa M, Murakumo Y, Imai T et al (2003) Cys611Ser mutation in RET proto-oncogene in a kindred with medullary thyroid carcinoma and Hirschsprung's disease. Eur J Hum Genet 11:364–368
20. Romeo G, Ceccherini I, Celli J et al (1998) Association of multiple endocrine neoplasia type 2 and Hirschsprung disease. J Intern Med 243:515–520
21. Brandi ML, Gagel RF, Angeli A et al (2001) Guidelines for diagnosis and therapy of MEN type 1 and type 2. J Clin Endocrinol Metab 86:5658–5671
22. Yip L, Cote GJ, Shapiro SE et al (2003) Multiple endocrine neoplasia type 2: evaluation of the genotype–phenotype relationship. Arch Surg 138:409–416 discussion 16
23. Miller CA, Ellison EC (2005) Multiple endocrine neoplasia Type 2B. In: Clark OH, Duh Q-Y, Kebebew E (eds) Textbook of endocrine surgery, 2nd edn. W.B. Saunders, Philadelphia, pp 757–763

24. Robertson DM, Sizemore GW, Gordon H (1975) Thickened corneal nerves as a manifestation of multiple endocrine neoplasia. Trans Sect Ophthalmol Am Acad Ophthalmol Otolaryngol 79:OP772–OP787
25. Carney JA, Go VL, Sizemore GW et al (1976) Alimentary-tract ganglioneuromatosis. A major component of the syndrome of multiple endocrine neoplasia, type 2b. N Engl J Med 295: 1287–1291
26. Samaan NA, Draznin MB, Halpin RE et al (1991) Multiple endocrine syndrome type IIb in early childhood. Cancer 68:1832–1834
27. Smith VV, Eng C, Milla PJ (1999) Intestinal ganglioneuromatosis and multiple endocrine neoplasia type 2B: implications for treatment. Gut 45:143–146
28. Cohen MS, Phay JE, Albinson C et al (2002) Gastrointestinal manifestations of multiple endocrine neoplasia type 2. Ann Surg 235:648–654 discussion 54–55
29. Lips CJ, Landsvater RM, Hoppener JW et al (1994) Clinical screening as compared with DNA analysis in families with multiple endocrine neoplasia type 2A. N Engl J Med 331:828–835
30. White ML, Doherty GM (2008) Multiple endocrine neoplasia. Surg Oncol Clin N Am 17:439–459, x
31. Wohllk N, Cote GJ, Bugalho MM et al (1996) Relevance of RET proto-oncogene mutations in sporadic medullary thyroid carcinoma. J Clin Endocrinol Metab 81:3740–3745
32. Elisei R, Romei C, Cosci B et al (2007) RET genetic screening in patients with medullary thyroid cancer and their relatives: experience with 807 individuals at one center. J Clin Endocrinol Metab 92:4725–4729
33. Neumann HP, Bausch B, McWhinney SR et al (2002) Germ-line mutations in nonsyndromic pheochromocytoma. N Engl J Med 346:1459–1466
34. Fialkowski EA, DeBenedetti MK, Moley JF et al (2008) RET proto-oncogene testing in infants presenting with Hirschsprung disease identifies 2 new multiple endocrine neoplasia 2A kindreds. J Pediatr Surg 43:188–190
35. Ogilvie JB, Kebebew E (2006) Indication and timing of thyroid surgery for patients with hereditary medullary thyroid cancer syndromes. J Natl Compr Canc Netw 4:139–147
36. Saad MF, Ordonez NG, Rashid RK et al (1984) Medullary carcinoma of the thyroid. A study of the clinical features and prognostic factors in 161 patients. Medicine (Baltimore) 63:319–342
37. Moley JF, DeBenedetti MK (1999) Patterns of nodal metastases in palpable medullary thyroid carcinoma: recommendations for extent of node dissection. Ann Surg 229:880–887 discussion 7–8
38. Gagel RF, Tashjian AH Jr, Cummings T et al (1988) The clinical outcome of prospective screening for multiple endocrine neoplasia type 2a. An 18-year experience. N Engl J Med 318:478–484
39. Niccoli-Sire P, Murat A, Baudin E et al (1999) Early or prophylactic thyroidectomy in MEN 2/FMTC gene carriers: results in 71 thyroidectomized patients. The French Calcitonin Tumours Study Group (GETC). Eur J Endocrinol 141:468–474
40. Rodriguez GJ, Balsalobre MD, Pomares F et al (2002) Prophylactic thyroidectomy in MEN 2A syndrome: experience in a single center. J Am Coll Surg 195:159–166
41. Wells SA Jr, Skinner MA (1998) Prophylactic thyroidectomy, based on direct genetic testing, in patients at risk for the multiple endocrine neoplasia type 2 syndromes. Exp Clin Endocrinol Diabetes 106:29–34
42. Kaufman FR, Roe TF, Isaacs H Jr et al (1982) Metastatic medullary thyroid carcinoma in young children with mucosal neuroma syndrome. Pediatrics 70:263–267
43. Gill JR, Reyes-Mugica M, Iyengar S et al (1996) Early presentation of metastatic medullary carcinoma in multiple endocrine neoplasia, type IIA: implications for therapy. J Pediatr 129: 459–464
44. Hundahl SA, Cady B, Cunningham MP et al (2000) Initial results from a prospective cohort study of 5583 cases of thyroid carcinoma treated in the United States during 1996. U.S. and German Thyroid Cancer Study Group. An American College of Surgeons Commission on Cancer Patient Care Evaluation study. Cancer 89:202–217
45. Sosa JA, Tuggle CT, Wang TS et al (2008) Clinical and economic outcomes of thyroid and parathyroid surgery in children. J Clin Endocrinol Metab 93:3058–3065

46. Machens A, Niccoli-Sire P, Hoegel J et al (2003) Early malignant progression of hereditary medullary thyroid cancer. N Engl J Med 349:1517–1525
47. Skinner MA, Moley JA, Dilley WG et al (2005) Prophylactic thyroidectomy in multiple endocrine neoplasia type 2A. N Engl J Med 353:1105–1113
48. Guillem JG, Wood WC, Moley JF et al (2006) ASCO/SSO review of current role of risk-reducing surgery in common hereditary cancer syndromes. J Clin Oncol 24:4642–4660
49. Simon S, Pavel M, Hensen J et al (2002) Multiple endocrine neoplasia 2A syndrome: surgical management. J Pediatr Surg 37:897–900
50. Bae SJ, Kim DJ, Kim JY et al (2006) A rare extracellular D631Y germline mutation of the RET proto-oncogene in two Korean families with multiple endocrine neoplasia 2A. Thyroid 16:609–614
51. Bethanis S, Koutsodontis G, Palouka T et al (2007) A newly detected mutation of the RET protooncogene in exon 8 as a cause of multiple endocrine neoplasia type 2A. Hormones (Athens) 6:152–156
52. Jimenez C, Dang GT, Schultz PN et al (2004) A novel point mutation of the RET protooncogene involving the second intracellular tyrosine kinase domain in a family with medullary thyroid carcinoma. J Clin Endocrinol Metab 89:3521–3526
53. Komminoth P, Kunz EK, Matias-Guiu X et al (1995) Analysis of RET protooncogene point mutations distinguishes heritable from nonheritable medullary thyroid carcinomas. Cancer 76:479–489
54. Pigny P, Bauters C, Wemeau JL et al (1999) A novel 9-base pair duplication in RET exon 8 in familial medullary thyroid carcinoma. J Clin Endocrinol Metab 84:1700–1704
55. Ercolino T, Lombardi A, Becherini L et al (2008) The Y606C RET mutation causes a receptor gain of function. Clin Endocrinol (Oxf) 69:253–258
56. Machens A, Schneyer U, Holzhausen HJ et al (2004) Emergence of medullary thyroid carcinoma in a family with the Cys630Arg RET germline mutation. Surgery 136:1083–1087
57. Modigliani E, Cohen R, Campos JM et al (1998) Prognostic factors for survival and for biochemical cure in medullary thyroid carcinoma: results in 899 patients. The GETC Study Group. Groupe d'etude des tumeurs a calcitonine. Clin Endocrinol (Oxf) 48:265–273
58. Brauckhoff M, Gimm O, Brauckhoff K et al (2001) Calcitonin kinetics in the early postoperative period of medullary thyroid carcinoma. Langenbecks Arch Surg 386:434–439
59. Fugazzola L, Pinchera A, Luchetti F et al (1994) Disappearance rate of serum calcitonin after total thyroidectomy for medullary thyroid carcinoma. Int J Biol Markers 9:21–24
60. Dottorini ME, Assi A, Sironi M et al (1996) Multivariate analysis of patients with medullary thyroid carcinoma. Prognostic significance and impact on treatment of clinical and pathologic variables. Cancer 77:1556–1565
61. Pellegriti G, Leboulleux S, Baudin E et al (2003) Long-term outcome of medullary thyroid carcinoma in patients with normal postoperative medical imaging. Br J Cancer 88:1537–1542
62. Traugott A, Moley JF (2005) Medullary thyroid cancer: medical management and follow-up. Curr Treat Options in Oncol 6:339–346
63. Machens A, Brauckhoff M, Holzhausen HJ et al (2005) Codon-specific development of pheochromocytoma in multiple endocrine neoplasia type 2. J Clin Endocrinol Metab 90: 3999–4003
64. Rodriguez JM, Balsalobre M, Ponce JL et al (2008) Pheochromocytoma in MEN 2A syndrome. Study of 54 patients. World J Surg 32:2520–2526
65. Pacak K, Eisenhofer G, Ahlman H et al (2007) Pheochromocytoma: recommendations for clinical practice from the First International Symposium, October 2005. Nat Clin Pract Endocrinol Metab 3:92–102
66. Unger N, Pitt C, Schmidt IL et al (2006) Diagnostic value of various biochemical parameters for the diagnosis of pheochromocytoma in patients with adrenal mass. Eur J Endocrinol 154: 409–417
67. Guller U, Turek J, Eubanks S et al (2006) Detecting pheochromocytoma: defining the most sensitive test. Ann Surg 243:102–107

68. Sawka AM, Jaeschke R, Singh RJ et al (2003) A comparison of biochemical tests for pheochromocytoma: measurement of fractionated plasma metanephrines compared with the combination of 24-hour urinary metanephrines and catecholamines. J Clin Endocrinol Metab 88:553–558
69. Lenders JW, Pacak K, Walther MM et al (2002) Biochemical diagnosis of pheochromocytoma: which test is best? JAMA 287:1427–1434
70. Raber W, Raffesberg W, Bischof M et al (2000) Diagnostic efficacy of unconjugated plasma metanephrines for the detection of pheochromocytoma. Arch Intern Med 160:2957–2963
71. Gerlo EA, Sevens C (1994) Urinary and plasma catecholamines and urinary catecholamine metabolites in pheochromocytoma: diagnostic value in 19 cases. Clin Chem 40:250–256
72. Gardet V, Gatta B, Simonnet G et al (2001) Lessons from an unpleasant surprise: a biochemical strategy for the diagnosis of pheochromocytoma. J Hypertens 19:1029–1035
73. Eisenhofer G, Lenders JW, Linehan WM et al (1999) Plasma normetanephrine and metanephrine for detecting pheochromocytoma in von Hippel-Lindau disease and multiple endocrine neoplasia type 2. N Engl J Med 340:1872–1879
74. Lairmore TC, Ball DW, Baylin SB et al (1993) Management of pheochromocytomas in patients with multiple endocrine neoplasia type 2 syndromes. Ann Surg 217:595–601 discussion 3
75. Brunt LM, Lairmore TC, Doherty GM et al (2002) Adrenalectomy for familial pheochromocytoma in the laparoscopic era. Ann Surg 235:713–720 discussion 20–21
76. Schuffenecker I, Virally-Monod M, Brohet R et al (1998) Risk and penetrance of primary hyperparathyroidism in multiple endocrine neoplasia type 2A families with mutations at codon 634 of the RET proto-oncogene. Groupe D'etude des Tumeurs a Calcitonine. J Clin Endocrinol Metab 83:487–491

Index